HANDBOOK OF
INTENSIVE CARE

HANDBOOK OF INTENSIVE CARE

R. S. ATKINSON
M.A., M.B., B.Chir., F.F.A.R.C.S.
Consultant Anaesthetist,
Southend Hospital

J. J. HAMBLIN
M.B., B.S., F.R.C.P.
Consultant Physician,
Southend Hospital

and

J. E. C. WRIGHT
M.B., B.S., F.R.C.S.
Consultant Cardiothoracic Surgeon,
The London Hospital and
The London Chest Hospital

Springer-Science+Business Media, B.V.

© 1981 R. S. ATKINSON
J. J. HAMBLIN
J. E. C. WRIGHT

Originally published by Chapman and Hall in 1981.
Softcover reprint of the hardcover 1st edition 1981

ISBN 978-0-412-14010-5   ISBN 978-1-4899-3238-9 (eBook)
DOI 10.1007/978-1-4899-3238-9

British Library Cataloguing in Publication Data

Atkinson, Richard Stuart
  Handbook of intensive care.

  1. Critical care medicine
  I. Title   II. Hamblin, J J
  III. Wright, J E C
  616   RC86.7

To   M.V.A.
           M.H.
           P.M.W.
           J.F-H.

Contents

		Page
	Contributors	viii
	Preface	ix
1.	The Intensive Care Unit	1
2.	Acid-Base, Water and Electrolyte Balance	6
3.	Shock	18
4.	Respiratory Failure	47
5.	The Airway	52
6.	Mechanical Ventilation	65
7.	Oxygen Therapy	79
8.	Specific Respiratory Problems	93
9.	Coronary Care	108
10.	Monitoring of the Cardiovascular System	132
11.	Pulmonary Embolism	144
12.	Trauma	156
13.	Renal Disease	175
14.	Metabolic Disorders	204
15.	Nutritional Care: Intensive Nutrition	230
16.	Poisoning	248
17.	Liver Disease	274
18.	Haematological Problems	296
19.	Neurological Problems	306
20.	Paediatric Intensive Care	332
21.	Acute Pancreatitis	343
22.	Psychiatric Problems of Intensive Care	348
23.	Regional Blocks	354
24.	Intravenous Techniques	358
25.	The Control and Management of Infection	363
	Index	379

Contributors

J. R. E. DATHAN, M.D., F.R.C.P.
Consultant Physician
Royal South Hants. Hospital
Southampton University Hospitals
(Chapter 13)

C. A. LAYTON, M.B., M.R.C.P.
Consultant Cardiologist
National Heart and Chest Hospitals
Southend Hospital
(Chapter 10)

G. B. RUSHMAN, M.B., B.S., F.F.A.R.C.S.
Consultant Anaesthetist
Southend Hospital
(Chapter 15)

Preface

The experience of active management of patients in the intensive care unit of a busy district general hospital has convinced us of the value of team work which, allied to enthusiasm and clinical expertise, provides the recipe for success. It is in this spirit that the present volume has been written and the authors are grateful to their colleagues who have given advice. In some cases this has been extended to the compilation of a special chapter and we are indebted to Dr. Dathan, Dr. Layton and Dr. Rushman for their contributions.

In this book we have attempted to set down the principles of intensive care as they concern the typical district general hospital without specialist units or the back up of research departments. In doing this we have tried to maintain simplicity and to give practical advice.

The book is not aimed at the specialist in intensive care who can draw on his own extensive experience, but rather at the junior doctor who takes his turn working in the intensive care unit. In particular we have considered the needs of those who require some information outside the parent speciality. We are also aware than in many British hospitals consultants assume a duty responsibility for patients in intensive care units and we hope that the information in this volume may be of some help to them. Trained nurses should also find this book of value.

We hope that this book will be regarded essentially as a practical manual, supported by such pathophysiological information as will help the practitioner make rational decisions.

ONE

The intensive care unit

The epidemic of poliomyelitis which occurred in Copenhagen in the summer of 1952 produced many cases of bulbar and respiratory paralysis. The combined efforts of physicians and anaesthetists were able to effect a marked reduction in mortality by the use of tracheostomy to secure a clear airway and by artificial inflation of the lungs to provide respiratory gas exchange (Lassen, 1953). In this situation the measurement of blood gases became recognised as of importance (Engell and Ibsen, 1952). The influence of this epidemic on the development of intensive care has been discussed by Ibsen (Ibsen, 1975), who was able to report on a series of 259 patients treated in an intensive therapy unit in 1958 (Ibsen and Kvittingen, 1958).

In the United Kingdom a number of respiratory units were set up, largely to provide respiratory support to patients with chronic respiratory failure secondary to neurological disease, and considerable experience was gained in the management of patients requiring mechanical ventilation (Spalding and Crampton Smith, 1963). The intensive therapy units as we know them today developed from such units and from the experience of some special units for patients who had undergone cardiac or neuro-surgery. The need for such units to provide treatment for a wide spectrum of medical and surgical conditions in patients in the district general hospital came to be recognized a few years later (Robinson, 1966; Jones, 1967). The World Congress of Anaesthesiologists held in London in 1968 included a symposium on the design and planning of intensive care units (Boulton *et al.*, 1970) which did much to promote interest in this field.

The development of critical care in the United States was rapid. For example, the respiratory unit at the Massachusetts General Hospital which opened in 1961 was soon treating 400 patients annually (Bendixen *et al.*, 1965).

The criteria for planning and equipping of intensive therapy units were put forward in a BMA Planning Unit Report (1967) and Hospital Building Note, Intensive Therapy Unit, No 27 (1970). There is general agreement that 1% of the acute bed complement of a hospital should be designated for intensive care and that this number should be increased up to 2% where there are special units in the hospital for cardiac or neuro-surgery. A unit of less than four beds is uneconomic and it may prove difficult to maintain medical and nursing standards with too many beds. It has been suggested that the optimal size is between 8 and 10 beds (Tinker, 1976).

Cardiac care units are usually separate entities, though they may share ancillary accommodation with intensive therapy units. The special problems of cardiac care are discussed in Chapter 9.

Paediatric patients are usually treated in the main hospital intensive therapy unit when their condition or the quality and quantity of nursing support precludes their management in the childrens' ward. The authors have experienced no major difficulties in this respect. Resources are seldom adequate for the establishment of a separate paediatric intensive care unit in the district general hospital, but regional centres can be set up to provide the special expertise which is advantageous in many neonatal conditions.

The intensive therapy unit should be provided with a patient area with rooms for supporting services. The patient area should have generous floor space, 200–300 sq ft per bed, to allow for the various apparatus that may be required. Isolation cubicles are advantageous in the prevention of cross-infection where provision of nursing staff allows, but the advantage has to be balanced against the need for full observation of all patients from the nursing station at all times. Most units compromise and have some beds in cubicles and some in open ward space. Isolation in cubicles is useful when a patient is highly infective or when his condition requires a high level of protection from cross-infection. Such cubicles can be supplied with fans to direct the flow of air out to the exterior (infected patients) or to provide clean air from the outside (non-infected patients).

Cross-infection is an ever present danger when debilitated patients are treated, particularly when the condition requires prolonged antibiotic therapy. Proper precautions should therefore be taken when medical and nursing procedures are carried out and these may include wearing of gowns, masks and overshoes. Too much emphasis on these aspects may, however, militate against proper observation and therapy, especially when nursing establishment is low.

The equipment which should be provided at each bed station will vary according to individual conditions and preference. A suggested minimum provision is listed in Table 1.1. Other apparatus which must be readily available includes mechanical ventilators, humidifiers, oxygen masks, cardiac monitors etc. It is advantageous for the unit to have its own X-ray apparatus. Resuscitation equipment is probably best kept on a special trolley and should include the means for inflating the lungs with oxygen, laryngoscopes, tracheal tubes, connections, defibrillator, etc. Monitoring equipment will probably include apparatus for central venous pressure measurement; direct arterial pressure measurement; measurement of respiratory volumes, etc. The ward must, of course, be equipped with that which is standard on the general medical and surgical ward and a number of stethoscopes should be available.

The drug cupboard should be stocked with all those agents in common use, including those used in resuscitation and a modest range of anaesthetic agents.

Full laboratory facilities with ability to provide rapid electrolyte and blood gas estimations are, of course, invaluable.

Table 1.1 Suggested minimum provision of equipment per bed space

Bed
    Light to move
    Brakes on wheels
    Control of height and tilt
    Cotsides available
    Bed head and foot removable
    Ability to attach orthopaedic appliances
Ripple mattress
Eight 13 amp sockets
Compressed oxygen
Compressed air
Suction (two sources)
Light
Wash basin
Locker
Sphygomanometer
ECG oscilloscope

Ancillary rooms should include a sister's and doctor's office which affords a full view of the ward as well as nurses' rest rooms, a small kitchen, clean and dirty utility rooms and a small laboratory. Storage space should be generous. A small relatives' room with bed allows relatives to stay near at hand when occasion demands. There should be provision for small group teaching of both medical and nursing staff.

The patient's psychological state should not be forgotten. Large windows with an outside view are a benefit to both patients and staff (Keep, 1972; Keep and James, 1980). The problems of disorientation are discussed in Chapter 22, but both calendar and clock should be in the patients field of vision. Clocks should have seconds hands to facilitate making of observations.

Occupational therapy should be available to those patients who may otherwise suffer boredom and depression. Radio and television are invaluable here. Sunblinds should be available to protect the patient from direct sun rays and screening facilities will allow a degree of privacy in an open ward. Venetian blinds collect dust and are best sited between two panes of glass. The room should be adequately heated to allow comfort for patients who are often exposed for therapeutic and monitoring purposes and this is particularly important when infants are treated (Brock, 1975).

The intensive therapy unit can be sited with advantage near to cardiac care units, operating theatres and accident centres and sometimes ancillary services can be shared. This is seldom feasible in British hospitals but should be considered when new buildings are planned. It should be noted that all these services provide a type of intensive care and there is often movement of patients from one of these sites to another.

MEDICAL STAFF

In the authors' opinion the intensive therapy unit should work under the direction of consultants with special interests and motivation who are placed in both administrative and clinical charge. It matters less the specialty of the consultant concerned, than that individual's interest and zeal. Usually, however, the departments of anaesthesia and acute medicine will provide the majority of the expertise required as so many of the problems are concerned with respiratory failure or metabolism. It is necessary for this consultant (or pair of consultants) to be in overall charge, though it is clear that they cannot be conversant with all aspects of intensive patient care. They must, therefore, be prepared to consult and liaise with other colleagues, not least those of the firm who were previously responsible for the patient care.

In our opinion, the method used in many hospitals, whereby the patient's previous clinical team continues to look after him in the intensive care unit, is less satisfactory. It is more important to develop unit policies and uniform therapeutic regimes where applicable and this can only be properly done when the unit has its own consultants in charge.

Junior staff must also work under supervision in the ITU. These should come from departments of anaesthesia, medicine and surgery, though the exact mix and method of rotation will depend on individual hospital arrangements. Junior staff must be on immediate call throughout the 24 hours and this should not be prevented by other duties such as outpatient clinics or operation lists. Some units expect a junior doctor to sleep on the ward each night and provision should certainly be made for this, although in the authors' opinion it is not always necessary.

There are certainly a good many routine tasks to be performed during daylight hours. These include taking of laboratory specimens, care of intravenous lines, supervision of humidifiers and ventilators and in our opinion the junior doctor on duty should be relieved of duties outside the ITU.

For future training purposes improved arrangements will have to be made to allow rotations between departments of anaesthesia, acute medicine, and perhaps medical measurement (Tinker, 1976).

Nursing staff

The proper provision of competent and motivated nursing staff is probably the greatest single factor in the operation of a successful ITU. Nursing procedures required are heavier and more intense than those obtaining on most general wards. The need is for one nurse per patient throughout the 24 hours and with allowances for sick leave and holidays the figure should be 4.25 per bed (Tinker, 1976). There should always be a sister on duty and if the unit is linked with other nursing areas a nursing officer should have overall charge.

A number of centres have been approved for the training of nurses in intensive therapy.

Other staff

A physiotherapist with special training in ITU work is invaluable though seldom available. The intensity and expertise of physiotherapy is very different from that pertaining on the ordinary ward and in practice this function has often to be taken over by the nursing staff.

Technical staff are also involved in ITU work in the maintenance and sterilization of equipment. In the future the manpower to do this may come from the scientific service envisaged in the Zuckeman report (DHSS, 1968) and may be based on medical physics departments.

REFERENCES

Bendixen, H. H., Egbert, L. D., Hedley-Whyte, J., Laver, M. B. and Pontoppidan, H. (1965), *Respiratory Care*, C. V. Mosby Co, St. Louis.

B.M.A. Planning Unit Report No. 1, *Intensive Care*, November, 1967.

Boulton, T. B., Bryce-Smith, R., Sykes, M. K., Gillett, G. B. and Revell, A. L. (eds) (1970), *Progress in Anaesthesiology*. Proceedings of the Fourth World Congress of Anaesthesiologists, London, 1968. *Excerpta Medica Foundation*, Amsterdam, pp. 477–491.

Brock, Lord (1975), The importance of environmental conditions, especially temperature, in the operating room and intensive care ward. *Br. J. Surg.*, **62**, 253.

Engell, H. C. and Ibsen, B. (1952), Continuous carbon dioxide measurement in respiratory air during anaesthesia in thoracic operations. *Acta chir Scand.*, **104**, 313.

Hospital Building Note, Intensive Therapy Unit, No. 27 (1970), London, H.M.S.O.

Ibsen, B. and Kvittingen, T. D. (1958), Arbejdet pa en anaesthesiologisk observationsafdeling. *Nord Med*, **60**, 1349.

Ibsen, B. (1975), From anaesthesia to anaesthesiology. *Acta Anaesth Scand*, suppl. 61.

Jones, S. E. (1967), The organisation and administration of the intensive care patient. *Postgrad Med. J.*, **43**, 339.

Keep, P. J. (1972), Stimulus deprivation in windowless rooms. *Anaesthesia*, **32**, 598.

Keep, P. J. and James, J. (1980), Windows in intensive therapy unit. *Anaesthesia*, **35**, 257.

Lassen, H. C. A. (1953), A preliminary report on the 1952 epidemic of poliomyelitis in Copenhagen with special reference to the treatment of acute respiratory insufficiency. *Lancet*, i, 37.

Robinson, J. S. (1966), The design and function of an intensive care unit. *Brit. J. Anaesth.*, **38**, 132.

Spalding, J. M. K. and Crampton Smith, A. (1963), Clinical practise and physiology of artificial respiration. Oxford. Blackwell.

Tinker, J. (1967), The staffing and management of intensive care units. *Brit. J. Hosp Med.*, **16**, 399.

TWO

Acid-base, water and electrolyte balance

ACID-BASE BALANCE

The hydrogen ion concentration of body fluids and tissues is the measure of acid base balance. One might as easily speak of acid base balance in terms of hydroxyl ion concentration since free hydrogen ions are mopped up by hydroxyl ions with the formation of water molecules,

$$H^+ + OH^- \rightarrow H_2O$$

but by convention hydrogen ion concentration is used as a reference. Hydrogen ion concentration was originally difficult to measure directly, and the concept of pH notation arose. pH is defined as the negative logarithm of the hydrogen ion concentration to the base 10 and thus varies inversely with the logarithm of the hydrogen ion concentration. The relationship between the two can be seen in Table 2.1.

Table 2.1 pH and hydrogen ion
concentration

pH	$[H^+]$ (nmol/l)
7.00	100
7.20	63
7.36*	44*
7.40*	40*
7.44*	36*
7.60	25
7.80	16
8.00	10

* physiological range

The relationship between hydrogen ion concentrations, bicarbonate concentration and concentration of carbonic acid forms one of the main buffering systems in the body. The reaction obeys the Law of Mass Action which states that in equilibrium the products of the concentration of the reagents on one side of the reaction is proportional to the product of the concentration of the reagents on the other side.

Thus, for the reaction:

$$H^+ + HCO_3^- \rightleftharpoons H_2CO_3$$
$$[H^+][HCO_3^-] = K \times [H_2CO_3]$$

where K is a constant and use of the square brackets indicates concentration.

This equation can be written in a number of ways. $[H_2CO_3]$ can be replaced by PCO_2 and assuming a solubility coefficient for CO_2 of 0.03 and other constants it may take the form:

$$[H^+] = 24 \frac{PCO_2}{[HCO_3^-]}$$

Alternatively, logarithmic notation can be used. $[H^+]$ becomes pH and the equation assumes the familiar form of the Henderson-Hasselbalch equation:

$$pH = pK + \log \frac{[HCO_3^-]}{[H_2CO_3]}$$

which again may be re-written

$$pH = pK + \log \frac{[HCO_3^-]}{0.03\ PCO_2}$$

In understanding the clinical significance of acid base changes in sick patients the three variables which are important are pH, PCO_2 and bicarbonate concentration. pK is the negative logarithm of the dissociation constant of carbonic acid and can be taken as 6.1 although it varies slightly with temperature and pH. Hypothermia is an important clinical state and when measuring pH a correction must be applied of 0.0147 of a pH unit per °C fall in temperature.

pH

pH is measured directly using the glass electrode which consists of a lattice of oxygen and silica atoms with metal cations in between. Hydrogen ions displace cations in a manner that can be measured as an electrical signal. It is necessary to make comparative measurements with known buffer solutions. Quality control studies suggest that significant variation of results can occur between different laboratories and that gross variations are more likely to result from departures from recommended procedure than from use of different types of apparatus. It is not justified to measure pH to more than 2 decimal places and this order of accuracy is quite satisfactory for clinical applications.

PCO_2

PCO_2 can be measured directly using the CO_2 electrode (Severinghaus and Bradley, 1958; Severinghaus, 1960). The glass electrode is separated from the test solution by a membrane permeable to carbon dioxide. The pH measured is related to PCO_2. PCO_2 can also be obtained using the Siggaard-Andersen nomogram (Andersen and Engel, 1960; Astrup *et al.*, 1960) or by indirect methods dependent upon rebreathing (Campbell and Howell, 1960).

Bicarbonate

Bicarbonate estimation can be made using the Siggaard-Anderson nomogram. Actual bicarbonate, standard bicarbonate, and total buffer base can be read off once the buffer line for the particular blood sample has been established.

Blood sampling

Blood samples must be taken with care.

Apparatus

The apparatus for pH and PCO_2 estimation is delicate and requires skilled operation and maintenance. It is necessary to leave apparatus clean after use and sampling electrodes must be flushed after use. Apparatus is now available which presents data in digital form and wholly automated equipment is now on the market.

Definitions

pH is the negative logarithm of the hydrogen ion concentration to the base 10.
Acidaemia. Hydrogen ion concentration above the normal range.
Alkalaemia. Hydrogen ion concentration below the normal range.
Respiratory acidosis. A rise in arterial PCO_2 which if uncompensated will lead to acidaemia.
Respiratory alkalosis. A fall in arterial PCO_2 which if uncompensated will lead to alkalaemia.
Metabolic (non-respiratory) acidosis. A process (other than rise of PCO_2) which if uncompensated will lead to acidaemia.
Base excess. The amount of acid or base in mmol per 1 required for titration back to pH 7.40 at PCO_2 of 40 mm Hg at a temperature of 38°C.
Standard bicarbonate. The concentration of bicarbonate at a PCO_2 of 40 mm Hg at 38°C, with haemoglobin fully saturated.

Other blood buffers

The bicarbonate system is the most important and the most widely studied but other important buffers include haemoglobin and plasma proteins.

Applications in the ITU

Many ill patients suffer disturbances of acid-base balance. *Respiratory* abnormalities are common when respiratory function is disturbed and in patients on IPPV. *Metabolic* abnormalities are common whenever tissue perfusion is compromised; they may also arise as a result of drug administration and due to the formation of acid substances as in diabetic ketosis and uraemia.

Whenever a primary pathological disturbance gives rise to acidosis or alkalosis the body attempts to correct this so as to keep pH within normal limits. Primary respiratory acidosis is therefore usually accompanied by metabolic alkalosis, respiratory alkalosis by metabolic acidosis. Primary metabolic acidosis is accompanied by respiratory alkalosis and vice versa. Where pathological circumstances prevent the occurrence of these compensating mechanisms the pH is likely to move outside the normal range. The hydrogen ion concentration range compatible with life has been stated to be 20 to 158 nmol per l (pH 7.70–6.80).

The situation in patients undergoing intensive therapy is often more complicated than this and mixed disturbances are likely to co-exist. Acidaemia may be both respiratory and metabolic in origin since respiratory failure may accompany both cardiovascular perfusion failure and renal failure. Interpretation may depend upon the sequence of clinical events so that careful evaluation is necessary before treatment is commenced. The aim of correction of acid-base imbalance is to restore the pH of the arterial blood to normal but at the same time energetic therapy must be directed towards the primary aetiological factors.

Correction of acid/base deficits

This is not necessary unless the base excess is outside the limits of + or − 5 mmol/l.

Respiratory changes can be reversed by alteration of ventilatory parameters in patients receiving IPPV, always provided that pathological changes in the lungs do not interfere with gas exchange. When $PaCO_2$ is high alveolar ventilation may be increased. Moderate depression of $PaCO_2$ levels below normal is unlikely to be associated with harm to the patient, but where hyperventilation is necessary to provide oxygenation and this results in gross falls of $PaCO_2$ deadspace can be added to the ventilator circuit in an attempt to bring levels back to normal.

Metabolic acidosis may be treated by administration of bicarbonate. This is most conveniently infused as the 8.4% solution of sodium bicarbonate which contains 1 mmol/ml. When the base deficit is known the dose of bicarbonate necessary to correct this in extracellular fluid may be calculated from the formula:

$$\text{body weight in kg} \times 0.3 \times \text{base deficit} = \text{required dose of } NaHCO_3 \text{ in mmol.}$$

Such calculations are at present an approximation since it depends on the assumption that the weight of extracellular fluid compartment is body weight × 0.3. No account is taken of intracellular fluid or the continuing pathophysiology giving rise to acidosis. Serial estimations may therefore be necessary with further doses of bicarbonate as required.

In the emergency situation (cardiac arrest) the following formula may be useful:

$$\text{dose of bicarbonate (mmol)} = \frac{\text{weight of pt (kg)}}{5} \times \frac{\text{duration of arrest (min)}}{2}$$

Table 2.2 Causes of acidosis

RESPIRATORY	Hypoventilation	Central respiratory depression
		Lung pathology
		Abnormalities of respiratory muscles
METABOLIC	Diabetic ketosis	
	Salicylate poisoning	
	Inadequate tissue perfusion	shock
		cardiac arrest
	Starvation	
	Renal failure	
	Lactic acidosis	
	Hyperchloraemic acidosis	

One disadvantage of sodium bicarbonate administration is that it is sometimes undesirable to administer sodium ions. This may be the case in the sick cell syndrome and in overt hypernatraemia. A possible alternative medication is THAM (tri-hydroxymethyl-amino-methane) though it is less effective than bicarbonate in the treatment of ventricular fibrillation and uptake to cells takes up to 6 hours. It corrects acidosis without the production of carbon dioxide and it is itself a diuretic, being eliminated unchanged in the urine over about 24 hours. It may depress respiration, exaggerate the hyperkalaemia or renal failure and cause a fall in blood sugar. It is irritant to veins (pH 10.2) and is given by intravenous infusion 150 mmol per hour (500 ml soln per hour) according to the formula:

ml 0.3M THAM required = base deficit (mmol per l) × body wt (kg)

Metabolic alkalosis

Correction is seldom required but if it is a similar formula can be used substituting an acid such as arginine hydrochloride for the alkali.

Correction of acid/base abnormalities is by the appropriate means as indicated above, but it is important to treat also the underlying pathological process and to pay attention to tissue perfusion.

Table 2.3 Causes of alkalosis

RESPIRATORY	Hyperventilation	Deliberate
		IPPV
METABOLIC	Bicarbonate administration	
	Pyloric stenosis	
	Injudicious use of diuretic (hypochloraemic alkalosis)	

FLUID AND ELECTROLYTE BALANCE

It is important to know the order of balance in the healthy individual before considering pathophysiological changes.

Water. Average figures for water *intake* may be taken as 2600 ml daily (1100 ml in food and 1500 ml in drink). The *output* of 2600 ml daily may be taken as 1500 ml in urine, 100 ml in faeces, 400 ml via the lungs, and 600 ml via the skin. The healthy individual can accept wide variations of these values by changes in urine output to compensate for changes in intake or altered losses by other routes.

Sodium. The total body sodium is over 105 grams, the greater proportion of which is found in the extracellular compartment. The normal range for serum sodium may be taken as 132 to 142 mmol/l, and comparable values exist in fluids such as bile, pancreatic juice, etc. Gastric juice contains about 60 mmol sodium per litre. A recent ileostomy may contain as much as 130 mmol sodium per litre in the fluids passed, though compensatory mechanisms reduce this value to about 50 mmol/l for an established ileostomy. The healthy individual consumes at least 100 mmol sodium per day and absence of intake may be important in patients unable to ingest food orally. (See Table 2.4.)

Table 2.4 Sodium concentrations of body fluids in mmol/l. (Mean figures)

Serum	142
Sweat	58.4
Gastric juice	59
Bile	145.3
Pancreatic juice	141.1
Intestinal juice	104.9
Ileal secretion (fresh ileostomy)	129.5
Colostomy	79.6
Formed stools	35
Urine	167.4
Intracellular fluid	7 (mmol/kg)

Potassium. The total body potassium is about 3200 mmol, the greater proportion of which is found in the intracellular compartment. The normal serum sodium level is 3.5 to 5.0 mmol/l and approximately the same concentration occurs in the secretions of the small gut and biliary system, though rather higher figures have been quoted for gastric juice (9.2) for recent ileostomy (11.2) and for caecostomy (7.9), though the loss in fluids from an established ileostomy may be significantly reduced (Johnston, 1966).

Chloride. The normal range for serum chloride is 98–106 mmol/l. Gastric juice contains 84, small bowel secretion 104, bile 100, pancreatic juice 77; while large fluids may contain 116 from a recent ileostomy, 21 from an old ileostomy and 42.5 mmol/l from a caecostomy (Johnston, 1966).

Water balance

Negative balance occurs when losses exceed intake. Accurate fluid balance charts are essential in the intensive care unit, but it is not possible to measure losses in expired gases (which rises with tachypnoea), loss in perspiration (increased in hot environments), direct losses (as in open heart surgery), and loss into body cavities and tissues (gut, lumen, pleural cavity, ascites). Fluid may also become translocated between intracellular and extracellular compartments.

Estimations of water balance are aided by serial estimations of packed cell volume, blood urea, etc, as changes occur as a result of concentration or dilution. Urinary volumes and central venous pressure monitoring are also significant.

Simple dehydration is best treated by intravenous infusion of water containing isotonic glucose. The oral or rectal route, though sometimes valuable, are not often applicable to the intensive care situation, but subcutaneous administration (with or without hyaluronidase) may occasionally be indicated, especially in children.

Water retention may occur in a variety of situations. These may be classified as:
   physical
   hormonal
   renal
   local

Oedema may occur as a result of cardiac failure or hypoproteinaemia. Inappropriate ADH excretion is considered below. Special considerations apply in liver failure (see Chapter 17) and in renal failure (Chapter 13).

Overinfusion of intravenous fluids must be considered also. The healthy kidney can eliminate excess fluid, but the diuresis which occurs may result in loss of electrolytes, especially potassium.

HYPONATRAEMIA

Hyponatraemia is a frequent finding in sick patients. The mechanisms by which this occurs must be considered carefully as correct treatment will depend upon appreciation of the underlying disorder of pathophysiology. It is important to note that a reduced serum sodium level does not necessarily indicate salt deficiency. Serum sodium levels are more a reflection of hydration than sodium metabolism.

Sodium depletion

Primary sodium deficiency is likely to occur if adequate replacement therapy is not given in post-operative cases, where there is loss of gastro-intestinal fluids or in the rare circumstances under which excessive salt is lost in the urine. To this must, of course, be added hypoadrenal states.

If sodium depletion is due to these causes the solution is replace the sodium, the calculation being based on accurate fluid balance charts.

Table 2.5 *Electrolyte contents of infusion fluids (mmol/1)*

	Na^+	K^+	HCO_3^- equiv	Cl_2^-	Ca^{2+}
Citrated plasma	150	12		55	
Normal saline (0.9%)	150			150	
4.3% Dextrose and					
0.18% saline solution	30			30	
Hartmann's solution	131	5	29	111	2
Sodium bicarbonate 1.4%	167		167		
Sodium lactate (M/6)	167		167		
M/6 Ammonium chloride				167	

The amount of Na^+ can be calculated as follows

$$Na^+ \text{ deficit (mmol)} = (140 - \text{plasma Na}) \times \text{body wt kg} \times 0.6$$

but this formula must only be used if there is clear evidence of sodium deficiency.

Salt-losing status

Excess renal loss of sodium occurs sometimes in analgesic renal disease, chronic pyelonephritis, especially during an exacerbation, and in advanced chronic renal failure, particularly if combined with dietary salt restriction.

Effects of sodium depletion

As the serum sodium falls due to excessive loss in body fluids without adequate replacement, hyponatraemia will result because fluid balance will generally be maintained by water, either by mouth or within appropriate infusion regimes. Sodium retention by the kidneys follows. This is followed by renal excretion of water and a shift of water into the cells so that the osmolarity of the extracellular fluid is maintained. The net result of these processes is hypovolaemia, circulatory insufficiency and a fall in renal perfusion with a rise in blood urea. The *clinical picture*, therefore, is due to extracellular fluid deficit with intracellular over-hydration.

The patient is drowsy and confused. Hypotension, often best demonstrated posturally, is frequent. Headache and vomiting are frequently complained of. The general appearance resembles dehydration with cold clammy skin, tachycardia and oliguria. Generalized muscular cramps and abdominal pain may be noted. Untreated, peripheral circulatory failure results.

It should be noted that hyponatraemia can result from renal disease, and itself cause uraemia. Diuretics may be mentioned at this point as sometimes contributing to this picture; this is particularly important in dealing with chronic liver disease (see Chapter 17). The situation is equally difficult in congestive cardiac failure where not only can over-enthusiastic use of diretics cause hyponatraemia, but they often cease to be effective if the serum sodium falls due to this or other factors (see below).

Water excess. Excessive overloading of the circulation with water to produce falls in serum sodium levels is unusual. It is probably most frequently seen in the mismanagement of acute renal failure (see Chapter 13). The controversy over the role of inappropriate secretion of ADH producing a dilutional hyponatraemia will be discussed below. If water overload is present it should be treated by restriction of fluid.

Other causes of hyponatraemia. The mechanisms described, however, cannot explain the frequent finding of hyponatraemia in a wide variety of different conditions. The spectrum of diseases in which it is a common finding is very large—meningitis, head injury, pneumonia, tuberculosis, lung abscess, carcinoma of lung and other sites, myxoedema, heart failure, liver failure and in post-operative patients without evidence of sodium loss. In many of these conditions it is short-lived, self-limiting and of little clinical significance.

It has been suggested that *inappropriate secretion of anti-diuretic hormone* (ADH) (Bartter, 1970) is the cause of the hyponatraemia—a dilutional situation. However, this has only definitely been shown to occur in oat cell carcinoma of the bronchus which is capable of producing many hormones to mimic endocrinological syndromes (often with severe electrolyte disturbance such as the 'chemical' Cushings syndrome). The criteria for diagnosis of inappropriate ADH secretion consist of:

(1) increased levels of ADH in serum
(2) hyponatraemia
(3) low plasma osmolality
(4) urine less than maximally dilute
(5) urine Na^+ greater than intake
(6) blood urea less than 3.5 mmol/l

These findings can be explained on other grounds and by other pathophysiological mechanisms based on a failure of the 'sodium pump' at a cellular level— the *sick cell syndrome* (Flear and Singh, 1973). It is suggested that changes in the permeability of cell membranes occur in such conditions as hypoxia and endotoxic shock so that if the normal 'sodium pump', which moves sodium ions out of cells into extracellular fluid, fails, osmolality changes will cause hyponatraemia. Regulation of the total solute of cells is the primary event in fixing the osmolality of body fluids.

There is good experimental and clinical evidence to support the 'sick cell' theory of the aetiology of hyponatraemia in many disease states.

Treatment

The treatment of hyponatraemia in this context is far more difficult than the relatively clear-cut condition of sodium deficiency or water excess.

It would be illogical and possibly highly dangerous to give large saline loads (particularly in congestive cardiac failure or hepatic fluid retention). However, if water excess can be established (and this is difficult) fluid restriction might help increase serum sodium concentration. The low serum should not be assaulted direct, in the majority of cases, but the cause of the condition, e.g. infection or shock. Volume expansion with whole blood (if haemorrhage is a factor) or salt free albumin is necessary to improve tissue perfusion; control of infection, and the other therapeutic manoeuvres used in shock (Chapter 3) have their place. Insulin-glucose regimes might sometimes be helpful.

HYPERNATRAEMIA

High serum sodium levels may be found as a result of:

    drug administration

    over-enthusiastic intravenous infusion

    dehydration

Treatment should be to withhold sodium and treat the underlying syndrome. 5% glucose may be infused intravenously.

Potassium balance

Potassium depletion may arise as a result of:

    diuretic therapy

    excessive losses from gastrointestinal tract

    hidden losses into body cavities (e.g. gut loops)

    deficient intake (inappropriate I.V. regimes)

    diuresis

    peritoneal dialysis

    diabetic ketosis

    adrenal hyperactivity (Cushing's syndrome; oat cell carcinoma)

    insulinoma

    familial periodic paralysis

    liver cirrhosis

    congestive cardiac failure

The causes of potassium depletion are therefore legion, but in the intensive care unit the physician could consider:

(1) The possibility of chronic deficiency before the acute illness.

(2) Observation of losses arising from the acute situation.

(3) The metabolic effects of the acute illness.

Diagnosis

(1) Lethargy, apathy, anorexia, nausea. Knowledge of the underlying pathophysiology of the acute or chronic illness.

(2) Serum estimation.

(3) ECG changes (which reflect intracellular levels). Depression of ST segment, lowering or inversion of T waves, prolongation of PR and QT intervals, appearance of U waves.

Treatment

(1) Oral. To be preferred when oral absorption is normal, e.g. KCl 2 g 6-hourly; K citrate 2.6 g 6-hourly. The effervescent potassium tablet (BPC) contained 6.5 mmol K^+.

(2) Intravenous. May be added to intravenous infusions (a) as a prophylactic routine or (b) as a therapeutic measure. Maximum dosage 20 mmol/h. May be dangerous if given too rapidly or in the presence of renal impairment.

HYPERKALAEMIA

This may arise as a result of:

(1) Renal failure

(2) Over enthusiastic administration

(3) After massive blood transfusion (stored blood may contain up to 25 mmol/l).

A pre-existing state of hyperkalaemia may be exacerbated (with potentially disastrous effects) by:

(1) Administration of suxamethonium (e.g. for tracheal intubation)

(2) Hypoxic episodes (serum K^+ may rise 50% in 5 min)

(3) Adrenaline, endogenous or exogenous

(4) Hypercapnia (K^+ may rise 0.5 mmol/l at P_aCO_2 150 mmHg, with a possible further rise on withdrawal of CO_2)

The *effects* are on the heart. The ECG may show tall peaked T waves with narrow base; diminished emplitude R wave, absence of P wave; widening of QRS; diphasic QRST. Ventricular fibrillation may supervene.

Treatment

(1) Avoid potassium administration.

(2) Correct hypoxia.

(3) Use of ion exchange resins.

(4) Administer glucose and insulin intravenously.

(5) Peritoneal dialysis (or haemodialysis).

(6) Administer bicarbonate.

(7) Calcium salts.

Chloride. Chloride ions are lost in body fluids and must be replaced as necessary.

Ureterosigmoidostomy. Implantation of ureters into the large bowel may result in reabsorption of chloride from the bowel, leading to a hyperchloraemic acidosis and hypokalaemia (*Lancet*, (1959), 7, 837).

Calcium. (See Chapter 14.)

Magnesium. The normal serum level is 1.5–2.5 mmol/l. Low levels may occur in ill patients on prolonged intravenous therapy. The clinical signs which may occur include tremor, twitching, tetany, muscle weakness, confusion and hallucinations. It may be suspected when the patient is failing to make progress despite adequate therapy. It may be given intravenously as magnesium chloride, 2 mmol/kg in 4 hours.

Zinc. Zinc deficiency may also be suspected in patient debilitated by prolonged illness and although the serum level cannot be conveniently estimated, oral therapy may be considered in the occasional patient who shows evidence of delayed healing.

REFERENCES

Andersen, O. S. and Engel, K. (1960), A new acid-base nomogram. An improved method for the calculation of the relevant blood acid-base state. *Scand. J. Clin. Lab. Invest.*, **12**, 177.

Astrup, P., Jorgensen, O. S., Andersen, O. S. and Engel, K. (1960), The acid-base metabolism. A new approach. *Lancet*, i, 1935.

Bartter, F. C. (1970), The syndrome of inappropriate secretion of antidiuretic hormone. *J. Roy. Coll. Phys. Lond.*, **4**, 264.

Campbell, E. J. W. and Howell, J. B. L. (1960), Simple rapid method of estimating arterial and mixed venous PCO_2. *Brit. Med. J.*, **1**, 458.

Flear, C. T., Singh, C. M. (1973), Hyponatraemia and sick cells. *Brit. J. Anaesth.*, **45**, 976.

Johnston, I. D. A. (1966), Review of parenteral feeding. *Proc. R. Soc. Med.*, **59**, 575.

Severinghaus, J. W. and Bradley, A. F. (1958), Electrodes for blood PCO_2, PO_2 determination. *Applied Physiol.*, **53**, 513.

Severinghaus, J. W. (1960), Methods of measurement of blood and gas carbon dioxide during anaesthesia. *Anesthesiology*, **21**, 717.

THREE

Shock

A clear understanding of the causes and pathophysiological sequence of events that lead to shock is essential if it is to be treated rationally and successfully. Although mortality from haemorrhagic shock has been dramatically improved by the liberal use and free availability of blood, plasma, and plasma substitutes, as surgery becomes more complex and employed in ever increasing age groups so the aetiology of shock becomes multifactorial and a rational protocol of treatment based upon reversal of the pathophysiological events is essential. It must be remembered that the characteristic alterations of the microcirculation are common to all forms of shock.

THE CAUSES AND CLASSIFICATION OF SHOCK

Shock may be classified according to haemodynamic considerations.

(1) Low cardiac output

(a) secondary to reduced venous return to the heart such as occurs in haemorrhage or fluid loss (hypovolaemic).

(b) due to cardiac insufficiency either because of intrinsic myocardial failure or secondary to pulmonary embolism or tamponade (cardiogenic).

(2) Normal or increased cardiac output

This form of shock is typically seen in association with bacteraemia. It is due to the opening of multiple arterio-venous shunts in the lungs and splanchnic areas. Under these circumstances tissue nutrition suffers. The heart has a limited ability to maintain this pathological work-load and this too will contribute to regional hypo-perfusion.

This haemodynamic classification can also be described as *cold* shock when when the cardiac output is low and the intense peripheral vasoconstriction has occurred; or *warm* shock with normal or raised cardiac output with reduced peripheral residance.

The cause of shock, therefore, can be expressed as those which originate in the pump mechanism or those which originate in the periphery.

THE CLINICAL FEATURES OF SHOCK

Shock is diagnosed by signs that tissue perfusion is reduced. If this is not

18

Table 3.1 Causes of shock

Cardiogenic		Circulation failure	
Primary	*Secondary*	*Hypovoloaemic*	*Normovolaemic*
Myocardial infarction	Tamponade	Haemorrhage	Bacteraemia
Gross arrhythmias	Caval obstruction	Plasma loss	Neurogenic shock
Myocardial failure	Pulmonary embolism	ECF loss	Anaphylaxis

recognized early tissue nutrition will become inadequate and organ failure rapidly ensues. The clinical features, therefore, that we recognize depend upon the impairment of function secondary to flow reduction.

(1) *The extremities* become cool as cutaneous vessels constrict in response to increased sympathetic activity. As the condition progressed, blanching occurs and the skin becomes sweaty. Eventually the skin becomes mottled and cyanosed due to capillary stagnation. Blood flow to the brain and other organs is maintained during the early stages of cutaneous vasoconstriction.

(2) *Blood pressure* It is only in the early stages of shock that the blood pressure remains normal or slightly raised. Coolness of the extremities will be the first indication of shock, and only for a while will cutaneous vasoconstriction be able to maintain the blood pressure as cardiac output drops. Thereafter a progressive fall will be recorded.

(3) *Pulse rate* will be raised from the onset. As the blood pressure falls the typical rapid thready pulse of shock will become obvious. It should, however, be noted that when intense vasoconstriction occurs absent peripheral pulsation may occur with near-normal intra-arterial pressure. It is also important to note that a healthy young adult can lose up to 25% of his blood volume with only minor changes in pulse and blood pressure (Shenkin *et al.*, 1944).

(4) *Renal function* As cardiac output falls renal blood flow falls proportionately more and urine output to less than 30 ml per hour. If untreated, tubular necrosis may occur with increasing oliguria, and the development of protein and casts in the urine.

(5) *The sensorium* Changes in the sensorium will occur early in shock and are an accurate reflection of the adequacy of arterial pressure. Anxiety and agitation are early features leading to apathy and coma as cerebral insufficiency progresses.

It is important to note that these changes are not presented as a dynamic sequence of changes as the rate of development will depend upon the aetiology of the shock; for example in bacteraemic shock the full picture can develop in minutes, whereas in haemorrhagic shock the clinical evolution will depend upon myocardial integrity among many other factors.

As can be seen from Table 3.1 above the end point of shock is impairment of

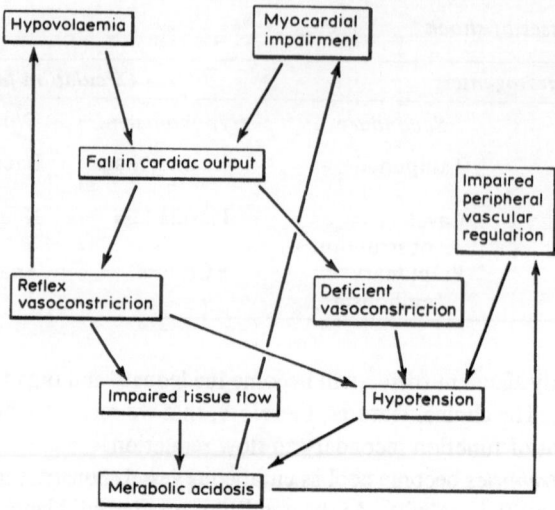

Fig. 3.1 *The pathophysiology of shock.*

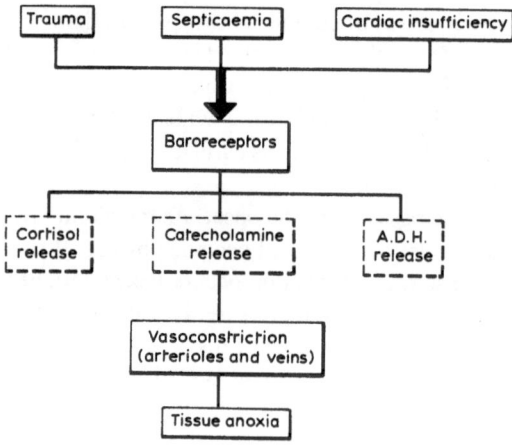

Fig. 3.2 *The great vessel baroreceptor system.*

tissue blood flow regardless of cause. The chain of events that leads to shock is independent of cause, originating in the baroreceptors of the great vessels.

Changes in body fluids

In the early stages of hypovolaemic shock there is movement of protein rich fluid from the interstitial fluid into the circulatory system. This probably occurs because, as a result of arteriolar constriction, there is a change of pressure gradient between the capillaries and extracellular space. Haemodilution occurs and the haematocrit serves as an index of the balance between loss of whole blood or plasma and gain of extravascular fluid. The haematocrit will fall and continue to decrease for several hours following untreated haemorrhage, but will rise when plasma loss has been heavy such as in burns.

Loss into pathological spaces

Large amounts of fluid can be lost into pathological spaces; this fluid is not lost from the body and does not appear in fluid balance charts, but it may contribute significantly to the hypovolaemia. Loss into the gut lumen, via fistulae or as a result of severe burns is well appreciated. More likely to be overlooked is the sequestration of fluid which occurs in traumatised tissues, which can be highly significant (Jenkins *et al.*, 1965).

Effects on tissues

As tissue hypoxia occurs anaerobic metabolism will result in the formation of lactic acid. Due to efficient buffer systems blood pH may show no change in the early stages of shock, and plasma lactate estimations will indicate the degree of cellular pH changes (Lemieux *et al.*, 1969).

The cell membrane

It has been shown that in haemorrhagic shock there is progressive loss of interstitial fluid greater than can be accounted for by movement into the intravascular compartment (Middleton *et al.*, 1969). There are changes in the resting cell membrane potential in skeletal muscle allowing entry of fluid to cells (Negberg *et al.*, 1968; Slonim and Stahl, 1968). The membrane potential remains depressed while hypotension persists and is associated with sodium potassium changes (Shires *et al.*, 1972). It would appear that cells, particularly skeletal muscle cells, form the principle site for fluid sequestration following severe shock. There is a reversal of normal ionic movement with sodium moving in, and potassium out, of the cells (Conway, 1957). These ionic changes affect the red cells and it has been suggested that red cell sodium estimations should accurately reflect the severity of the shock state (Cunningham *et al.*, 1971).

Capillaries

Less than half the capillary circulation is open under normal conditions (Hardaway, 1965), the remainder opening when required. The initial response to tissue hypoxia is capillary dilation, an effect which is enhanced by tissue metabolites, particularly lactic acid. As perfusion is progressively reduced as a result of stagnation and sludging, anaerobic metabolism occurs with the production of increasing amounts of lactic acid.

TREATMENT OF SHOCK

Regardless of cause, the treatment of shock must be based upon the reversal of the sequence of pathophysiological effects outlined in the previous section:

$$BLOOD\ PRESSURE = FLOW \times RESISTANCE$$

Table 3.2 The treatment of shock*

Hypovolaemia	Fluid and volume replacement	Blood plasma
		Plasma substitutes
		Electrolyte solutions
		Vaso-active drugs alpha blockers
Impaired tissue perfusion		Steroids
		Positive inotropic agents
Infection		Antibiotics
Metabolic changes		Oxygen
		Bicarbonate
		Steroids

* Cardiogenic shock is discussed in Chapter 9).

To raise the blood pressure treatment must be directed towards increasing perfusion rather than resistance.

Fluid and volume replacement

This must always be the first priority if irreversible changes in the microcirculation leading to tissue hypoxia are to be avoided. The first question, therefore, is 'what fluid, and how much?' The fluid chosen will most often be dictated by clinical circumstances. The need, of course, is for a fluid that will be retained in the vascular compartment.

(1) Blood

Blood will be indicated in all cases of haemorrhagic shock. If delay occurs before whole blood is available plasma, or one of its substitutes, as described below, will be used.

Transfusion of whole blood, especially if large quantities have to be given rapidly, can be hazardous, and the complications of massive blood transfusion are described in a later section.

Acid-citrate-dextrose (ACD) blood stored for three weeks will provide at least 70% of live cells (Bunn *et al.*, 1969; Valerie, 1971). Expansion of plasma volume without increase in oxygen transport will not prevent tissue hypoxia and therefore whole blood is the ideal solution for the treatment of haemorrhagic shock.

(2) Plasma

(a) *Dried Pooled Plasma* is still available, but is being replaced by Plasma Protein Fraction. A bottle of dried plasma contains the dried solids of 400 ml citrated plasma.

(b) *Plasma Protein Fraction* (PPF) will eventually replace dried pooled plasma. It is supplied as a 4.5 G% protein solution in bottles, each containing 400 ml. It exerts a similar colloid osmotic pressure as reconstituted dried plasma. This solution is free from the risk of transmitting serum hepatitis.

(c) *Fresh Frozen Plasma* (FFP) is of great importance as it contains those factions of plasma essential for the control of coagulation (see Chapter 18). As the problem of disseminated intravascular coagulation becomes more relevant in the evolution of many shock conditions, so this substance should be regarded as an essential part of the infusion regime after haemorrhage.

Plasma preparations (Dried Pooled Plasma and PPF) are given without regard to the blood group of the recipient. The principal disadvantage of plasma is that it affords negligible oxygen carrying capacity. It has also been shown that dispersal from intravascular to extravascular fluid compartments occurs relatively rapidly, up to 500 ml per hour. In addition the albumin in the circulation may be degraded.

(3) Plasma substitutes (Ingleman *et al.*, 1969; Howard *et al.*, 1956; Rickets, 1973)

An ideal plasma substitute should have an osmotic pressure comparable to that of plasma, remain in the circulation long enough to effect its function and then be disposed of by metabolic degradation or excretion. Except for its physical properties it should be inert. (Tinker, 1979.)

No such ideal agent exists as yet. It should, of course, be remembered that they do not provide oxygen carrying capacity and contain no clotting factors.

There are three types of substitute available:

(a) *The Dextrans* which are long-chain polysaccharides. They are available in differing molecular weights, and their properties (and disadvantages) are related to this.

Dextran 40 (Rheomacrodex): This is generally used as a 10% solution to provide a short lived but definite increase in the circulating volume, and it may produce a dramatic improvement in flow through small vessels. It causes dis-aggregation of red cell rouleaux which may have been causing sludging. Urine viscosity is increased with high concentrations and cases of acute renal failure have been described.

Dextran 110: this remains longer in the vascular compartment but may prolong the bleeding time.

Dextran 70: this is probably the best of the dextran plasma substitutes and a molecular weight of about 70 000 seems to be about the right compromise in terms of freedom from serious side effects and a reasonable survival in the circulation.

(b) *The Gelatin solutions* are produced by the hydrolysis of crude collagen.

(c) *Hydroxyethyl starches* are only just becoming available for clinical use and their place has not yet been established.

Disadvantages of plasma substitutes. They interfere with cross matching of blood, and it is essential that samples for cross matching must be taken before they are given. The laboratory must always be informed if blood is sent for cross matching after dextrans have been given.

A further important problem with all the plasma substitutes is the incidence of sometimes severe anaphylactoid reactions. The overall incidence is 0.03% (which is less than the incidence of adverse reactions to blood transfusion) (Ring and Messmer, 1977).

If plasma or plasma substitutes are used the haemoglobin level should not be allowed to drop below 9.0 g%. Tissue oxygenation also depends on the viscosity of the blood reaching the capillaries and the ideal haematocrit should be about 30% (Messmer, 1975).

(4) Electrolyte solutions

Electrolyte solutions are poor volume expanders because of rapid transfer to the extracellular space, but they may be indicated in refractory shock as replacement for the loss of extracellular fluid into the cells. Normal saline or Hartmann solution is an effective replacement fluid when intravascular stagnation, rather than blood loss, occurs such as in bacteraemic shock.

How much fluid?

Estimation of blood loss is desirable, but often difficult. The use of complicated formulae for estimating the amount of blood lost into crushed limbs; (blood volume estimations by dye or isotope dilution techniques; nomograms and similar techniques) are often misleading in the dynamic situation of haemorrhage. The amount of blood needed to treat haemorrhagic shock is the amount necessary to restore basic measurements to normal. Of these the most sensitive indicator is the central venous pressure and blood should be infused rapidly to raise the CVP to 5–10 cm H_2O and then given as required to maintain that level. Confirmation of recovery occurs as the pulse rate falls, blood pressure rises and skin temperatures return towards normal. Constricted limb veins fill as the circulatory volume deficit is corrected and it may then be considered that an adequate transfusion has been given.

Under certain circumstances blood loss can be measured directly, as when a haemothorax is treated by intrapleural drainage and *accurate* replacement can then be undertaken. But even under these circumstances other factors such as extravasation into traumatised tissue and loss of extracellular fluid must be taken into account and reliance placed upon CVP and the clinical observations described above. It should be remembered that gastro-intestinal haemorrhage may occur spontaneously in critically ill patients. (See page 28.)

In non-haemorrhagic shock plasma expansion will always be required if the

CVP is below 10 cm H_2O. If the problem is one of dehydration saline or Hart-mann's solution will be indicated, under other circumstances where haemo-concentration has occurred, such as in severe burns, plasma or plasma substitute should be given in sufficient quantities to raise the CVP to 10 cm H_2O. In bacteraemic shock increasing the CVP to 15–20 cm H_2O may push cardiac output to optimum levels.

Where a CVP line is not in use observation on pulse, blood pressure and venous tone will at best provide an indication as to the adequacy of volume replacement, but they are relatively insensitive and delayed indicators of the state of the circulation.

Drug therapy

Therapy with vaso-active drugs should not be considered until adequate fluid and volume replacement has been achieved. If, after this, regional blood flow remains impaired and hypotension persists, the use of these drugs should be considered. It cannot, however, be over-emphasized that these pharmacological agents are no substitute for aggressive fluid and volume replacement.

Secretion of catecholamines is an integral part of shock, particularly in cardiogenic shock (*Lancet*, 1969). The beta adrenergic effect is seen as an increase in force of myocardial contraction and heart rate. The alpha adrenergic effect is seen as peripheral vasoconstriction. Whereas the beta effect is beneficial the alpha effect may be harmful and the two should be differentiated both in diagnosis and treatment.

It is, of course, possible to increase the blood pressure and venous pressure by constriction of arterioles and veins by means of an alpha-stimulating drug but this will inevitably further reduce tissue perfusion. Instead of shrinking the circulatory space to fit the available blood volume, it is preferable to augment the volume to fit the space.

Table 3.3 Catecholamines used in shock

Catecholamine	Beta-1 receptors	Beta 2 receptors	Alpha receptors	Dopamine receptors	Dosage range (ng/kg/min)
Dopamine	++	0	+ → ++	++	1–30
Adrenaline	++	++	+ → ++	0	0.06–0.18
Noradrenaline	++	0	++	0	0.01–0.07
Isoprenaline	++	++	0	0	0.02–0.18
Dobutamine	++	+	+	0	2–40

(From Tinker, 1979.)

(1) Adrenaline

Adrenaline has both an alpha and beta stimulating adrenergic effect. Overall it augments vasoconstriction and its use in shock is dangerous. The vasoconstriction it produces may be sufficiently severe to produce gangrene of the extremities.

(2) Isoprenaline

This is mainly a beta-adrenergic stimulant, both inotropic and chronotropic in its effect, but it is also a vasodilator. It is given in a drip containing 5 mg in 500 ml 5% glucose and is indicated in cardiogenic shock as it produces both increased cardiac output and increased tissue perfusion. Isoprenaline increases myocardial contractility, and serum potassium must be monitored and kept between 4.5 and 5.0 mmol/l. The drip should normally be regulated to maintain a systolic blood pressure around 100 mm Hg. Tachycardia and cardiac arrhythmias may occur.

(3) Dopamine

This is an immediate precursor of noradrenaline and is now available in a proprietary preparation (Intropin). It is probably superior to isoprenaline in terms of renal blood flow and left ventricular function. In common with other drugs of this nature its use in patients with ischaemic heart disease must be very cautious. There is, as with isoprenaline, a risk of tachydysrhythmias, and owing to its effects on myocardial oxygen requirements and coronary perfusion, myocardial ischaemia can be worsened.

It has a short plasma half-life and has to be given by intravenous infusion. For details of the dosage of dopamine see page 25 (Chapter 9).

(4) Dobutamine

This is derived from isoprenaline. Its spectrum of activity can be seen from the table. It differs from dopamine by not stimulating the heart by noradrenaline release.

(5) Noradrenaline, methoxamine, angiotensin

These pressor agents all cause a rise in blood pressure by producing intense vaso-constriction and their use in shock is illogical and dangerous.

Of the catecholamines discussed above it seems likely that dopamine is the agent of choice.

(6) Alpha blocking agents

This group of drugs produces vasodilation by blocking the vasoconstrictive action of catecholamines. Organ perfusion may therefore be improved, but at the price of a drop in blood pressure and more volume replacement will often be required. If these drugs are used (also isoprenaline) the CVP and blood pressure must be watched very carefully. The prime indications for their use are:
  (1) persistent shock
  (2) Elevation of CVP
  (3) pulmonary congestion

(a) *Phenoxybenzamine* (Dibenzyline). It is given by intravenous infusion 1 mg per kg body weight in 500 ml 5% glucose. The full effect may take half an hour to develop with a duration of action of several hours.

(b) *Phentolamine* (*Rogitine*) has to be given by a continuous drip as it has a short duration. The dose is 1–2 mg per minute. Its effect can be reversed promptly by the use of pressor drugs since it acts as a competitive inhibitor at the alpha-receptor.

(c) *Chlorpromazine* (Largactil). (Collins *et al.*, 1962). This drug has a moderate alpha-blocking action together with a depressant effect on the nervous system. Although its effects and onset of action are variable it remains a useful agent, especially in distressed patients with the secretion of large amounts of endogenous catecholamines and inappropriate vasoconstriction.

It is given slowly by intravenous infusion, 1 mg every five minutes, monitoring the CVP and blood pressure until a response is observed.

Alpha blocking agents should only be used when refractory shock occurs and their use is accompanied by a very real risk of overexpansion of the vascular capacity at a time when circulatory volume is reduced, thereby, further prejudicing the perfusion of vital organs. Rapid volume replacement is almost always necessary, a CVP line is therefore mandatory.

(7) Steroids

The role of steroids in the treatment of shock remains controversial a decade after their introduction. In bacteraemic shock their role is perhaps more clearly defined, but in hypovolaemic or cardiogenic shock there remains dispute as to their value (Dietzman and Lillehei, 1968; Dietzman *et al.*, 1969; Lillehei *et al.*, 1967).

The actions of high-dose steroids in shock It is important to appreciate that massive doses of corticosteroids are used for their pharmacologic effects and not as replacement therapy. These effects have generally been demonstrated in experimental animals and it is unwise to extrapolate these results to man:
   (a) Positive inotropic effect
   (b) Decrease of peripheral resistance
   (c) Stabilisation of lysozomes
   (d) Preservation of integrity of small vessels, preventing leakage from microcirculation.
   (e) Reduction in platelet adhesiveness. (Sambi *et al.*, 1962; Wilson and Fisher, 1968; Repogle *et al.*, 1966.)

It is therefore suggested that the microcirculation is enhanced by a combination of vasodilation, increase in cardiac output, whilst protecting cells from the damaging effects of proteases produced when cell membranes are damaged.

Commercial preparations of methyl-prednisolone and dexamethasone are available pre-packed in syringes in the high dosages required.

Table 3.4 Steroid and dosage

Steroid	Dosage (24 hours)
Hydrocortisone	50–100 mg/kg
Methyl-prednisolone (Solu-medrone)	15– 30 mg/kg
Dexamethasone (Decadron)	2– 6 mg/kg

The use of steroids in shock. This form of therapy is no substitute for adequate fluid and volume replacement therapy. In bacteraemic shock (*vide infra*), their use is justifiable in the early phases of treatment but in hypovolaemic states due to blood or fluid loss, and in cardiogenic shock, they should not be used unless conventional and aggressive use of the other vaso-active drugs discussed above has failed to improve the clinical state.

Therapy with steroids should be continued for 72 hours and it has been shown that no tailing-off process is required as no adrenal suppression occurs. Nor is there evidence that the long-term effects of steroids on wound healing or gastro-intestinal bleeding occur with acute short-term high dose therapy.

(8) Positive inotropic agents

The use of positive inotropic agents is theoretically attractive, and routine digitalisation has been suggested. *Digoxin* is the only inotropic agent which does not increase myocardial oxygen demand. However, digoxin does not increase the cardiac output as much as isoprenaline in acute shock. Digoxin is safe in the absence of arrhythmias, and in the presence of a normal serum potassium. Caution must be used if the patient has been on digoxin previously. Rapid digitalisation is achieved by giving 1.5 mg intravenously as an infusion in 5% dextrose over 3 to 6 hours. *Cedilanid* (Lanatocide-C) is a useful alternative cardiac glycoside and is given intravenously 400 mcg in 2 ml. *Glucagon* is claimed to exert a positive inotropic effect, but in clinical use results have been disappointing. The intravenous dose is 800 mcg–1.6 mg. The use of glucagon and insulin/glucose regimes is discussed in Chapter 9.

(9) Gastro-intestinal haemorrhage

Erosions, ulceration and very often haemorrhage of the upper gastrointestinal tract are common complications of severe trauma, major surgery, sepsis, and shock states of any cause. This is also a frequent problem in patients suffering from renal or hepatic failure. It is likely that increased gastric acid secretion is an important factor. The H2 receptor antagonist cimetidine should therefore be given in this group of high risk cases (although it would be naive to imagine that this drug could arrest bleeding from erosion of a major vessel).

The drug is given (under these circumstances) by intravenous infusion in a dose of 60–150 mg/h.

Reversal of metabolic changes

Although *acidosis*, due to tissue hypoxia is a result, not a cause of shock, it is a reflection of the severity of shock state, and a measure of tissue hypoperfusion. Moreover, lactic acidosis exerts a deleterious effect on myocardial function. Therefore if the measures above are not successful in restoring adequate tissue perfusion intravenous sodium bicarbonate should be given. The amount required can be determined using the following formula:

$$\text{Dosage (mmol)} = 0.3 \times \text{Body Weight (kg)} \times \text{Base Deficit (mmol)}$$

Equally important is the consideration of *hypoxia*—it has been stated that the most frequent single cause of death in shock is failure to achieve adequate ventilation. (See below—lung changes in shock.)

Other therapeutic measures

(1) Analgesic agents

Relief of pain is an essential part of the drug therapy of shock. Morphine remains the drug of choice, although it should be remembered that it may depress respiration and cause a fall in the blood pressure. Generally small incremental doses are preferred to single large doses. When peripheral vessels are constricted intramuscular or subcutaneous injection will result in erratic absorption, and therefore morphine should be given intravenously (1–2 mg intravenously as indicated). Diamorphine may cause less nausea and vomiting, it has excellent analgesic properties and the risk of addiction is not great when used under these acute circumstances.

(2) Posture in shock

Elevation of the legs 15–20° aids venous return to the heart and prevents pooling in the dependant limbs. Head down tilt is no longer considered advantageous since prolonged 10° Trendelenberg position has been shown to cause a fall in arterial pressure, and there is also a risk of cerebral oedema, retinal detachment and even brachial plexus lesions (Taylor and Weil, 1967).

BACTERIAL SHOCK

The importance of this syndrome justifies special attention. It has been shown that 70–90% of patients who develop bacteraemic shock are already in hospital when infection occurs. The widespread abuse of broad-spectrum antibiotics may contribute to the syndrome's apparently increasing incidence.

The diagnosis of bacteraemic shock

A high index of suspicion is the most valuable tool for the clinician in making the diagnosis. Special attention should be paid to susceptible patients.

The incidence is particularly high in neonates and in the aged.

Frequently the first symptom will be a rigor, although elderly or debilitated

*Table 3.5 Pre-disposing factors in bacter-
aemic shock*

Urinary tract infection, obstruction or
    instrumentation
Peritonitis
Abdominal surgery, especially to gall
    bladder or colon
Renal failure
Infected intravenous or dialysis lines
Diabetes mellitus
Skin sepsis and burns
Extensive pneumonia
Septic abortion
Broadspectrum penicillin antibiotic therapy
Blood dyscrasias
Steroid therapy
Cytotoxic therapy
Tampon shock syndrome

patients may show neither rise in temperature nor leucocytosis. At this stage, urine flow may be normal with a high or normal specific gravity, but unless treated oliguria will develop rapidly. Many patients will develop the haemo-dynamic changes of shock rapidly without obvious indication of infection. In these cases a sudden drop in blood pressure, rise in pulse rate, or change in the sensorium should alert suspicion. Jaundice occurs in about 10% of cases. Dis-seminated intravascular coagulation is frequently associated with meningococcal septicaemia, but can occur in any bacteraemic state. (This syndrome is discussed in Chapter 18.) It must always be considered when abnormal bleeding, purpura or gangrene of the extremities is noted. It is associated with a drop in platelet count, prolonged prothrombin time, and low fibrinogen concentration.

The diagnosis is therefore made on clinical grounds, in susceptible patients and confirmed by taking blood cultures. *Treatment cannot be delayed until results of blood cultures are available.* It is safer to treat a patient who is not, in fact, suffering from a septicaemia than to allow the diagnosis to lapse for several hours.

Pathophysiological changes in bacteraemic shock

It is generally accepted that endotoxin produced by the organism is an impor-tant cause of the syndrome. The site of action of bacterial products may be on the heart or blood vessels; but whatever mechanism is involved the final pathway is that common to all forms of shock—failure of the microcirculation leading to tissue hypoxia. Because of the potency of the endotoxin these changes can develop in minutes, rather than hours, as in hypovolaemic shock.

The effects of bacteraemic, or endotoxic, shock on the cardiac output are variable. Often, at least in the initial stages, the clinical picture is that of 'warm shock' with a normal or increased cardiac output, and warm extremities.

However, despite this apparently paradoxical situation, tissue nutrition is threatened because the cardiac output is not reaching the cells. It is bacteraemic shock that pathological a/v shunting in the lungs and other organs has been demonstrated. If not treated effectively at this stage the condition will rapidly progress to the low output state described in the preceding sections.

The organisms involved in bacteraemic shock

Earlier beliefs that the endotoxic shock situation is only associated with Gram Negative organisms have been shown incorrect, and it is now recognized that the syndrome can result from infection with Gram Positive organisms, anaerobes, or even fungi (McMurdoch *et al.*, 1968). The recently described toxic shock syndrome associated with the use of tampons is due to *Staphylococcus aureus* toxin (Editorial 1980).

In most series the commonest organism has been *Escherichia coli*, with *Klebsiella/Enterobacter* species, *Pseudomonas aeruginosa* (*pyocyanea*) and *Proteus* species as other common causes. When blood cultures are taken particular attention should be paid to anaerobic culture as, unless this is done, infection by anaerobic organisms such as *Bacteroides* will be missed.

The treatment of bacteraemic shock

The essentials of treatment are exactly the same as with other forms of shock, i.e. maintenance of regional perfusion by fluid and volume replacement, the use of vaso-active drugs if indicated, and the correction of metabolic changes; but the additional factor relevant in this context is the use of antibiotics.

It is important to appreciate that the syndrome produced by gram-negative and gram-positive organisms, whether endotoxin-producing or not, is the same and the treatment identical. It has been stated that warm hypotension is a feature of gram-positive sepsis and that peripheral shut-down cyanosis and cold hypotension occurs in gram-negative infection, but such differentiations are not helpful in the clinical situation. However cardiac output is a more reliable indicator of prognosis (Weil and Nishijima, 1978). A high cardiac output carries a better prognosis as does a respiratory alkalosis (pH 7.5) as compared with a metabolic acidosis (pH 7.3).

The use of antibiotics in bacteraemic shock

It has already been emphasized that there is no time to wait for the result of blood cultures and bacteriological sensitivities, treatment must be instituted immediately.

Often there will be some indication as to the nature, and possibly sensitivities of the infecting organisms. Any bacteriological report from septic lesions antedating the septicaemic may provide important sensitivity results. Many Intensive Care Units have an endemic organism, often *Pseudomonas* or *Proteus*, which may infect vulnerable patients. The particular circumstances of the case will often indicate the likely organism and therefore the appropriate antibiotic.

Table 3.6 Some clinical associations with infecting organisms

E. coli	Urinary tract surgery or instrumentation Bowel surgery Abdominal sepsis
Klebsiella/Enterobacter	Bowel surgery Abdominal surgery Previous treatment with broad-spectrum penicillin
Pseudomonas	Blood dyscrasias Steroid therapy
C. Welchii	Septic abortion/severe trauma
Staphylococcus Streptococcus	Skin sepsis Bone or soft tissue infection

The choice of antibiotic will depend upon the likely nature of the infecting organism in the clinical context of individual patients; or on the basis of sensitivity reports from septic lesions in the patient. Often, however, it is unwise to assume the nature of the organism, and therefore combination chemotherapy is used until bacteriology reports are available. Anaerobic organisms, such as *Bacteroides*, may be missed on preliminary blood cultures, or the result delayed. The need, therefore, is for a chemotherapeutic regime that is likely to be effective against aerobic gram-negative or gram-positive organisms, and anaerobic infections, usually bacteroides.

The AMINOGLYCOSIDE group of antibiotics are the agents of choice under these circumstances. GENTAMICIN is the drug of choice. This drug has the advantage of activity against *Pseudomonas, Aeruginosa* and some gram-positive organisms, notably *staph-aureus*, in addition to its activity over *E. coli* and the *Klebsiella* group. It will, therefore, be effective in the majority of bacteraemic states.

Gentamicin should be given immediately in a dosage of 3–5 mg/kg body weight per day in 8 hourly divided doses. The route of administration is by intravenous injection—however it should not be added to infusion bottles to run in over several hours. Unless it is given as bolus injection effective serum levels are not achieved.

Caution, however, is necessary as gentamicin is ototoxic and nephrotoxic and it must be used in reduced dosage if renal impairment is present.

The aim of therapy is to achieve levels of at least 8–12 μg/ml. Toxic changes are likely to develop if serum levels rise above 15 μg/ml.

Assays of gentamicin levels must be performed regularly if there is any renal impairment. If the drug is being given intravenously the level should be checked 15 minutes after administration; one hour after intramuscular injection. It is essential that adequate serum levels are obtained, and gentamicin assays should

Table 3.7 Dosage of gentamicin

Blood urea (mmol/l)	Creatine clearance (ml/min) (GFR)	Dose and frequency
7	70	80 mg* 8 hourly
7–16	30–70	80 mg* 12 hourly
10–30	10–30	80 mg* daily
32+	5–10	80 mg* every 48 hours
Dosage for children 2 mg/kg/24 h		*60 mg if body weight < 60 kg.

be done to confirm this. Blood urea estimations should be performed daily (Noone *et al.*, 1974).

Kanamycin and *colomycin* have similar toxic effects but the spectrum of activity does not extend to include *Pseudomonas* with kanamycin or *Staphylococcus aureus* with colomycin.

Table 3.8 Narrow-spectrum antibiotics effective against gram-positive organisms

Antibiotic	Dose
Lincomycin*	600 mg 12 hourly by intravenous infusion in 250 ml of 5% dextrose
Fucidic acid (Fucidin)	500 mg 8 hourly (oral). Children 25–50 mg/kg/24 hours (an intravenous preparation is available)
Flucloxacillin	250 mg 6 hourly (children 125 mg). can be given orally, intravenously or intramuscularly.
Clindamycin*	150–300 mg 6 hourly. oral only.

* Also effective against Bacteroides *infection.*

It should be noted that clindamycin and lincomycin if used in combination with gentamicin must be given with an interval between the two drugs. There is an antagonistic action if clindamycin or lincomycin are used in combination with antibiotics acting on the cell wall (penicillin or cephalosporin).

Anaerobic sepsis

Bacteraemia with anaerobic organisms is increasingly recognized. Their isolation may be delayed and therefore in cases where there is a high risk of anaerobe infection an appropriate antibiotic should be given pending bacteriological confirmation.

The organisms involved are usually bacteroides (which are sensitive to clinda-mycin and lincomycin), but many other pathogens have been described includ-ing *B. melaninogenicus, B. fragilis, Peptostrep anaerobius* and, of course, the *clostridia.*

Patients particularly at risk from this group of pathogens are those who have undergone major bowel or genital tract surgery.

It is important to recognize that an anaerobic infection will often be associated with the more easily recognizable aerobic infection.

The antibiotic with the broadest spectrum of activity against anaerobes is metronidazole (Flagyl). This is given intravenously in a dosage of 500 mg 8 hourly, each infusion being over a period of twenty minutes.

This drug should be considered as an ingredient of the primary therapy in all cases where anaerobic infection is a possibility.

Cephalosporins

Table 3.9 The cephalosporins

Drug	Route	Adult dose (with normal renal function)
Cephaloridine (Ceporin)	i.m. i.v.	0.5–1.0 g 8 hourly
Cephalothin (Keflin)	i.m. i.v.	2–6 g/24 h (8 hourly).
Cephalexin (Keflex Ceporex)	oral	250–500 mg 6 hourly
Cephradine (Velosef)	i.v. i.m. oral	250–500 mg 6 hourly
Cephazolin (Kefzol)	i.m.	500 mg–1 g 6–8 hourly
Cefamandole (Kefadol)	i.v. i.m.	500 mg–2 g 4–8 hourly
Cefuroxime (Zinacef)	i.v. i.m.	750 mg–1.5 g 6–8 hourly
Cefoxitin (Mefoxin)	i.v. i.m.	3–12 g/daily (4–8 hourly)
Cefaclor (Distaclor)	oral	250 mg–750 mg 8 hourly

The cephalosporins are useful broad-spectrum bactericidal antibiotics. The newer members of the group have an enhanced spectrum of activity and are, in this context, to be preferred to the older ones. All of them are effective against

34

the common gram-positive cocci and many gram negative species. Cefoxitin, cefuroxime and cefamandole are also effective against many strains of *Klebsiella*, *Enterobacter* and *Proteus*, also some anaerobic organisms such as bacteroides. The group is not effective in *Pseudomonas* infection.

The cephalosporins should always be used with caution in patients with impaired renal function as they are all, to a greater or lesser extent, nephrotoxic. This is particularly so if they are used in conjunction with the aminoglycoside antibiotics or high dose frusemide therapy (Noone *et al.*, 1973).

Each manufacturer supplies a formula to work out dosage in renal failure.

The cephalosporins have a particular value in patients who are sensitive to penicillin.

The 'second generation' cephalosporins (cefamandole, cefaroxime and cefoxitin) are now important antibiotics for the primary treatment of septicaemia of uncertain nature, pending results of bacteriology.

Carbenicillin (Pyopen) is effective against *Pseudomonas* and *Proteus*, but un-fortunately several strains are resistant. Large amounts are required to achieve bacterocidal levels (20–25 g daily, in divided doses). The sodium salt is used and in elderly patients salt and water retention can cause problems (this may also be an important consideration when renal function is impaired).

Semi-synthetic broad-spectrum penicillins for parenteral administration. Three important penicillins have recently become available for the treatment of severe infections. Their use should be restricted to severe infections where no other antibiotic is likely to be helpful or in the initial treatment of overwhelming infection before bacteriological diagnosis has been made. Under these circum-stances they are best used in conjunction with an aminoglycoside.

(1) *Ticarcillin* (Ticar)

The range of sensitivity includes streptococcus species, *Pseudomonas* and *Proteus* species, *E. Coli*, *H. influenzae*, penicillin sensitive staphylococci, *Clostridium* and importantly, anaerobes, including bacteroides. The drug is administered as a disodium salt which implies potential hazards in terms of salt and water overload.

(2) *Mezlocillin* (Baypen)

The range of activity embraces that of carbenicillin and ampicillin. In com-parison with ticarcillin it is twice as active against bacteroides and more active against *Klebsiella*, *H. influenzae* and gram-positive Streptococci. It contains 1.85 mmol/g of sodium as compared with 5.2 mmol/g in ticarcillin.

(3) *Azlocillin* (Securopen)

This acylureido semisynthetic penicillin is particularly effective in *Pseudo-monas areuginosa* infection, where it is 4–8 times as active as carbenicillin. As the monosodium salt it is less likely to produce sodium overload. As with the two antibiotics described above beta-lactamase producing strains of gram-positive organisms are likely to be resistant. The range of activity is, in general, similar to mezlocillin and ticarcillin.

The dosage of these agents is given below. *NOTE* these drugs will often be administered in conjunction with aminoglycosides or the newer cephalosporins and under these circumstances the two drugs must not be mixed together in the same syringe or infusion fluid.

Ticarcillin	15–20 g daily (4–8 hourly)
Mezlocillin	15–20 g daily (6–8 hourly)
Azlocillin	15–20 g daily (8 hourly)

NOTE These doses are for adults with normal renal function. When the creatinine clearance is less than 30 ml/min the total daily dose should be approximately 50% of the above dose, each dose at 12-hourly intervals. These drugs are administered by intravenous infusion, in bolus doses infused over 10–20 minutes. Mezlocillin can be given by intramuscular injection but the dose should not exceed 2.0 g 6–8 hourly.

Chloramphenicol has serious side-effects, notably aplastic anaemia, which may not in all cases be dose-related. It remains the drug of choice, despite the risks, for septicaemia due to invasive salmonella infections. Occasionally, in the presence of renal impairment, it might be justified to use chloramphenicol for gram-negative sepsis, as it is not nephrotoxic. Daily blood counts must be performed on any patient on chloramphenicol.

Broad-spectrum penicillin combinations. (magnapen, ampiclox). The majority of staphylococci found in hospital are resistant to ampicillin. Furthermore, this drug is not effective against many *Enterobacter/Klebseilla* species, and if given for gram-negative infection there is a grave risk of superinfection with organisms of this group. *There is, therefore, no place for the use of combination preparations containing Ampicillin.* If staphylococcal infection is considered likely cloxacillin should be given; with lincomycin or fucidic acid if combination chemotherapy is considered desirable.

If ampicillin is used, it must be given with an antibiotic effective against *Klebsiella/Enterobacter*, e.g. gentamicin.

Summary of antibiotic use in bacteraemic shock

(1) Treatment must be commenced before positive bacteriology.

(2) If necessary treatment can be changed later.

(3) Combination chemotherapy should be used if the nature of the organism is unknown:

Gentamicin + mezlocillin/cefamandole + metronidazole.

(4) If gram-negative infection is probable:

Gentamicin ± ampicillin.

(5) Gram-positive infection probable:

Lincomycin/fucidic acid/cloxacillin ± cephalosporin.

(6) *Pseudomonas* infection—azlocillin ± colomycin.

(7) Anaerobic infection—Metronidazole.

(8) Do *not* use magnapen or ampiclox.

Treatment with antibiotics must be continued for a minimum of 10–14 days. After the initial acute phase the drugs can usually be given by mouth. Once results of bacterial sensitivities are known treatment should be continued with a single appropriate antibiotic. There is no place for multiple antibiotics at this stage, and bacteraemic shock, although a serious clinical emergency, is no excuse for polypharmaceutical panic.

Steroids

The role of steroids in massive doses in endotoxic shock is more clearly defined than in hypovolaemic shock (Christy, 1971). They should be given early in treatment in the dosage suggested in Table 3.6 above.

Treatment of underlying disease

Surgical treatment for any localized collection of pus is essential in the management of bacteraemic shock.

CARDIOGENIC SHOCK

Shock associated predominantly with pump failure is discussed on page 124.

NEUROGENIC SHOCK

Shock in relation to head and spinal cord injuries is essentially a condition of hypotension with normovolaemia. Blood pressure may be unstable following transection of the spinal cord, when sympathetic outflow is interrupted; a situation analogous to that of spinal analgesia. Hypothermia is an important feature of neurogenic shock.

Acute hypotension, usually in association with bradycardia can also occur as a result of nervous reflex with vagal efferents. This can occur when pressure is exerted on the carotid sinus, when mesentery is stretched or when sphincters are dilated. Certain vagotonic drugs can cause a similar effect, (e.g. halothane, suxamethonium), and administration of atropine can ameliorate or prevent their occurrence.

ANAPHYLACTIC SHOCK

This occurs when there is a massive release of histamine in response to an allergen. It develops extremely rapidly—the patient collapses and develops signs of laboured breathing with bronchospasm, urticaria, hypotension and possibly laryngeal oedema (Macaulay, 1972).

Treatment

(1) Adrenaline 1 mg subcutaneously repeated in 15 minutes if necessary.

(2) Antihistamines (e.g. promethazine 50 mg or chlorpheniramine (Piriton) 10 mg) given intravenously.

(3) Maintenance of airway: this may involve tracheal intubation, but rarely tracheostomy.

(4) Administration of oxygen.

(5) Steroids intravenously (e.g. hydrocortisone 100 mg intravenously).

Once an individual has suffered acute anaphylaxis strict precautions are necessary to prevent further exposure to the allergen. In hospital practice, the majority of cases will occur in the X-ray department when contrast media are given intravenously.

MONITORING RESPONSE TO THERAPY

Pulse and blood pressure

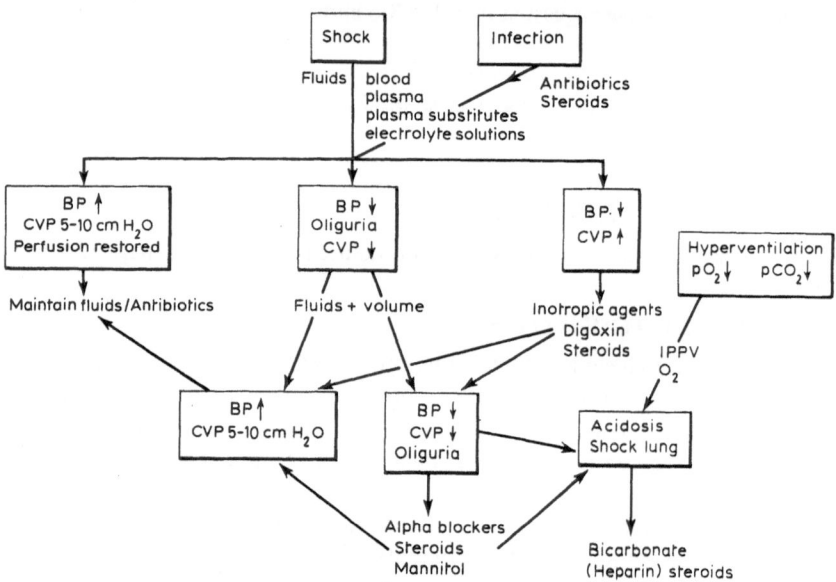

Fig. 3.3 An outline of the treatment of shock.

Broadly speaking, if treatment is successful, the blood pressure will rise and the pulse rate fall. These parameters should be measured every 15 minutes. However, it is unwise to regard the blood pressure as a reliable guide to the progress of shock therapy. Blood pressure reflects changes in cardiac output, circulating volume and peripheral resistance, and therefore the cardiac output and blood pressure are not directly proportional; moreover, as has been emphasized above, tissue perfusion can be inadequate even if the arterial blood pressure is relatively normal when severe vasoconstriction has occurred.

Direct measurement of the cardiac output is not yet available as a routine procedure in the District General Hospital.

If a direct arterial line has been placed, to monitor blood pressure (see Chapter 10), the radial artery may give fallacious results due to arterial constriction and the femoral artery is preferred. In this site damage to the artery from flushing the line is unlikely to occur.

Central venous pressure

The technique of inserting a central venous line, and its complications are described in Chapter 10). The normal heart will pump all the blood it receives from the venous system. Pump failure results in a rise in pressure, hypovolaemia in a fall. The CVP will provide invaluable information as to fluid requirements during therapy. A falling CVP will generally indicate the need for more volume expansion. If the CVP rises, in association with deteriorating tissue perfusion, aggressive therapy with positive inotropic agents will be indicated.

It should be noted that intermittent positive pressure ventilation, by its effect on intrathoracic pressure may itself cause a rise of up to 5–10 cm H_2O. During IPPV there is a reversal of the respiratory swing transmitted to CVP. It is important to verify that respiratory swing is present, whether respiration be spontaneous or passive, since this is an indication of correct siting of the central catheter.

Temperature readings

Tissue perfusion can be related to the colour and temperature of the skin of the extremities. As shock develops the skin temperature drops, and at the same time central core temperature rises because skin heat loss is reduced. If a thermocouple is affixed to a digit and the temperature monitored, dramatic drops in temperature can be recorded, to as low as 12–15°C. As peripheral perfusion improves with therapy, the skin temperature will rise.

Urine flow

The changes in the renal circulation in shock are profound and the kidney is very vulnerable to hypovolaemia. In the initial phases there exists a mechanism for maintaining glomerular filtration rate despite a fall in arterial blood pressure. As the GFR falls when the compensatory mechanisms cease to be effective there will be a concomitant fall in the excretion of solutes, usually accompanied by an increase in ADH secretion leading to oliguria with highly concentrated urine. Renal damage can be strongly suspected if urine osmolality is near to plasma osmolality, urine sodium excretion is over 50 mmol/l.

Urinary output should be measured on an hourly basis and if less than 30 ml/h, despite adequate fluid and volume replacement as monitored by the CVP line, steps must be taken to protect renal function.

Intravenous 20% mannitol 250 ccs should be infused over 30 minutes. This may reduce the swelling in the hypoxic cells in the nephron by virtue of its action as an osmotic diuretic, and thereby exert a protective effect on the kidney; however, it is also noted that if no diuresis occurs as a result of the infusion, then the probability is high that renal damage has occurred. This infusion should not be repeated because of the risks of inducing pulmonary oedema.

Frusemide given intravenously can also be used at this stage to assess renal integrity. The role of high dose frusemide therapy in acute renal failure is discussed in Chapter 13).

Other measurements

(1) Blood gas analysis will demonstrate hypoxaemia and base deficit, which will need correction.

(2) Lactic acid estimations. It has been claimed that serial estimations of lactic acid, and also the lactate/pyruvate ratio, provide a useful indication of the severity and progress of shock. An initial value of less than 10 mmol/l lactate which drops with treatment may indicate a better prognosis.

(3) Serial haemoglobin, packed cell volume, urea and electrolyte estimations are essential.

THE LUNG IN SHOCK

The importance of disorders of pulmonary function and structure in shock merits special discussion. Oxygen therapy is of vital importance in the therapy of shock, and every effort should be made to assure a PaO_2 of at least 70 mm Hg. Where clinical evidence of pulmonary insufficiency is present at the time of admission following trauma mortality rates are high. The pattern of respiration is one of rapid shallow respiration; the tidal volume being low but the minute volume close to normal. At this stage the PaO_2 may be normal but within a few hours this will fall to below 70 mm Hg, and this is associated with a drop in the P_aCO_2. The clinical picture is one of respiratory distress, tachypnoea, cyanosis, refractory hypoxaemia and poor lung compliance. Although the chest X-ray is often normal in the earlier stages, by this time it will show bilateral diffuse shadows.

There are many factors which contribute to respiratory insufficiency in shock, which are listed below.

Post-mortem examination of the lungs of patients who have died following traumatic shock reveals only minor changes within the first eighteen hours. Petechial haemorrhages, scattered areas of atalectasis in dependant areas are found, and on microscopic examination pulmonary venous and capillary engorgement with thrombo-emboli in the small vessels. After 18 hours the changes become more evident and may proceed to haemorrhagic consolidation of entire lobes with severe pulmonary venous congestion, scattered thrombo-emboli, interstitial oedema and peribronchial and perivascular haemorrhage. After 72 hours the lungs often resemble liver with microscopic finding of hyaline

Table 3.10 *The phases of post-traumatic respiratory insufficiency (Moore* et al., *1969)*

Phase I	Period of shock Spontaneous hyperventilation and hypocapnia
Phase II	Early respiratory distress Hypoxia due to shunting of 10–20% cardiac output Hyperventilation and hypocapnia
Phase III	Gross hypoxia: mechanical ventilation required Chest X-ray shows shock lung
Phase IV	Terminal anoxaemia with final CO_2 retention

Table 3.11 *Factors which contribute to respiratory insufficiency in shock*

1. Fluid overload and lowered surfactant.
2. Physical exhaustion : inactivity : airways obstruction.
3. Aspiration pneumonia.
4. Fat embolism and fatty acid toxicity.
5. Blood transfusion with stored blood.
6. Oxygen toxicity.
7. Haemorrhagic shock.
8. Septic or endotoxin shock.
9. Acidosis and hypoxia.
10. 'Shock lung' as the result of microembolism by platelet aggregates.

(Wardle, 1974.)

membrane in alveoli, diffuse haemorrhage and consolidation, and bronchopneumonia. Sequestration of polymorph leucocytes in pulmonary capillaries has also been described (Blaisdell and Stallome, 1970; Ratcliffe *et al.*, 1971).

The aetiology of 'shock lung' as a specific entity remains uncertain but (Hardaway, 1970), there is considerable evidence that it is due to microembolisation of the lungs secondary to disseminated intravascular coagulation. This would explain many of the features, and the importance of DIC in the pathophysiology of shock is only recently being appreciated.

Diagnosis

Shock lung should be suspected in any patient with hypovolaemic shock with hyperventilation, refractory hypoxaemia and hypocapnia.

Treatment

(1) Elevation of PaO_2. This may involve mechanical ventilation of the lungs using a volume cycled apparatus and perhaps positive end expiratory pressure (Chapter 6).

(2) Control of oxygen administration to prevent further insult of oxygen toxicity (Chapter 7).

(3) Regulation of intravenous fluids to prevent overload; the use of diuretics.

(4) Treatment of secondary infection with specific antibiotics for specific infections.

(5) Steroids—which may reduce capillary permeability and maintain the integrity of the alveolar epithelium.

(6) Heparin—where not contra-indicated because of haemorrhage; or alternatively, low molecular weight dextran to reduce platelet aggregations.

THE COMPLICATIONS OF MASSIVE BLOOD TRANSFUSION

If large quantities of stored blood have to be given over a short period of time, consideration must be given to the complications of the procedure. The problem of *circulatory overload* will be avoided by careful monitoring of the CVP. If the patient develops signs of acute pulmonary oedema, with cyanosis, dyspnoea, elevation of the JVP and basal crepitations, the intravenous infusion must be slowed and an intravenous diuretic given, e.g. frusemide 40 mg. If conscious, the patient will complain of chest tightness and may develop a cough, which may be accompanied by haemoptysis.

The problems of stored blood

Circulatory arrest is a complication of massive blood transfusion and several factors are thought to contribute to this (Ludbrook and Wynn, 1958).

Temperature

Blood must be rewarmed before administration. This can be achieved by the use of thermostatically controlled water baths, or by ultrasonic equipment. If cold blood is transfused to a shocked patient who is already in an unstable thermoregulatory state selective cardiac hypothermia may result. The oxygen dissociation curve of blood is shifted to the left in hypothermia and this will be aggravated by the shift already present in acid-citrate-dextrose (ACD) stored blood (Valtis and Kennedy, 1954). Rapid rewarming of stored blood will cause haemolysis, therefore the practice of dumping blood containers in hot, or even warm, water is to be avoided. Not only will there be a risk of haemolysis but slow rewarming will encourage growth of any bacteria that may be present. (Blood that has been rewarmed must be discarded if not used, Leading Article *Lancet*, 1966.)

Calcium

Each 540 ml (1 pint) of stored blood contains 120 ml of acid-citrate-dextrose solution as an anticoagulant. Citrate, when infused, may depress ionised calcium levels in the recipient's blood. It is therefore advisable to give calcium if large quantities of ACD blood have to be given rapidly. (2.5 ml of 10% calcium chloride or 10 ml of 10% calcium gluconate with each pints.) It has been suggested that these measures are unnecessary, even harmful (Howland *et al.*, 1965).

pH

Stored blood has a pH of 6.58–6.72, which increases the longer it is stored. As patients with shock will already be liable to acidosis, bicarbonate should be administered (50 ml of 8.4% sodium bicarbonate with every 5 pints).

Potassium

The serum potassium of stored blood may rise to 11 mmol/l. However, with rewarming much of the potassium returns to the red cells. But it should be remembered that a vulnerable myocardium is at risk when exposed to high concentrations of potassium.

Haematological complications

Platelets and some labile clotting factors are not stable in stored blood and when massive transfusions are given a bleeding diathesis may develop. In shock this may be compounded by the presence of intravascular coagulation at the same time. Thrombocytopaenia occurs when more than 5000 ml of stored blood is given over 48 hours and usually reverts to normal within 2 to 3 days. The effects on platelets and clotting factors can be minimized by using blood that has been stored for as short a time as possible. About 10–20% of blood given in massive transfusions of this nature should be fresh (Krevans and Jackson, 1955).

Particular caution is necessary when the patient has severe liver disease, because the liver is the site of citrate metabolism, and under these circumstances calcium should be given (as above).

Mis-matched transfusions

When large quantities of blood have to be given rapidly extra care is essential in the cross-matching and checking of blood, as it is these circumstances that mistakes can occur. The problem of mis-matched transfusion is discussed in Chapter 18.

Microembolisation

It has been suggested that the hypoxia associated with trauma is related to the amount of blood transfused (Hissen and Swank, 1965). A factor may be the debris present, particularly when blood is more than 48 hours old. This could be of particular relevance to the development of the 'shock lung' syndrome. It would, therefore, be reasonable to suggest that transfused blood should be filtered. The ideal filter should not interfere with the rate of transfusion, should not damage the normal cellular components of blood and remove particles to a size of 20 μm (Mason *et al.* 1975).

INFECTION FROM INTRAVENOUS FLUIDS (Meers *et al.*, 1973; Makie *et al.*, 1973)

If a patient who is receiving intravenous fluids becomes shocked, where the clinical situation is otherwise inappropriate, the possibility of bacterial contamination of intravenous fluids must be considered. The organism responsible may be unusual and not always rapidly identified by the laboratory. The remnants of any suspect container must be retained for bacteriological examination. Suspicion should be alerted if the fluid is cloudy or opalescent. All containers must be checked for their integrity.

REFERENCES

Blaisdell, F. W. and Stallome, R. J. (1970), The mechanisms of pulmonary damage following traumatic shock. *Surg. Gyn. Obst.*, 130, 15.

See *British Medical Journal* (1977), Editorial. Dopamine in cardiac failure and shock. *Brit. med. J.*, 2, 1563.

Bunn, H. F. *et al.* (1969), Haemoglobin function in stored blood. *J. Clin. Invest.*, 48, 311.

Christy, J. H. (1971), Treatment of Gram Negative Shock. *Am. J. Med.*, 50, 77.

Collins, V. J., Jaffee, R. and Zahony, I. (1962), Shock: a different approach to therapy. *Illinois med. J.*, 122, 350.

Conway, E. J. (1957), Nature and significance of concentration relations of potassium and sodium ions in skeletal muscle. *Physiol. Rev.*, 37, 84.

Cunningham, J. N., Shires, G. T. and Wagner, Y. (1971), Changes in intracellular sodium and potassium content of red blood cells in trauma and shock. *Amer. J. Surg.*

Dietzman, R. H. and Lillehei, R. C. (1968), The nature and treatment of shock. *Brit. J. Hosp. Med.*, 1, 300.

Dietzman, R. H., Ersek, R. A., Lillehei, C. W., Casterada, A. R. and Lillehei, R. C. (1960), Low output syndrome. Recognition and Treatment. *J. Thorac. Surg.*, 57, 139.

Editorial (1980), Toxic shock and tampons. *Brit. med. J.*, 281, 1161.

Hardaway, A. M. (1970), *J. clin. Path.*, 23, Suppl. 4, 110.

Hardaway, R. M. (1965), Microcoagulation in Shock. *Amer. J. Surg.*, 110, 298.

Hissen, W. and Swank, R. L. (1965), Screen Filtration pressure and Pulmonary Hypertension. *Am. Journal Physiology*, 209, 715.

Howard, J. M. *et al.* (1956), Studies of dextrans of various molecular sizes. *Ann. Surg.*, 143, 369.

Howland, W. S., Schweiger, O., Boyan, P. C. (1965), The effect of buffering on the mortality of massive transfusion. *Surg. Gyn. Obst.*, 121, 177.

Inglemon, B., Gronwall, A., Gelin, L-E. and Eliasson, R. (1969), Properties and applications of dextrans. *Acta Acad. Reg. Sci. Upsaliensis*, 12, 1.

Jenkins, M. T., Giesecke, A. H. and Shires, G. T. (1965), Electrolyte Therapy in shock: management during Anaesthesia. In *Clinical Anaesthesia—Clinical*

Management of the Patient in Shock. ed Lerkin, L. R. Blackwell, Oxford.

Krevans, J. R. and Jackson, D. P. (1955), Haemorrhagic disorder following massive whole blood transfusions. *J. Am. Med. Ass.*, **159**, 171.

Leading Article (1966), Warm blood for massive transfusion. *Lancet*, i, 1193.

Leading Article (1969), Catecholamines and myocardial infarction. *Lancet*, ii, 1051.

Lemieux, M. D., Smith, R. N. and Couch, N. P. (1969), Surface pH and redose potential of skeletal muscle in graded haemorrhage. *Surgery*, **65**, 457.

Lillehei, R. C., Dietzman, R. H. and Block, J. H. (1967), Hypotension and low cardiac output syndrome following cardiopulmonary bypass. In *Cardiac Surgery* ed. Norman J. C., Appleton Centenary Crofts, New York.

Ludbrook, J. and Wynn, V. (1958), Citrate intoxication—A Clinical and Experimental Study. *Brit. Med. J.*, 2, 523.

Macaulay, D. B. (1972), Acute anaphylaxis. *Brit. J. Hosp. Med.*, 8, 273.

Makie, G. D., Goldmann, D. A., Rhame, F. S. (1973), Infection Control in Intravenous Therapy. *Ann. Int. Med.*, **79**, 867.

Mason, K. G., Hall, L. E., Lamoy, R. E. and Wright, C. B. (1975), Evaluation of blood filters, dynamics of platelets and platelet aggregates. *Surgery*, 77, 235.

McMurdoch, J., Spiers, C. F., Pullen, H. (1968). The bacteraemic shock syndrome. *Brit. J. Hosp. Med.*, 1, 347.

Meers, P. D., Calder, M. W., Mayhar, M. M. and Laurie, G. M. (1973), Intravenous infusion of contaminated dextrose-solution—The Devonport Incident. *Lancet*, ii, 1189.

Messmer, K. (1975), *Surg. Clin. N. Am.*, **55**, 659.

Middleton, E. S., Matthews, R. and Shires, G. T. (1969), Radiosulphate as a measure of the extracellular fluid in cute haemorrhagic shock. *Am. Surg.*, **170**, 174.

Moore, F. D., Lyons, J. H., Pierce, E. C., Morgan, A. P., Drinker, P. A., MacArthur, J. P. and Dammin, G. J. (1969), *Post-traumatic respiratory insufficiency.* London, W. B. Saunders.

Negberg, S., Nalmas, H. and Rochert, H. (1968), Shock reactions in skeletal muscles. III: The electrolyte content of tissue fluid and blood plasma before and after induced haemorrhagic shock. *Am. Surg.*, **168**, 243.

Noone, P., Pattison, J. R., Shafi, M. S. (1973), Renal failure in combined gentamicin and cephalothin therapy. *Brit. med. J.*, 2, 776.

Noone, P., Parsons, T. M. C., Pattison, J. R., Slack, R. C. B., Hughes, K. and Garfield-Davies, D. (1974), Experience in monitoring Gentamicin therapy during treatment of Serious Gram Negative sepsis. *Brit. med. J.*, 1, 477.

Ratcliff, N. B., Wilson, J. W., Mikat, E., Hackel, D. B. and Graham, T. C. (1971), The lung in haemorrhagic shock. IV: The role of neutrophilic polymorphonuclear leucocytes. *Am. J. Path.*, **65**, 325.

Repogle, R. L., Gazzaniga, A. B. and Gross, R. E. (1966), Use of corticosteroids during cardiopulmonary bypass: possible lysozyme stabilisation. *Circulation*, 33. (Supp. I), 86.

Ricketts, C. R. (1973), Blood Substitutes. *Brit. J. Anaesth.*, **45**, 958.

Ring, J. and Messmer, K. (1977), *Lancet*, i, 466.

Sambi, M. P., West, M. H. and Udhoji, V. N. (1962), Increase in cardiac output—a pharmacologic effect of corticosteroids. *Circulation*, 26, 780.

Shenkin, H. A. *et al.* (1944), On the diagnosis of haemorrhage in man: A study of volunteers bled in large amounts. *Am. J. Med. Sci.*, **208**, 421.

Shires, G. T. *et al.* (1972). Alterations in cellular membrane function during haemorrhagic shock in primates. *Am. Surg.*, **176**.

Slonim, M. and Stahl, W. M. (1968), Sodium and water content of connective versus cellular tissue following haemorrhage. *Surg. Forum*, **14**, 53.

Taylor, J. and Weil, M. H. (1967), Failure of the Trendelenberg position to improve circulation during clinical shock. *Surg. Gyn. Obst.*, **124**, 1005.

Tinker, J. (1979), A pharmacological approach to the treatment of shock. *Brit. J. Hosp. Med.*, **21**, 261.

Valeri, C. R. (1971), The Viability and Function of Preserved Red Cells. *New Eng. J. Med.*, **284**, 81.

Valtis, D. J. and Kennedy, A. C. (1954), Defective gas transport function of stored red blood cells. *Lancet*, i, 119.

Wardle, E. N. (1974), Post-traumatic respiratory insufficiency: What is 'Shock Lung'? *J. Roy. Coll. Physcns Lond.*, **8**, 251.

Weil, M. H. and Nishijima, H. (1978), *Am. J. Med.*, **64**, 920.

Wilson, R. F. and Fisher, R. R. (1968), The haemodynamic effects of massive steroids in clinical shock. *Surg. Gyn. Obst.*, **127**, 769.

Respiratory failure

Respiratory failure may be considered to occur when gas exchange in the lungs becomes inadequate as a result of pathophysiological changes. No blood gas values can be quoted as determining the onset of failure and exhaustion of the patient is an important factor to consider.

Respiratory failure is not in itself an indication for intensive therapy. There must be reasonable hope that such failure is reversible before the patient is submitted to the uncomfortable, expensive and sometimes prolonged regime of mechanical ventilation, which is not itself without complications. The decision to ventilate or to withhold therapy is not always easy and the clinician must weigh up the prognosis in the individual patient.

CAUSES OF RESPIRATORY FAILURE

The causes of respiratory failure are legion and it is necessary to restrict discussion to those conditions likely to benefit from treatment in the intensive care unit. In general the aim is to treat the disease process while maintaining function by mechanical ventilation. Difficulties in achieving adequate gas exchange may arise when the source of failure lies within the lungs themselves.

Some important causes of respiratory failure can be listed.

Diseases of the central nervous system

(1) *Poliomyelitis.* Respiratory inadequacy can arise as a result of paralysis of the muscles of respiration, with inability to swallow saliva in the bulbar form of the disease. Nowadays rare in the U.K.

(2) *Polyneuritis.* Peripheral neuritis involving the motor nerves can also cause paralysis of respiratory muscles. The tidal volume may become inadequate to maintain gas exchange in the lungs and failure to cough may result in sputum retention.

(3) *Guillain-Barre syndrome.* This condition is considered in detail in Chapter 19. Paralysis of respiratory muscles may result in respiratory failure which may be associated with sputum retention. The autonomic system may also be involved with resultant blood pressure disturbances, dysrhythmias, excessive sweating and gastrointestinal disturbances.

(4) *Head injury.* Breathing may be stertorous and may be associated with muscle spasms and bouts of hyperventilation resulting in increased oxygen utilization. In other cases respiration may become shallow or frank apnoea may develop. Such patients may be extremely sensitive to respiration depressant drugs. For a full discussion see Chapter 12.

(5) *Spinal cord injury.* Depending on the level of injury, the nerve supply to respiratory muscles may be interrupted with resultant fall in tidal volume.

(6) *Intracranial haemorrhage.* Sudden rise in intracranial tension may result in respiratory inadequacy or apnoea. Subarachnoid haemorrhage in a previously fit young adult may not be diagnosed until tracheal intubation and IPPV have been instituted, but the prognosis is almost hopeless once apnoea has occurred and it is not justified to continue IPPV in the deeply comatose areflexic patient for an indefinite period. The diagnosis of brain death is discussed in Chapter 12.

(7) *Meningitis and encephalitis.* These conditions may result in respiratory inadequacy. The prognosis is not always hopeless and IPPV should be undertaken when there is a chance of successful treatment.

Diseases involving muscles

(1) *Myasthenia gravis.* See Chapter 19. IPPV may be indicated during exacerbations of the disease or in crisis.

(2) *Myotonia.* Patients with myotonia are susceptible to respiratory depressant drugs and may require ventilatory support in some circumstances, as in the post-operative period.

Lung diseases

(1) *Acute exacerbations of bronchitis.* When these occur in the patient with obstructive airways disease IPPV may be indicated. See Chapter 8.

(2) *Bronchospasm.* In severe cases, when the patient is becoming exhausted IPPV may be indicated. See Chapter 8.

(3) *Post-operative respiratory insufficiency.* IPPV may be carried out electively following major surgery or it may become evident that the patient requires temporary ventilatory support.

(4) *Trauma.* Damage to the chest wall or the presence of pneumo- or haemothorax may compromise respiration. Conditions such as fat embolism and shock lung are considered elsewhere. See Chapter 12.

(5) *Rare causes of block of oxygen transfer at alveolar level.*

Poisoning

This subject is considered in Chapter 16. In appropriate circumstances tracheal intubation and IPPV are necessary.

Tetanus

Muscle spasms may interfere with pulmonary ventilation and treatment by muscle relaxant drugs and IPPV may become necessary. Additional problems are posed when autonomic discharges occur. See Chapter 19.

Status epilepticus

Frequent muscle spasms lead to hypoxia and exhaustion. When it proves impossible to control the patient with anticonvulsant drugs it may be necessary to administer muscle relaxant drugs. Respiration must then be maintained artificially.

Iatrogenic causes

Respiratory inadequacy may occur as a result of patient sensitivity or as a result of frank misuse. Accidents with techniques can also result in apnoea (e.g. total spinal block). IPPV is necessary until recovery occurs.

Neonatal

The respiratory distress syndrome of the newborn may be severe enough to warrant IPPV. Chest infections in small babies may result in respiratory failure.

DIAGNOSIS OF RESPIRATORY FAILURE

The diagnosis of respiratory failure rests primarily on *clinical observations*, supported by simple bedside measurements of lung function and the laboratory estimation of blood gases.

Clinical features

These will vary according to the causation of the respiratory failure. The history, physical examination and the clinical course of the disease are all important. The patient may attempt to compensate for inadequate gas exchange by a rise in respiratory rate or by the use of accessory muscles of respiration, but as he fails to do this he is likely to exhibit sweating and he may become cyanosed. Cyanosis is, however, a late sign and may not occur at all. It should be remembered that the patient has 5 g of reduced haemoglobin in the circulating blood before cyanosis is detectable by the observer. The plethoric or polycythaemic patient readily becomes cyanosed, but the anaemic may never become cyanosed or only when arterial PO_2 is very low. The healthy subject does not become cyanosed until one third of his circulating haemoglobin is reduced and this corresponds to an arterial oxygen tension of about 5 kPa (38 mmHg).

When the lungs are healthy respiratory insufficiency is likely to result from an inadequate respiratory excursion. It may be obvious that respiration is shallow and breath sounds may be distant. Added sounds may be heard when bronchial secretions are retained. The tidal volume, minute volume and vital capacity become reduced. The need for ventilatory support is assessed after observation of the patient over a period of time.

When the respiratory tract is diseased, two types of respiratory failure may occur. In the first, tidal excursion is reduced and there may be evidence of sputum retention as well as of major pathological changes in the lung parenchyma. The patient is unable to maintain satisfactory gas exchange. In the second type the patient makes increased effort to overcome a disability but eventually becomes exhausted. The primary cause may be bronchospasm, inhalation of a foreign body, bilateral recurrent laryngeal nerve palsy or obstructing carcinoma. The patient may be able to compensate for a time, but eventually he becomes exhausted with a falling arterial oxygen tension and hypercarbia. The indication for IPPV is often exhaustion.

The need for IPPV is often obvious clinically and laboratory tests, radiology, etc., play little part in determining the initiation of IPPV. Blood gases, chest X-ray and ECG may of course offer additional information and also serve for comparison with subsequent measurements during the course of the patients illness.

Lung function tests

These have some part to play in the management of the acute situation. Tidal volumes can often be recorded using an instrument such as the Wright's anemometer mounted on an anaesthetic facemask, though it is necessary to ensure an airtight fit with the face. The patient may be too exhausted to co-operate in the measurement of vital capacity, forced expiratory volume or peak flowrate. The patient in pain may also fail to co-operate adequately. In any case, single readings are less valuable than serial measurements and it is misleading to quote actual figures as an indication of respiratory failure, though tidal volumes of less than 300 ml or vital capacity of less than 1000 ml in the adult may give rise for concern. Lung function tests are, however, valuable to assess progress in some circumstances, and the vital capacity measured serially during the recovery phase may be valuable in the patient with neurological disease.

Blood gas estimation

Rapid and accurate estimations of arterial oxygen and carbon dioxide tensions are a useful adjunct in the assessment of respiratory failure. Trends are more important than single estimations, particularly in terms of response to therapy, and the diagnosis of respiratory failure must always be made on clinical and not on laboratory findings. Arterial oxygen tensions above 6.6 kPa (50 mmHg) are usually acceptable since this represents saturation of the major part of the circulating haemoglobin with oxygen. The A-aDO$_2$, the difference between alveolar and arterial oxygen tensions is also important. The difference is magnified when pure oxygen is administered and an acceptable range for A-aDO$_2$ is

7 to 27 kPa after the subject has respired 100% oxygen for 15 minutes. Arterial carbon dioxide tensions are important in the management of respiratory failure. Levels above 8 kPa (60 mmHg) suggest the need for ventilatory support.

FIVE

The airway

Preservation of the airway is fundamental to survival. It is threatened in the comatose patient but also in a variety of pathological situations.

Coma

As the depth of coma increases the muscles of the tongue and pharynx become relaxed and the tongue tends to fall back against the posterior pharyngeal wall. Some individuals are particularly likely to suffer respiratory obstruction if they become unconscious, the bull-necked or those with nasal obstruction being cases in point, but any patient may require airway support. The tongue tends to drop away from the posterior pharyngeal wall when the patient is placed in the lateral or prone positions. The latter makes clinical observation difficult, but the lateral position is generally the safest one for unconscious patients.

The comatose patient is always likely to suffer regurgitation of stomach contents with subsequent pulmonary aspiration. This is also due to relaxation of the cardiac sphincter at the lower end of the oesophagus. Many comatose patients suffer this complication during transport or before admission to hospital and once again the lateral position helps to avoid the possibility of aspiration to the lungs as regurgitated material is more likely to flow out of the mouth. The prone position, on the other hand, may cause a rise of intra-abdominal pressure with an increased likelihood of regurgitation.

Congenital abnormalities

Congenital abnormalities of the jaw and other congenital conditions such as choanal atresia may cause respiratory obstruction in the newborn. It may be necessary to nurse the infant in a face down position and to hold the tongue forwards by means of a tongue stitch or tongue forceps. Laryngoscopy and tracheal intubation may be difficult or impossible in this situation. The newborn may also be unable to suck when the nose is blocked.

Infection and oedema

Acute infection and its associated oedema may threaten the airway. Ludwig's angina or the oedema of allergic reactions may produce acute distress. Chronic inflammation may produce late problems as a result of scar tissue formation as in tracheal stenosis.

The lower airways

These may become obstructed due to foreign bodies, aspiration of stomach contents or blood clot, bronchospasm and oedema.

Obstruction to the upper airways can be relieved by the use of pharyngeal airways, tracheal intubation or tracheostomy.

Pharyngeal airways

These have a limited use in the ITU since their insertion does not by itself guarantee airway patency. They are, however, useful in some patients in light coma. The appropriate size for the patient must be selected and the airway inserted carefully so as not to initiate gagging reflexes. Use of topical analgesic ointment may sometimes be justified. Pharyngeal airways are also useful to act as bite-blocks for some patients with orotracheal tubes in place or in some patients having epileptic fits.

Indications for tracheal intubation

There are three main indications:

(1) Preservation of the airway.

(2) To facilitate removal of secretions from the tracheo-bronchial tree. Sputum retention occurs in debilitated patients or when the cough reflex is ineffective.

(3) As an adjunct to mechanical ventilation of the lungs. See Chapter 6.

TRACHEAL TUBES

Tracheal tubes may be passed by the oral or nasal routes or via a tracheostomy.

Material of the tube

Rubber tubes may be irritant on prolonged use and the disposable plastic tubes are associated with less laryngeal injury (Hedden *et al.*, 1969). Early plastic tubes were thought to promote irritation should chemicals seep out of the material used but modern tubes are tested to prevent this complication. Sterilization with ethylene oxide can cause problems in this way if proper aeration has not been allowed for elimination of the agent.

Cuff hazards

Traumatization of the mucous membrane of the trachea by an overdistended cuff is a serious problem as it may result in subsequent scarring and stenosis. Much thought has been given to this problem and various remedies suggested have included intermittent deflation and reflation, inflation during the inspiratory phase of the respiratory cycle only (Kirby *et al.*, 1970), and the use of double cuffs (Carroll *et al.*, 1974). Current thought favours the use of large floppy cuffs (Grillo *et al.*, 1971; Cooper and Grillo, 1972; Carroll, 1973; Carroll *et al.*, 1974). These cuffs have a large volume and a large diameter and occlude the trachea over a large area of mucous membrane exerting a relatively low pressure. Cuff pressure can be measured using an aneroid gauge; the pressure needed to permit adequate capillary blood flow in the mucous membrane of the trachea has been stated to be 1.0 to 2.4 kPa (20–25 cm H_2O) (Carroll *et al.*, 1974). Overinflation is to be avoided as excessive pressure may otherwise be exerted and it is possible for the cuff of some types of tube to herniate over the tip of the tube to cause obstruction (Cooper and Grillo, 1972; Carroll *et al.*, 1974). The best advice is to inflate the cuff carefully until the leak is abolished and to put in no more. The volume of air used should be recorded as an increasing requirement may suggest tracheal dilatation. The Lanz tube has recently been recommended (Leigh and Maynard, 1979) as the pilot balloon has a pressure control valve and pressure does not become excessive with overinflation.

The practice of pre-stretching high pressure cuffs (Geffin and Pontoppidan, 1969) can no longer be justified as complications have been reported following use of this technique (Martinez and Kalter, 1971; Lawson, 1973) and low pressure cuffs are now available.

Tube length

Accidental endobronchial intubation (more commonly on the right side) is all too easy, especially when the tube has been passed in emergency situations by unskilled operators. It is essential to confirm that there is good air entry to both lungs and this is best achieved by auscultation. If there is any doubt the tube should be withdrawn. Some manufacturers place a black line on the tube just above the cuff and it is suggested that this line should be visible above the cords on direct laryngoscopy when the tube is correctly positioned. Others mark the tube length in cm at the level of the incisor teeth so that when the tube is changed the new one can be cut to the correct length. The practice of leaving an excessive amount of tube outside the mouth is to be deprecated since the tube may accidentally slip further in subsequently. The opportunity should always be taken to look for the level of the tip of the tube when chest X-rays are viewed as this provides an additional check.

Tube diameter

The correct size of tube should be used. Tubes too large in diameter cause trauma; too small a tube may be associated with airflow resistance and to the need for excessive cuff inflation. The over-distended cuff may in turn compress the tube which may have become softened at body temperature.

Tube shape

The tube of conventional shape is likely to cause trauma to the posterior part of the larynx and the arytenoids are particularly vulnerable (Lindholm, 1969). Patient movement increases the likelihood of damage. Some thought has been given recently to the ideal shape of tube for prolonged orotracheal intubation.

Tube fixation

Accidental displacement of a tracheal tube is not only inconvenient but it may threaten life. There should be a unit policy with regard to technique of secure fixation. In general, an orotracheal tube should be fixed to the upper lip rather than the more mobile lower lip, while a nasotracheal tube is easier to render secure. When necessary, the patients hands must be bandaged to prevent him pulling out the tube and adequate sedation prescribed when appropriate. The connections to the ventilator or humidifier must be such that traction does not pull out the tracheal tube.

Crusting of secretions

This must be prevented by provision of adequate humidification (see Chapter 6).

Oral or nasal tubes?

In surgical practice the anaesthetist usually prefers oro- to naso-tracheal tubes since the former route allows passage of a tube of generous internal diameter under direct vision without trauma. This can be performed in the presence of profound relaxation. Nasotracheal tubes, on the other hand, are limited in diameter by the size of the nasal passage and their passage may involve trauma to structures such as the turbinates as well as the carriage of infected material to the trachea.

The situation in the ITU is very different. The conscious patient usually finds the nasotracheal tube to be more comfortable than the orotracheal tube which is an encumbrance in the mouth. It is not always easy to use a laryngoscope in the semi-conscious or awake patient and it is not always desirable to induce anaesthesia or profound muscular relaxation. Those skilled in the act of blind nasal intubation can often pass the nasal tube with or without topical analgesia and/or sedation in the patient whose jaw is not relaxed. Nasal tubes offer comfort, convenience and easier fixation without kinking, but where they are not satisfactory, as in the presence of nasal obstruction, oral tubes are to be preferred. Oral tubes are in fact often more convenient in the deeply unconscious patient when many of the considerations in favour of the nasal route do not apply.

Technique of tracheal intubation

The technique used will vary according to the clinical situation and the degree of urgency. The procedure is not without hazard, especially in the hypoxic subject, and it should nearly always be possible to administer oxygen by bag and mask to relieve hypoxia until the preparations for tracheal intubation are complete.

A variety of laryngoscopes and tracheal tubes with connections should be available in the intensive care environment together with provision for pharyngeal and bronchial suction.

Pre-oxygenation is strongly recommended. Vagal reflexes may be initiated by laryngeal manipulations and sympathetic discharges are also common as evidenced by ventricular dysrythmias. The patient is protected by full oxygenation which should be given for at least five minutes by bag and mask. The use of atropine should be considered if bradycardia or pharyngeal secretions are thought to present a problem. An indwelling intravenous needle should whenever possible be in place before the procedure is commenced.

Some techniques:

(1) The deeply unconscious patient. The jaw is usually well relaxed and laryngeal reflexes inactive so that technical problems rarely present.

(2) Semi-conscious or comatose patients with masseter tone or spasm. Laryngoscopy may be difficult and carry a risk of trauma unless a muscle relaxant is administered. The muscle relaxant may itself produce complications such as regurgitation of stomach contents and drugs of this group should never be used unless the administrator is confident of maintaining artificial ventilation in the apnoeic patient. Blind nasal intubation is worthy of consideration in this type of patient, again always providing the operator possesses the necessary skill. It is easier to perform when the patients respiratory excursion is increased as in some unconscious subjects following head injury. Any disadvantage of rise of intracranial pressure as a result of intubation is usually more than offset by the advantages of rapidly establishing a clear airway, though when clinical circumstances dictate the use of IPPV it may be wiser to carry out intubation with the aid of a muscle relaxant.

(3) Awake intubation. Some patients are co-operative and will accept laryngoscopy and tracheal intubation after application of topical analgesia. This is particularly true when the subject is ill or exhausted. Patients who are less co-operative may require sedation, suitable drugs being diazepam or the neurolept agents. The anaesthetist must, however, beware of causing respiratory depression unless he is prepared to proceed at once to IPPV. Conventional general anaesthesia, using intravenous induction agent and muscle relaxant can, of course, be used when conditions are appropriate. It is seldom justified to cause distress to the patient by insisting on awake intubation when there is no contra-indication to brief general anaesthesia.

Nasal intubation is best preceded by application of local analgesic drugs to the nasal mucous membrane. Judicious spraying with 4% cocaine will produce vasoconstriction and lessen the risk of epistaxis. Otherwise 4% lignocaine may be used, with or without adrenaline to promote vasoconstriction.

Toleration of tubes

Tracheal tubes are tolerated surprisingly well by the majority of sick patients. Fit patients, such as those regaining consciousness following a drug overdose will frequently extubate themselves. Restless patients may require physical restraint when preservation of the airway is essential. The use of sedative drugs requires careful evaluation in the particular clinical situation.

Humidification

This subject is considered in more detail in Chapter 5, but the importance of humidification must be stressed when mouth and nose are by-passed by a tracheal tube. In the authors' experience the blower humidifiers are the best method of introducing moisture to the inspired gases of the spontaneously breathing patient. They may be connected to the tracheal tube by means of a T-piece arrangement, and it is important that the open end does not become obstructed by bedclothes, etc. Condenser humidifiers can also be used, but they add weight and cause strains to the tube connections with the possibility of displacement.

Duration of intubation

How long can a patient be managed by oro- or nasotracheal intubation before recourse is made to tracheostomy? There are no hard and fast rules concerning this and the subject has caused controversial debate. Since there are complications associated with the use of oro-, naso-tracheal and tracheostomy tubes the advantages and disadvantages of each must be considered in the individual patient context. However, some general principles may be enunciated:

(1) In small children and infants the hazards of tracheostomy, especially outside specialized paediatric units, are increased and tracheal intubation is generally preferred. The tracheal tube can be changed at intervals.

(2) When the prognosis is considered bad, particularly when the patient is unconscious, there is less indication to proceed to tracheostomy.

(3) When the need for a tracheal tube is considered to be short there is little indication for tracheostomy. In cases of doubt the operation may be postponed for a few days.

(4) When it is clear that long term respiratory support is required there is little point in delaying conversion to tracheostomy and the operation should be carried out at the earliest convenient time. Management of the patient with tracheostomy is easier than that of the patient with oro- or naso-tracheal tubes on many counts. It is more comfortable for the conscious patient to have mouth and nose free of tubes; oral hygiene is better maintained, drinking and eating is easier and can usually be managed without tube feeds; and the patient can be put on and off the ventilator more easily at the time of weaning. In the authors' view, the advantages of tracheostomy are overwhelming during provision of respiratory support for more than a week.

(5) When unexpected difficulties arise during intubation, conversion to tracheostomy should be considered. These include the need for frequent tube change, kinking of the tube, failure of the patient to tolerate it, etc.

(6) It must be recognized that in the occasional patient, tracheostomy is virtually impossible. This may be so in the presence of large goitre or malignant tumour in the neck.

TRACHEOSTOMY

There are three main advantages of tracheostomy as compared to tracheal intubation:

(1) The system is simpler, less likely to kink or obstruct, and the tube is easier to replace if it becomes dislodged.

(2) It is more comfortable for the awake patient and less irritating to the confused patient. The awake individual can eat and drink, and with suitable arrangements even talk.

(3) It is simpler to achieve removal of tracheobronchial secretions by suction.

Surgical technique

Tracheostomy is best performed under general anaesthesia with a tracheal tube *in situ*. Emergency tracheostomy carried out on an anxious, confused, ill patient under local analgesia should be necessary on only rare occasions when prior tracheal intubation is impossible. The biggest risk of the operation lies in its performance under less than ideal conditions. It cannot be stressed too much that tracheostomy should be a major and planned step in a schedule of treatment for a particular patient.

There are certain pre-requisites for tracheostomy:

(1) The presence of a competent surgeon, anaesthetist and nurse, with an assistant for the surgeon.

(2) An intubated anaesthetised patient in the correct position, i.e., supine with shoulders slightly raised and neck extended.

(3) A sterile operation field.

(4) A complete set of instruments.

(5) A powerful suction apparatus, with catheter that will traverse the selected tube.

(6) The correct tracheostomy tube with connections to the mechanical ventilator if in use.

Tracheal intubation prior to tracheostomy is only contra-indicated in the presence of severe facial injuries or laryngeal obstruction which cannot be relieved.

Size of tracheostomy tube

Table 5.1 Recommended sizes of tracheostomy tubes

Age (yrs)	Recommended size (FG)
2	16–18
2–5	20
5–10	22–24
10–14	26–30
Adult male	36
Adult female	32

The French gauge (FG) is used and the sizes according to age are suggested in Table 5.1.

$$FG = \frac{\text{mm external diameter} \times 10}{3}$$

The operation

A horizontal 'collar' incision is made 1 cm above the manubrium. In adults it should be 5 cm long. The platysma muscle is cut transversely and the strap muscles separated vertically. The easiest way to avoid loss of direction is to constantly palpate the trachea. It is rarely necessary to divide the thyroid isthmus and if encountered it usually means that the dissection is too high.

The pre-tracheal fascia is divided and the trachea exposed. Adequate retraction is now essential and this should be undertaken by the assistant.

The tracheal incision must be below the first tracheal ring. If the first ring is damaged cricoid inflammation and subsequent laryngeal stenosis may occur.

It is common practice to use a Bjork flap (Bjork, 1960). This is a ∩ shaped incision starting at the third ring, dividing it and the second. The resultant flap is sewn back to the skin edge below. It should be wide enough to allow easy passage of the selected tube. This flap allows easy insertion of the tube at the time of operation and easy replacement subsequently. It needs no subsequent correction and when the tracheostomy is no longer required it will readily heal over a few days.

Once the flap has been sewn back the orotracheal tube may be withdrawn above the operation site, but it should remain between the cords until the tracheostomy tube is in position so that the situation can easily be restored should any difficulties arise.

Low tracheostomy is to be avoided. It has no advantages, is more difficult to perform and increases the risk of bronchial intubation.

In children, a vertical slit is preferred to the Bjork flap. This may reduce the danger of subsequent tracheal stenosis or collapse, though this remains unproven (Nelson, 1957).

Technical difficulties may contra-indicate tracheostomy in certain circumstances, as in the presence of goitre, the fixed neck in flexion, or when oedema or surgical emphysema obscures the field. Oro- or naso-tracheal intubation may then be continued for as long as a tracheal tube is required.

The tracheostomy tube

The disposable plastic tube is now preferred for patients undergoing intensive care as it is now well established that plastic is less irritant to the tracheal mucosa than rubber (Salt *et al.*, 1960). These tubes are usually sterilized by gamma radiation in the factory and a warning should be given against the use of ethylene oxide which may be difficult to remove from the plastic (Cunliff and Wesley, 1967).

The tube should be cuffed to prevent soiling of the tracheobronchial tree and to facilitate mechanical ventilation. The hazards inherent in the use of cuffs have been discussed on p. 53. In children, however, a non-cuffed tube is often appropriate as the presence of a cuff may require use of a smaller diameter tube than otherwise.

Once the tracheostomy tube is in place the cuff is inflated with the minimum volume of air necessary to make a seal. The two tapes are fixed to the flange and tied to prevent displacement of the tube. A simple dressing is placed beneath the flange over the sutured skin wound.

The external orifice of the tube should be at right-angles to the skin. The risk of the inner end of the tube pressing on and ulcerating the tracheal mucosa is thus minimized. When a mechanical ventilator is used the tubing must not be allowed to exert traction on the tracheostomy tube.

Tracheobronchial toilet

This is an essential procedure, not only for patients with retained secretions, but for all patients with a tracheostomy tube *in situ*. The presence of the tube causes an increase in secretions and a diminution in the normal clearance mechanisms. The explosive cough process has also been rendered inactive.

Tracheobronchial aspiration is an important procedure which requires attention to detail. Its effectiveness may make the difference between a successful outcome and early bronchopneumonia. The catheter used should be soft and flexible and without sharp edges. An example of a satisfactory design is the Toronto catheter which has an angulated tip and side holes (Fairley, 1963). It is best used with a device such as a Y-connector which allows a measure of control over the degree of suction applied (Plum and Dunning, 1956).

Tracheal suction should be carried out as an aseptic procedure and the operator should wear gloves. The catheter is connected to the Y-piece before it is completely removed from its package. It is passed through the tracheal tube with no suction applied (i.e. the open end of the Y-piece not occluded) and when the tip is considered to be in one of the main bronchi suction is applied as the catheter is withdrawn. It should not be left in place for more than a few seconds in case hypoxia should occur due to gases being sucked out internally from the lung (Berman and Stahl, 1968). The use of the angled tip should make possible entry to both main bronchi.

The frequency of aspiration is dictated by need. It may be necessary every few minutes or only every few hours. Usually noisy respiration serves as an adequate indicator, but even when respiration is quiet and easy aspiration is advised every few hours.

Difficulty in passing the suction catheter may be due to crusting inside the tube as dried secretions collect. When this happens the tube should be changed. Other difficulties are usually attributable to malposition of the tube and it is essential that this be corrected so as to allow easy passage of the catheter for the full extent of the bronchial tree.

Five to 10 ml of physiological saline injected down the tube prior to aspiration may help to loosen thick secretions. The use of larger quantities, although sometimes recommended, may cause hypoxia and even death (Boccles, 1970).

An effective method of removing secretions is to produce an artificial cough. This can be achieved when the lungs are inflated manually using an anaesthetic bag. The pressure is released suddenly and at the same time the chest is squeezed. The secretions are then aspirated and the process repeated if necessary. This procedure may also serve to prevent the atelectasis which can occur following endobronchial suction (Brandstater and Muallem, 1969).

Changing the patients position is also of value in preventing the accumulation of secretions. However, it should be remembered that postural changes are not always well tolerated by very ill patients who may not be able to correct haemodynamic changes brought about as a result of movement. Also, changes in position can adversely affect lung function (Hedley-Whyte, 1968).

Complications of tracheostomy

Mechanical. The following points should be checked if any mechanical malfunction is suspected:

(1) If a mechanical ventilator is in use is it working satisfactorily? If not, ventilate by hand.

(2) If a mechanical ventilator is in use is it connected to the tracheal tube?

(3) If ventilation is inadequate the cuff may be under-inflated or leaking.

(4) The cuff may be over-inflated and compressing the tube or obstructing its end.

(5) Is the tube in the trachea? If not, remove and replace under direct vision.

(6) Is the tube occluded? Passage of a catheter usually indicates a patent tube, but this is not an infallible test and if there is doubt it should be replaced.

(7) Is the tube angled correctly? The end of the tube may be occluded by pressure on the lateral tracheal wall.

(8) Is the tube too long? Auscultation should be carried out to see whether air is entering both lungs. A penetrated X-ray is a useful check.

(9) Does the patient need tracheobronchial suction? Many problems are solved by this simple procedure.

Haemorrhage

Primary haemorrhage is due to inadequate haemostasis at the time of tracheostomy. It can result in obstruction of the trachea by clots. The source must be found and dealt with after clots have been sucked out.

Haemorrhage can also occur as a result of damage to mucosa caused by bronchial toilet.

Rarely, a large and often fatal haemorrhage can occur from a major vessel near the tracheostomy site. This is due to secondary infection with ulceration of the vessel wall. It is essential to keep the tracheostomy site clear and well drained, not allowing infected material to accumulate.

Infection

Contamination of the tracheostomy tube is inevitable. It occurs within hours of insertion (Rogers and Osterhouts, 1970). However, the major pathogens are introduced by contact from carriers or infected areas. Thus the very great importance of scrupulous technique while performing tracheobronchial toilet must be stressed.

Prophylactic antibiotics may encourage infection rather than prevent it (Petersdorf *et al.*, 1957). They may also result in the emergence of resistant strains or lead to superadded fungal infections due to the suppression of normal flora. It is best to perform routine cultures of sputum and to treat specific infections as they arise. Antibiotics can never be a substitute for meticulous care.

Ulceration and stenosis

Mucosal ulceration can occur at cuff level (Cooper and Grillo, 1969) and lower down the bronchial tree due to suction injuries (Thambiran and Ripley, 1966). There are a number of possible mechanisms by which ulceration can occur (Davidson *et al.*, 1971). Aspiration of gastric contents to the region above the cuff may also be important (Leverment and Pearson, 1977). Late stenosis is a not infrequent complication. It can occur at the level of the tracheostome, or more frequently at the site of the cuff (Pearson *et al.*, 1968). The sequence of events is mucosal ulceration, secondary infection, granulation tissue formation and subsequently scarring. Several months may pass before clinical symptoms arise and the condition is often misdiagnosed as asthma. This is probably because distress does not usually arise until the tracheal diameter is 6 mm or less.

Bronchoscopy at this stage reveals a tight but often short tracheal stricture. Dilatation relieves the immediate distress, but surgical resection is almost always required as a definitive procedure.

Discontinuation of tracheostomy

When the need for a tracheostomy is gone the tube can be removed and the tracheostome left to heal. No secondary procedure is needed to close the defect which usually heals in about ten days. During this time the patient can occlude the defect with his finger, allowing him to cough and talk.

Sometimes it is not easy to decide the exact time when a tracheostomy can be dispensed with. During this time a speaking tube can be inserted which allows suction to be performed at will, but permits speech. Otherwise a plastic tube can be fenestrated and a latex bung used to occlude the mouth of the tube when suction is not required. In the intensive therapy unit this is often preferable to the metal speaking tube which has an inner tube with a simple flap valve but which has a propensity to become occluded by secretions or crusts due to its small diameter.

After a few days of such manoeuvres it becomes apparent when the right time has come to remove the tube permanently.

REFERENCES

Berman, I. R. and Stahl, W. M. (1968), Prevention of hypoxic complications during endotracheal suctioning. *Surgery*, **63**, 586.

Bjork, V. O. (1960), Partial resection of the only remaining lung with the aid of respirator treatment. *J. Thoracic Surgery*, **39**, 179.

Boccles, J. S. (1970), *Status asthmaticus*. *Med. Clin. N. Am.*, **54**, 443.

Brandstater, B. and Muallem, M. (1969), Atelectasis following tracheal suction in infants. *Anesthesiology*, **31**, 468.

Carroll, R. G. (1973), Evaluation of tracheal tube cuff designs. *Crit. Care Med.*, **1**, 45.

Carroll, R. G., McGinnis, G. E. and Grenvik, A. (1974), Performance characteristics of tracheal cuffs. *Int. Anesthesiol. Clin.*, **12**, 111.

Cooper, J. D. and Grillo, H. C. (1972), Analysis of problems related to cuffs on intratracheal tubes. *Chest*, **62** (suppl), 21.

Cunliff, A. C. and Wesley, F. (1967), Hazards from plastics sterilised by ethylene oxide. *Brit. med. J.*, **2**, 575.

Davidson, I. A., Cruickshank, A. N., Duthie, W. H., Bargh, W. and Duncan, J. G. (1971), Lesions of the trachea following tracheostomy and endotracheal intubation. *Proc. Roy. Soc. Med.*, **64**, 886.

Fairley, H. B. (1963), Respiratory insufficiency. *Int. Anesth. Clin.*, **1**, 351.

Geffin, B. and Pontopiddan, H. (1969), Reduction of tracheal damage by the prestretching of inflatable cuffs. *Anesthesiology*, **31**, 462.

Grillo, H. C., Cooper, J. D., Geffin, B. and Pontopiddan, H. (1971), A low-pressure cuff for tracheostomy tubes to minimise tracheal injury. A comparative clinical trial. *J. Thorac. Cardiovasc. Surg.*, **62**, 898.

Hedden, M., Ersoz, C. J., Donnelly, W. H. and Safar, P. (1969), Laryngotracheal damage after prolonged use of orotracheal tubes in adults. *J. Am. Med. Ass.*, **207**, 703.

Hedley-Whyte, J. (1968), Control of the uptake of oxygen. *New Eng. J. Med.*, **259**, 1152.

Kirby, R. R., Robinson, E. J. and Schulz, J. (1970), Intermittent cuff inflation during prolonged positive pressure ventilation. *Anesthesiology*, **32**, 364.

Lawson, D. R. (1973), Pre-stretched cuffs on tracheostomy tubes. *Brit. J. Anaesth.*, **45**, 234.

Leigh, J. M. and Maynard, J. P. (1979), Pressure on the tracheal mucosa from cuffed tubes. *British Medical Journal*, **1**, 1173.

Leverment, J. N. and Pearson, F. G. (1977), Tracheal damage associated with cuffed tracheostomy tubes. Aspiration of gastric content as a cause of local damage in tracheostomised dogs. *Anaesthesia*, **32**, 601.

Lindholm, C. E. (1969), Prolonged endotracheal intubation. *Acta Anaesthesiol Scand.* (suppl), **33**, 1.

Martinez, L. E. and Kalter, R. D. (1971), Extensive tracheal necrosis associated with a prestretched tracheostomy tube cuff. *Anesthesiology*, **34**, 488.

Nelson, T. G. (1957), Tracheostomy: a clinical and experimental Study. *Am. Surgeon*, **23**, 660.

Pearson, F. G., Goldberg, M. and da Silva, A. J. (1968), Tracheal stenosis complicating tracheostomy with cuffed tubes. *Arch. Surgery*, **97**, 380.

Petersdorf, R. G., Curtin, J. A., Halprich, P. D., Peeler, R. N. and Bennett, I. L. (1957), A study of antibiotic prophylaxis in unconscious patients. *New Eng. J. Med.*, **257**, 1001.

Plum, F. and Dunning, M. F. (1956), Technics for minimising trauma to the tracheobronchial tree after tracheostomy. *New Eng. J. Med.*, **254**, 193.

Rogers, L. A. and Osterhouts, S. (1970), Pneumonia following tracheostomy. *Am. Surgeon*, **36**, 39.

Salt, R. H., Parkhouse, J. and Simpson, B. R. (1960), Improved material for Radcliffe tracheostomy tubes. *Lancet*, **2**, 407.

SIX

Mechanical ventilation

TYPES OF VENTILATOR

Classification has been attempted according to various schemes which include:

Type of activation

(1) Electrical. Mains or battery.

(2) Powered by gas supply. Compressed air or oxygen from pipe-line sources or a compressor. The gas supply may be independent of the gas circuit to the patient or may provide inspiratory gas following enrichment or dilution to obtain the desired FIO_2.

(3) Manual. Provision for emergency manual is essential whatever type of mechanical ventilation is used.

Generators (Mapleson, 1962)

(1) *Pressure generators.* Inspiratory gas flow is terminated when a pre-set pressure is reached. This pre-set pressure is then responsible for cycling (or the change from inspiratory to expiratory phase). Such a system compensates for small leaks in the gas circuit though large leaks may cause cessation of function as the pre-set pressure is not reached. Examples of such ventilators include the Engstrom, East Radcliffe and Barnet. In some cases the pressure varies during the inspiratory phase. For example, the Engstrom generates a pressure increase towards the end of inspiration; the Minivent, on the other hand, is associated with a pressure fall as the volume of the elastic reservoir bag decreases.

Many of these ventilators have given excellent service in intensive care units. A drawback is the changes in tidal volume (and minute volume) which occur when compliance changes (as in bronchospasm).

(2) *Flow generators.* Flow is usually generated by a mechanically driven piston which is set to deliver a predetermined volume of gas. In the presence of an obstruction pressure builds up to ensure that the predetermined volume is delivered (within the limits of a safety blow-off valve), but there is no compensation for leaks in the circuit. Flow generators are useful in the presence of changing compliance over short time periods, as may occur in the presence of bronchospasm. The pressure and volume patterns have been illustrated diagrammatically (Robinson, 1971). The Cape Ventilator and the Oxford Penlon are examples of this type of apparatus.

Cycling

This is the term used to describe the mechanism by which the inspiratory phase is terminated.

(1) *Time cycling.* The East Radcliffe apparatus makes use of simple gears as on a bicycle chain. Servo-ventilators and the Barnet incorporate electronic timing mechanisms.

(2) *Pressure cycling.* This has been described under *Pressure generators.*

(3) *Volume cycling.* See *flow generators.*

The characteristics of an ideal intensive care ventilator have not yet been met in commercial models as some of the possible design features are contradictory. However, the following basic desiderata are generally accepted:

(1) The apparatus should supply a maximum inspiratory flow rate of up to 80 l per min.

(2) It should be possible to use air or oxygen or any combination of the two so that $F1O_2$ is known.

(3) Adequate humidification of inspired gases must occur.

(4) It should be possible to monitor inspiratory pressures, tidal volumes and the temperature of inspired gases.

(5) The apparatus should be robust, easily moved in position, with warning systems and provision for manual use in an emergency.

(6) The cost of the apparatus should be reasonable.

(7) It is desirable that gas loss by internal compliance changes in ventilator tubing should be minimal (Bushman, J. A. and Collis, J. M. 1967; Loh, L. and Chakrabarti, M. K. 1971). Non-expanding tubes made of plastic are better than corrugated rubber hose in this respect.

(8) Patient cross-infection must be prevented by use of autoclavable circuits, bacterial filters, disposable tubing.

(9) There should be a facility for nebulisation of drugs into the inspiratory gas stream (e.g. bronchodilators and antibiotics).

(10) There should be facilities for the application of positive and expiratory pressure (PEEP).

(11) Patient triggering is desirable in some circumstances. The device should be sensitive to 0.5 cm H_2O pressure difference or 5 to 10 ml volume displacement and delay in delivery of gas should not exceed 0.2 sec. Too great a sensitivity is not desirable since activation might otherwise occur from the action of the heart.

(12) Provision of simple controls, easily understood by nursing staff.

(13) The facility of intermittent mandatory ventilation (IMV) is useful.

Other factors are more controversial:

Waveform. It is technically possible to produce almost any desired waveform during the inspiratory phase but authoritative opinion is lacking as to the value of the different types in the variety of clinical circumstances which may exist. Pressure generators produce a rapid inflationary stroke giving rise to an essentially square waveform. Flow generators produce a triangular waveform. Servo-ventilators have been designed to produce a variety.

Sighing. The idea that an occasional deep breath or sigh would prevent miliary atelectasis in the lungs and assist in the reduction of A-a DO_2 differences has not gained general acceptance. Provided the lungs are properly ventilated such complications should not develop and air trapping by airways closure should be overcome instead by the use of PEEP. The sighing facility is nevertheless provided on some servo-ventilators and deep inspiration can then be set to occur at a predetermined frequency.

Negative pressure. Some years ago this was thought to be of value in causing a reduction in mean intrathoracic pressure during IPPV. It is now appreciated that even levels of -5 cm H_2O can cause air trapping and the technique has become unpopular. Positive pressure during expiration (PEEP) is indeed nowadays applied without deleterious effects on venous return to the heart although PEEP does sometimes result in a fall of cardiac output.

Positive End Expiratory Pressure (PEEP). (Cheney *et al.*, 1967; Seed *et al.*, 1970; Adams *et al.*, 1969). PEEP is valuable in a variety of clinical situations where the A-a DO_2 is large and where acceptable values of PaO_2 cannot be obtained even with high FIO_2. Provision of the PEEP facility by simple controls is therefore advantageous. The corollary to this is the abandonment of the use of negative pressure during the expiratory phase which is seldom advocated as it may result in air trapping, especially in the older patients in whom the closing volume of the lungs may infringe the tidal volume, particularly when FRC is reduced. The effect of PEEP is to cause an increase in FRC and one mechanism by which it acts may be by raising it above closing volume. PEEP may be valuable in patients with both the infant and the adult respiratory distress syndrome.

PEEP is not, however, without its disadvantages. Complications include alveolar rupture, pneumothorax, surgical emphysema and air embolism, though these are rare (Kumar *et al.*, 1973). The raised intrathoracic pressure may hinder venous return to the heart and therefore cardiac output. The overall oxygen availability to the tissues might not be improved. There is little evidence that PEEP removes water from the lungs in the patient with pulmonary oedema. It may be that antidiuretic hormone secretion is increased and water retained (Baratz *et al.*, 1977). When PEEP is applied a close watch should be kept on the cardiovascular signs and efforts made to ensure that hypovolaemia is not present. PEEP is best avoided in patients with obstructive airways disease (Sugarman *et al.*, 1972) and status asthmaticus (Ashbaugh and Petty, 1973). The effects of PEEP have been reviewed by Stoddart (Stoddart, 1979).

Sterilization of ventilators

The problems of cross-infection in the intensive therapy units are discussed elsewhere (Chapter 25). The patient circuits of ventilators may easily become contaminated with organisms which may then be discharged into room air or into the respiratory tracts of patients (Phillips and Spencer, 1965).

The problems of sterilization arise from the complex design of some ventilators and the relative inaccessibility of the gas circuit. Chemical methods have been favoured in the past using agents such as formalin (Sykes, 1964), alcohol (Spencer *et al.*, 1968) and the disinfectant fluids (Meadows *et al.*, 1968; Nancekievill and Goya, 1969a and b). Ethylene oxide, though expensive and potentially explosive, has probably been the most effective chemical agent for use in a wide variety of mechanical apparatus (Smith and Young, 1968). It has good powers of penetration but takes several hours to exert a bactericidal effect. It must be used as a mixture with carbon dioxide at a relative humidity of 30–50%. Unfortunately its very powers of penetration carry a disadvantage in that time must be allowed for aeration of equipment if toxic manifestations on patient tissues are not to occur. At least six post-sterilization vacuum pullings after completion of sterilization of apparatus have been recommended (Thomas and Longmore, 1969).

The most satisfactory method for sterilizing of patient circuits is use of the autoclave. When ventilator design allows for easy removal this is a very satisfactory method, though more than one patient circuit must be available if IPPV is to continue without interruption.

Bacterial filters can also be used to prevent entrance of organisms to the ventilator. Resistance, however, develops if condensation is allowed to occur and this requires a heating mechanism (Helliwell *et al.*, 1967). Also filters require to be changed at frequent intervals. There is evidence that bacteria can travel against the direction of the gas stream (Babington *et al.*, 1971) and filters are necessary on both inspiratory and expiratory limbs of the patient circuit.

Sterilization of humidifiers

The warm moist environment of the humidifier encourages bacterial colonization. Realization of this problem led to the use of increased temperatures (60°C) in humidifiers to produce a kind of 'pasteurization' (Phillips and Spencer, 1965). Hot water humidifiers can also be boiled at intervals when not in patient use, usually by cutting the thermostat out of circuit temporarily. More serious problems arise in humidifiers which do not utilise heat as a source of vapourisation and the possible bacterial colonisation in nebulisers and ultrasonic humidifiers should not be overlooked.

Other methods suggested for the discouragement of bacterial growth in humidifiers include the addition of small amounts of disinfectant and the use of copper as an antibacterial agent.

Humidification. The aim of humdification is to prevent drying and crusting of secretions in the respiratory tract. Problems are likely to occur when the upper airways are by-passed by the use of tracheal tubes and dry gases are supplied. It is necessary to supply air saturated with water vapour at body temperature or to supply water in the form of fine droplets.

Blower-humidifiers. Air becomes saturated with water vapour when it is blown over the surface of warm water in a suitable container. The temperature is usually kept at 60°C by use of a thermostat for reasons given above and it follows that some condensation is likely to occur as the gases cool on their way along the delivery tube to the patient. The temperature at the tracheal tube should be around 37°C and this can be verified by the use of a small monitoring thermometer in the connection. A water trap should be used to collect and remove condensed water.

Nebulisers. Nebulisers act by breaking up of water into fine droplets to form a mist. They may work on a Venturi principle when production depends upon gas flow and some 55% of droplets are formed within the desired range (0.5 to 5.0 μm), but more efficient is the ultrasonic nebuliser when water is dropped on to a vibrating piezo-crystal to produce 95% droplets below 5 μm.

Size of droplets is important because the larger droplets are deposited before reaching the patient's airways and the smaller ones are carried into the bronchial tree. It is not clear, however, what is the optimal droplet size, nor how far into the air passages actual droplets should reach.

Nebulisers are also valuable as a means for the administration of drugs such as bronchodilators and antibiotics.

The regulation of ventilation

Patient acceptance of mechanical ventilation may be easy or difficult according to circumstances. The means available may be summarised as follows:

(1) *Administration of drugs to depressed spontaneous respiration.* The drugs most valuable here are the opiates and their derivatives. IPPV is easier to institute if the respiratory centre is depressed and this can be achieved with a background of intramuscular morphine or diamorphine (there is some evidence that the latter has less side effects) and the intravenous short acting potent narcotic analgesics such as phenoperidine and fentanyl. Dosage should be generous enough to achieve the desired effect, always provided the cardiovascular system is not depressed.

(2) *Use of sedatives and tranquillizers.* These drugs are useful in the anxious patient who may panic and become difficult to manage. Sedation may be pushed to actual anaesthesia in some circumstances as when intravenous thiopentone (perhaps in combination with a muscle relaxant) is used to accomplish tracheal intubation or tracheostomy. Other drugs which may be useful include

intravenous diazepam or droperidol (often in combination with fentanyl) and intramuscular phenothiazine drugs, of which the authors have most experience with promazine finding it to be without undesirable side effects.

(3) *Hyperventilation.* There is no doubt that lowering of $PaCO_2$ by hyperventilation represents one of the best ways of gaining control of respiration by IPPV in the conscious patient. Hyperventilation produces also some clouding of consciousness and analgesia in susceptible patients, but if excessive inflation pressures are used harmful effects may occur.

(4) *Muscle relaxants.* The patient's respiratory effort can readily be abolished by the use of muscle relaxants. It is seldom advantageous to reverse any muscle relaxant used in the operating theatre if IPPV is to be continued. Deliberate paralysis in the conscious patient may, however, cause distress while in the context of head injury it may mask the level of consciousness and other useful signs. When muscle paralysis is thought to be the method of choice, however, information can be gained from monitors (McDowell, 1976). Unless the intensive therapy unit is well staffed and equipped the danger of accidental disconnection in the paralysed patient must always be considered.

Initiation of mechanical ventilation

Manual ventilation should always be continued until the mechanical ventilator has been assembled and checked. The apparatus must be clean, with sterile tubing, the humidifier connected, the desired oxygen flow running, and the machine must be switched on and tested for leaks. The rate and pressure or volume controls must be correctly adjusted before attachment to the patient.

The patient may be apnoeic or breathing spontaneously, unconscious or alert. The conscious patient has often required sedation for tracheal intubation and this aids acceptance of IPPV. Manual control by hyperventilation prior to use of mechanical apparatus often aids smooth transfer.

An intravenous line should always be established prior to initiation of IPPV. This allows administration of drugs and fluids. Fall in blood pressure is not uncommon after the patient has been sedated and mechanical ventilation commenced. This may be due to a variety of factors including:

(1) The direct depressant effects of sedative drugs in an ill patient. All the potent sedatives and analgesics may have a depressant effect on the cardiovascular system in the clinical circumstances.

(2) Alteration in the inspiratory and mean intrathoracic pressures with consequent diminished venous return. This may be more important if PEEP has been instituted.

(3) Hypovolaemia. The patient with incipient respiratory failure has frequently had diminished fluid intake over a period of several days. The intake of food and drink is likely to have been much less than normal, particularly if the patient has been nursed at home. The effects of drugs and change in intrathoracic

pressure may be enough to cause significant fall in cardiac output in the hypo-volaemic patient.

(4) Sudden fall in $PaCO_2$ consequent upon institution of IPPV. There is good evidence that this is a major cause of fall in cardiac output and arterial pressure.

The causes of hypotension are often multiple and it is usually some hours before the ability to control arterial pressure is restored. During this period the cardiovascular system is vulnerable to changes affecting reflex maintenance of the cardiac output and the patient must be observed closely with frequent monitoring of arterial blood pressure and central venous pressure. Should undue hypotension occur this should be treated by:

(1) Reduction of inspiratory pressure, minute volume and perhaps rate if any of these are considered more than absolutely necessary in the clinical situation. This is likely to result in reduction of means intrathoracic pressure and a less sharp fall in $PaCO_2$.

(2) Avoidance of injection of sedative or analgesic drugs unless these are strictly necessary, and then slowly in reduced dosage.

(3) Infusion of intravenous fluids to correct dehydration and/or electrolyte imbalance. The CVP monitor is useful here.

(4) Avoidance of sitting or head up positions while hypotension persists.

A watch must also be kept on urinary output which should usually be monitored by indwelling urethral catheter. In the presence of hypotension and/or hypovolaemia urinary excretion may be inadequate.

Maintenance of IPPV

Once the patient has accepted mechanical ventilation, IPPV can usually be maintained by the use of moderate hyperventilation using minute volumes of the order of 10 to 15 l/min in the average patient. Lowering of $PaCO_2$ removes the normal stimulus for inspiration, but if this value becomes unnecessarily low, dead space volume can be added to the patient circuit if it is undesirable to reduce ventilation.

The use of drugs is often valuable during the first few days of mechanical ventilation:

(1) Opiates can be used to depress respiratory drive. Suggested dosage—diamorphine 5 mg i.m., morphine 10 mg i.v., phenoperidine 1 mg i.v.

(2) Sedatives and tranquillizers, particularly if the patient is apprehensive and he is not accepting ventilation for this reason. Suggested dosage—promazine 25 mg i.m. 6-hourly, diazepam 5 to 10 mg i.m. or i.v., droperidol 5 to 10 mg i.m. or i.v. These drugs should be used for limited periods in regular dosage in case cumulation or side effects occur.

(3) Muscle relaxants are not recommended unless patient observation is continuous by staff unskilled to observe accidental disconnection of breathing tubes. They may, however, be indicated for other purposes (e.g. to control epileptiform fits), or, should the above measures fail (often a sign of worsening prognosis with gas exchange becoming increasingly inadequate).

Other measures which may be needed include:

(1) Intravenous line for fluid administration and perhaps for intravenous nutrition if alimentary methods fail.

(2) Urethral catheter, at least until it is clear that the patient can urinate unaided.

(3) Nasogastric tube for tube feeds (or in other circumstances for aspiration) until such time as the patient can swallow. Many patients learn to take an adequate soft diet with tracheostomy tube on IPPV or even with nasotracheal tube in place. Should tracheal soiling occur due to material entering the laryngeal aperture tube feeding must be resumed. Oral thrush is a complication which sometimes prevents natural swallowing. Alkali should be given regularly if patients are not fed for any reason. Cimetidine has also been used.

General nursing care is important

(1) Care of mouth hygiene.
(2) Pressure points. A ripple bed is valuable.
(3) Chest suction and physiotherapy.
(4) Passive or active movements in all joints to prevent stiffening.
(5) Maintenance of communication with the patient. Reassurance.

Tracheal suction

This is necessary at regular intervals to remove tracheobronchial secretions. At the same time it is important to prevent contamination with pathogenic organisms. This is best achieved by scrupulous attention to no-touch technique; the nurse or doctor should wear a clean plastic glove when touching the tracheal connecting tubes and the hands should not touch the suction catheter tip which is used once only and then discarded.

A variety of suction catheters are available. Since they are used as disposable items cost is an important factor. Catheters should be non-traumatic and smooth-tipped. Special designs such as the Aero-Flow catheter are more expensive but may be useful in special cases, while the catheters which are angled to facilitate passage into left or right main bronchi may also have a place. In the typical case, the authors have found the simple rubber or plaster catheter satisfactory, though occasionally trauma occurs on frequent suction as evidenced by aspiration of fresh blood.

Tracheal suction may be used in combination with vigorous physiotherapy and postural drainage (see below) and instillation of saline is often helpful to liquify tenacious secretions.

Bronchoscopy to remove bronchial plugs may be necessary when ordinary methods of tracheal suction fail, but it is not without hazard if it means interruption of IPPV. The Sanders injector principle is useful for maintaining tidal volume when the bronchoscope is in position, but there is a danger of acute hypoxia if any delay is experienced during its insertion. The fibreoptic broncho-scope can be threaded down the lumen of a tracheal tube and is the only instrument which can be used for bronchoscopy without interruption of ventilation. Experience has yet to prove, however, that all tenacious plugs can be removed.

Dangers of tracheal suction
(1) Trauma (see above).
(2) Acute hypoxia as a result of interruption of IPPV.
(3) Reflex vagal bradycardia or cardiac arrest; this can occur in the hypoxic patient. Pre-oxygenation with high FIO_2 for a few minutes may prevent unnecessary hypoxia.

Physiotherapy during IPPV
This must often be vigorous and combined with postural drainage if the airways are to be cleared of secretions and bronchial plugs.
(1) Posture. Affected lung uppermost or prone position.
(2) Squeezing of the chest during expiration, and shaking.
(3) Use of skin vibrator (milder cases).
These measures may exhaust the patient temporarily and cause increased hypoxia. For this reason vigorous physiotherapy should be combined with hand bag-and-mask ventilation with pure oxygen. When the patient is in pain appropriate analgesia should be administered. Manual hyperventilation with chest squeezing and shaking should be followed by tracheal suction.

Chest physiotherapy requires intelligent application in the knowledge of the clinical situation and chest radiography. When properly carried out it can result in significant clinical improvement with aeration of previously collapsed segments of lung.

Monitoring during IPPV
Blood pressure, pulse, temperature. The usual measurements must be made at regular intervals—4-hourly. Variations or trends away from normality may indicate development of complications. Pyrexia, increasing pulse rate, rise of blood pressure or hypotension, must have a cause and this should be sought for.

Inflation pressure, respiratory rate and volume. Changes in these parameters may indicate changing lung compliance, intensification or relaxation of bronchospasm, or reflect changes in the course of lung disease. They also act as a check that the mechanical ventilator is working satisfactorily without leaks.

Humidifier temperature. The thermostat is usually set at $55°C$ on hot water humidifiers. Departures from the preset temperature may indicate failure of the heater or thermostat. Monitoring of temperature at the catheter mount is also helpful.

Fluid and electrolyte balance. Proper fluid balance charts should be kept and daily electrolyte estimations obtained in patients not on normal diet. The doctor should be alert for conditions such as the 'sick cell syndrome' (see Chapter 2).

White cell estimation. Leucocytosis is commonly seen with infection.

Arterial blood gases. Daily blood gases act as a useful check on clinical progress and the adequacy of ventilation.

Chest X-ray. This should normally be carried out daily to assess clinical progress. Clinical auscultation of the chest should not be neglected, but some signs are not always easy to detect during IPPV (e.g. the signs of pneumothorax).

Bacteriology. Regular culture of sputum for bacteriology and sensitivity.

COMPLICATIONS OF MECHANICAL VENTILATION

Lung complications

(1) Inadequate gas exchange as a result of
    (a) ventilator malfunction or disconnection
    (b) Accidental endobronchial instrumentation
    (c) changes in pulmonary status
(2) Pneumothorax and surgical emphysema. This may result from trauma (e.g. fractured ribs) or from breakdown of an area of consolidation.
(3) Cross-infection and development of resistant organisms.
(4) Late complications as a result of trauma to the larynx and trachea.

Other complications

(1) Restlessness and mental confusion as a result of cerebral hypoxia.
(2) Cardiovascular problems secondary to initiation of IPPV.
(3) Perforation of gastric or duodenal ulcer, especially in patients on steroids, which may be masked by analgesia caused by hyperventilation.

WEANING FROM MECHANICAL VENTILATION

The decision to commence weaning is a clinical one depending upon improvement in the pathological process requiring IPPV.

Some workers place reliance on triggered ventilators, blood gas estimations, etc., but the authors have found it simple to detain the ventilator for some minutes and to observe spontaneous respiration. This is best done at a time when the patient is not under the influence of respiratory depressant or sedative drugs and when experienced staff are present to offer the necessary encouragement and to observe the need to recommence IPPV if necessary.

The patient can be allowed to breathe spontaneously for increasing periods, depending upon the clinical situation, but IPPV should be recommenced should distress develop as evidenced by dyspnoea, rising respiratory rate, tachycardia or fatigue. When the patient is able to breathe spontaneously during the daylight hours it is time to consider removal of the mechanical ventilator altogether.

The tracheostomy tube should be kept in place for a few days until the need for respiratory assistance and tracheal aspiration has clearly passed. Once spontaneous respiration is established the tracheostomy tube may be fenestrated to allow speech, and later it may be removed and the wound allowed to heal.

The time scale of weaning will vary according to the clinical situation. Short-term ventilation, as in the case of drug overdose, will usually be followed by rapid recovery of spontaneous respiratory function. The weaning period may extend over several days in the case of respiratory failure secondary to acute or chronic chest infection and there may be at least 24 hours required between major steps.

Intermittent mandatory ventilation

This concept may aid in the weaning of the patient when difficulties arise (Downs *et al.*, 1973a, b, c, d; Margand and Chodoff, 1975; Lawler and Nunn, 1977; Hewlett *et al.*, 1977). The apparatus is pre-set to deliver mandatory breaths at set intervals. The frequency may be gradually diminished over a period of time until the patient can breathe spontaneously all the time. Such devices can be incorporated into electronic timing mechanisms as on Servo ventilators and special precautions may be needed where PEEP is also being used (Dittmann *et al.*, 1977). However, the place for intermittent mandatory ventilation in clinical practice is not yet defined (Stoddart, 1979).

PROCEDURE SHOULD EFFICIENT VENTILATION FAIL

This may be due to an apparatus failure or a sudden change in the condition of the patient. Whenever a patient is treated by mechanical ventilation a separate circuit for manual IPPV should be immediately available. Should any respiratory crisis occur hand ventilation should be instituted while the problem is identified and the cause corrected. The following check list may be of value:

Apparatus failure

(1) *Failure of driving power.* Check sources of power; electricity, mains or battery; compressed gas, pipe-line, compressor or cylinder.

(2) *Failure of the integral parts of the ventilator.* Likely to require expert advice from the manufacturer.

(3) *Leaks in the circuit.* Disconnection. Failure of one-way valves. The humidifier is a common source of leaks and should be checked. Leaking tracheal connections; failure of tracheal cuff to inflate satisfactorily. May be evidenced by failure to achieve inflation pressure.

(4) *Obstruction in the circuit.* Kinks. Condensed water. Incorrect connections. Inflation pressure is often high but observed stroke volume low.

Patient changes

(1) *Gross obstruction.* Mechanical factors include blockage of tracheal tube by secretions and crust, haemorrhage. Inappropriate position of tube, impingement on carina, etc. It may be necessary to change the tracheal tube, to undertake tracheal suction and lavage, to check whether humidifier functioning. Note that tracheostomy tubes can obstruct because of bevel approximation to tracheal wall, or actual displacement of the tip into soft tissues of the neck.

(2) *Compliance changes.* Due to changes in bronchospasm, spasm of chest wall muscles, blockage of small air passages etc. Consider whether inspiratory pressure should be increased. Should drugs be given so that the patient does not breathe 'out of phase' with the ventilator? Are bronchodilators indicated?

(3) Look for *gross pathology changes* in the patient. These include pneumothorax, collapse of major lung segment. Treat as appropriate.

The humidifier. This should be checked routinely. Is water present? Are there any connector leaks? Is the temperature satisfactory?

It is clearly necessary that patients receiving mechanical ventilation should be observed continuously. Alarm systems are available to give warning of pressure variations in the circuit outside preset values, but nothing can replace personal observation by the nursing staff. This not only gives early warning of any deterioration in the quality of lung ventilation but also aids the confidence and morale of conscious patients.

REFERENCES

Adams, A. P., Morgan, M., Jones, B. C. and McCormick, P. W. (1969), A case of massive aspiration of gastric contents during obstetric anaesthesia. *Brit. J. Anaesth.*, 41, 176.

Ashbaugh, D. G. and Petty, T. L. (1973), Positive end expiratory pressure: physiology indications and contraindications. *J. of Thoracic and Cardiovascular Surgery*, 65, 165.

Babington, P. C. B., Baker, A. B. and Johnston, H. H. (1971), Retrograde spread of organisms from ventilator to patient in the expiratory limb. *Lancet*, 1, 61.

Baratz, R. A., Philbin, D. M. and Patterson, R. W. (1977), Plasma antidiuretic hormone and urinary output during continuous positive pressure breathing in dogs. *Anesthesiology*, 34, 510.

Bushman, J. A. and Collis, J. M. (1967), The estimation of gas losses in ventilator tubing. *Anaesthesia*, 22, 664.

Cheney, F. W., Honbein, T. F. and Crawford, E. W. (1967), The effect of expiratory resistance on the blood gas tensions of anesthetized patients. *Anesthesiology*, 28, 670.

Dittman, M., Pike, P. M. H. and Wolff, G. (1977), The Basle PEEP weaner. *Anaesthesia*, 32, 559.

Downs, J. B., Klein, E. F., Desantels, D., Model, J. H. and Kirby, R. R. (1973), Intermittent mandatory ventilation: A new approach to weaning patients from mechanical ventilators. *Chest*, 64, 331.

Downs, J. B., Perkins, H. M. and Sutton, W. W. (1974a), Successful weaning after five years of mechanical ventilation. *Anesthesiology*, **40**, 602.

Downs, J. B., Perkins, H. M. and Model, J. H. (1974b), Intermittent mandatory ventilation. An evaluation. *Arch. Surg.*, **109**, 519.

Downs, J. B. and Mitchell, L. A. (1974c), Intermittent mandatory ventilation following cardiopulmonary bypass. *Crit. Care Medicine*, **2**, 39.

Downs, J. B., Block, A. J. and Vennum, K. B. (1974d), Intermittent mandatory ventilation in the treatment of patients with chronic obstructive pulmonary disease. *Anesth. Analg. Curr. Res.*, **53**, 437.

Helliwell, P. J., Jeaves, A. L., Watkin, R. R. and Gibbs, F. J. (1967), The Williams bacterial filter. *Anaesthesia*, **22**, 497.

Hewlett, A. M., Platt, A. S. and Terry, V. G. (1977), Mandatory minute volume. A new concept in weaning from mechanical ventilation. *Anaesthesia*, **32**, 163.

Kumar, A., Pontoppidan, H., Falke, K. S., Wilson, R. S. and Lara, M. B. (1973), Pulmonary barotrauma during mechanical ventilation. *Critical Care Medicine*, **1**, 181.

Lawler, P. G. P. and Nunn, J. F. (1977), Intermittent mandatory ventilation. *Anaesthesia*, **32**, 138.

Loh, L. and Chakrabarti, M. K. (1971), The internal compliance of ventilators. *Anaesthesia*, **26**, 414.

Mapleson, W. W. (1962), The effect of changes of lung characteristics on the functioning of automatic ventilators. *Anaesthesia*, **17**, 300.

Margand, P. M. S. and Chodoff, P. (1975), Intermittent mandatory ventilation; an alternative weaning technique. A case report. *Anesth. Analg. Curr. Res.*, **54**, 51.

McDowall, D. G. (1976), in *Recent Advances in Anaesthesia and Analgesia–12* (eds Hewer, C. L. and Atkinson, R. S.), Churchill Livingstone, Edinburgh, London and New York.

Meadows, G. A., Richardson, J. C., Fish, E. and Williams, A. (1968), A method of sterilisation for the East-Radcliffe ventilator. *Brit. J. Anaesth.*, **40**, 71.

Nancekievill, D. G. and Goya, H. (1969a), Disinfection of the East-Radcliffe ventilator (A bacteriological study of a modified picloxydine technique). *Anaesthesia*, **24**, 42.

Nancekievill, D. G. and Goya, H. (1969b), Decontamination of the Cape Ventilator. *Anaesthesia*, **24**, 359.

Phillips, I. and Spencer, G. (1965), Pseudomonas aeruginosa cross-infection due to contaminated respiratory apparatus. *Lancet*, **2**, 1325.

Robinson, J. (1971), Chapt. 9 in *General Anaesthesia*, I, 3rd edn. (ed Gray, T. C. and Nunn, J. F.) Butterworths, London.

Seed, R. F., Sykes, M. K. and Finlay, W. E. I. (1970), The effect of variations in end-expiratory inflation pressure on cardiorespiratory function before and after open-heart surgery. *Brit. J. Anaesth.*, **42**, 488.

Smith, R. M. and Young, J. A. (1968), Simplified gas sterilisation: a new answer for an old problem. *Brit. J. Anaesth.*, **40**, 909.

Spencer, G. *et al.* (1968), Disinfection of lung ventilators by alcohol aerosol. *Lancet*, **2**, 667.

Stoddart, J. C. (1979), in *Recent Advances in Anaesthesia and Analgesia–13*, (eds Hewer, C. L. and Atkinson, R. S.), Churchill Livingstone, Edinburgh, London and New York.

Sugarman, H. J., Rogers, R. M. and Miller, L. D. (1972), Positive end expiratory pressure: indications and physiological considerations. *Chest*, **62**, 86.

Sykes, M. K. (1964), Sterilising mechanical ventilators. *Brit. Med. J.*, **1**, 561.

Thomas, L. C. and Longmore, D. B. (1971), Ethylene oxide sterilisation of surgical stores. *Anaesthesia*, **26**, 304.

SEVEN

Oxygen therapy

A significant proportion of patients treated in the intensive care unit require oxygen therapy at some time. Proper understanding of the pathophysiological changes associated with arterial hypoxaemia and tissue hypoxia, coupled with knowledge of the principles of oxygen administration and the ability to monitor arterial oxygen tension, will result in rational therapy.

It is not possible to discuss all aspects of respiratory physiology within the confines of this volume, but certain features particularly related to oxygen carriage require mention.

The oxygen cascade

This concept has been used to describe the decreasing tension of oxygen as the gas passes through the various physiological body compartments to reach the tissue cells. Typical figures for the tension of oxygen in normal individuals breathing air at sea level are; atmospheric air 20, alveolar gas 13, arterial blood 12.5, capillary blood 6.8 and mixed venous blood 5.3 kPa, while the tension at mitochondrial level is considered to be less than 1.5 kPa.

Alveolar oxygen tension

Alveolar gases are fully saturated with water vapour (tension 6.5 kPa at $37°C$) and nitrogen tension does not vary. The remaining value after subtraction from barometric pressure may be taken as 20 kPa and this is occupied by oxygen and carbon dioxide in alveolar gas. There is a relationship between the two which can be expressed in various forms as an *alveolar air equation*. For example, it can be written:

$$P_AO_2 = P_IO_2 - \frac{P_ACO_2}{R}$$

where R is the respiratory exchange ratio (carbon dioxide elimination/oxygen uptake). R is normally 0.8 and the equation can then be re-written:

$$P_AO_2 = P_IO_2 - 1.25 \times P_ACO_2$$

This concept may be important in clinical situations where carbon dioxide retention is present. It can also be expressed graphically for different inspired oxygen tensions (Fig. 7.1). For more detailed explanations the reader is referred

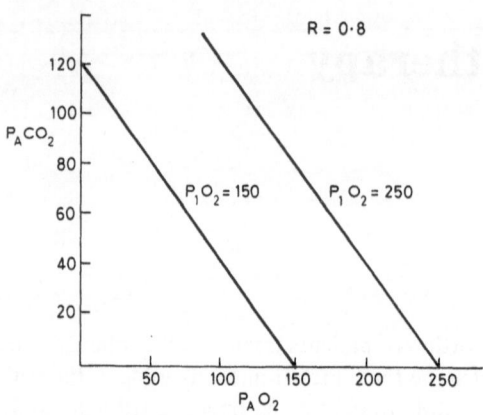

Fig. 7.1 O_2-CO_2 *Diagram showing the relationship between* $P_A O_2$ *and* $P_A CO_2$ *at varying* $P_I O_2$.

to other texts (Comroe, Forster, Dubois, Briscoe and Carlsen, 1962; Nunn, 1969; Sykes, McNicol, and Campbell, 2nd ed. 1976).

Oxygen carriage in the blood

With a haemoglobin concentration of 15 g%, an oxygen tension of 100 mmHg and 97% saturation, the oxygen content of arterial blood can be taken as 19.8 vol%. The greater part of this is carried in combination with haemoglobin, but 0.3 ml is in simple solution in the plasma. Venous blood at an oxygen tension of 5.3 kPa has a content of about 15 vol%.

Oxygen therapy is likely to be of most benefit when haemoglobin saturation has fallen, but even when haemoglobin is already fully saturated a significant rise in oxygen carriage can be achieved by increase of the amount carried in the plasma (see Table 7.1). This is particularly so with hyperbaric oxygenation.

Table 7.1 Oxygen carriage in blood (vols %)

	Breathing air	Breathing 100% O_2	Breathing O_2 at 2 atm.	Breathing O_2 at 3 atm.
Oxygen combined with haemoglobin	19.5	20.1	20.1	20.1
Oxygen in solution	0.3	1.0	4.2	6.5
Total	19.8	22.0	24.3	26.6

The oxygen dissociation curve for haemoglobin

This shows the relationship between oxygen tension and saturation. In acidosis the curve is shifted to the right and flattened. The effect of this, however, is not so serious as might be expected since full saturation is still obtained in the normal range of oxygen tension whereas more oxygen is given up to the tissues at low tension. Oxygen delivery may therefore actually be improved unless arterial oxygen tension is already low, in which case correspondingly lower values for saturation will be present.

Oxygen availability

The oxygen available to the tissues is the product of arterial oxygen content and cardiac output (Freeman and Nunn, 1963). The former depends on haemoglobin content and the degree of its saturation with oxygen which is in turn related to P_aO_2. The available oxygen can be expressed as

$$\left\{ \frac{1.39 \times Hb \times S_aO_2 + 0.003 \times P_aO_2}{100} \right\} \times \frac{Qml}{100}$$

where 1.39 represents the oxygen capacity of haemoglobin in ml/g and 0.003 the ml of oxygen dissolved in plasma per mm Hg per 100 ml whole blood. For a healthy subject this might be taken as

$$\left\{ \frac{1.39 \times 15.0 \times 97 + 0.003 \times 100}{100} \right\} \times \frac{5000}{100}$$

which gives a value approximating to 1000 ml/min.

Coefficient of utilization

The normal body consumption of oxygen at rest is about 250 ml/min so that considerable reserve exists, particularly where cardiac output can be increased. The coefficient of utilization can be expressed as a percentage, relating oxygen consumption to the oxygen available. A normal value might be 250/1000 or 25%. The coefficient will rise when reserve is reduced as when haemoglobin percentage, oxygen saturation, oxygen tension or cardiac output falls, or when there is a rise in body consumption as with exercise, shivering or fever when cardiac output fails to increase as a compensatory mechanism.

THE AIM OF OXYGEN THERAPY

Although oxygen is required at cellular level and many factors are concerned in the transport of oxygen to the tissues, the immediate aim of oxygen therapy is to increase the amount of the gas in arterial blood. The only practical port of entry for oxygen is via the lungs. Increased tension of oxygen in inspired gas should result in a rise in oxygen tension in alveolar gas and then in P_aO_2. Difficulties arise when lung function is grossly impaired as a result of disease. It is therefore necessary to examine some of the causes of arterial hypoxaemia and the ways in which oxygen uptake is impaired.

Causes of arterial hypoxaemia

Hypoventilation

Oxygen administration does not compensate for inadequate alveolar ventilation except in the very short term and it is necessary to institute effective ventilation by manual or mechanical means. Depending upon clinical circumstances it may be necessary to use oxygen enriched air or even pure oxygen for a time.

Ventilation-perfusion disturbances

In healthy lung tissue alveolar ventilation with gas and perfusion with capillary blood are reasonably well matched so that there is efficient oxygen uptake and carbon dioxide elimination. In pathological lung tissue there may be gross disturbances in ventilation perfusion relationships. Alveoli may be well ventilated but under-perfused or well perfused but receive little or no ventilation. Gas exchange is impaired with increase in physiological dead space and arterial hypoxaemia. Oxygen therapy will result in correction of hypoxaemia unless it is very gross, though unless respiratory control is normal there is a danger that relief may result in underventilation and progressive retention of carbon dioxide. The patient with chronic obstructive airways disease may exhibit these character-istics and it is in these circumstances that controlled doses of oxygen may be required.

Airways closure

The concept of airways closure, though not universally accepted, serves to explain some of the causes of arterial hypoxaemia. During expiration there comes a time when small airways collapse and cause air trapping. The volume of air in the lungs when this takes place can be measured and is known as the *Closing volume* of the lungs (CV). Should the CV impinge on the tidal volume (TV) ventilation perfusion disturbances are probable and arterial hypoxaemia occurs. CV increases with advancing age, with adoption of the recumbent posture and in cigarette smokers. When the functional residual capacity (FRC) is reduced as after abdominal operations CV may also encroach on TV and this has been put forward as an explanation of post-operative hypoxaemia. Oxygen administration will cause a rise in the oxygen tension of those alveoli that are ventilated and perfused and will produce a rise in P_aO_2.

Right-to-left shunts

When shunts are present a proportion of blood which should pass through the lungs fails to receive oxygen. Since the blood which does reach the alveoli is almost fully saturated increase in P_AO_2 will have little effect. However, the small rise in oxygen combined with haemoglobin together with the greater increase in oxygen dissolved in the plasma (see Table 7.1) may be significant as it may amount to about 10% increase in oxygen carriage in that volume of blood which reaches the alveoli and such an increase could in some circumstances be life-saving. If 50% of blood is shunted through the lungs without partaking in gas exchange, it is likely that pure oxygen will fail to correct the low P_aO_2. Since it is difficult to provide an inspired percentage of more than 60% oxygen therapy has little effect in practice with shunts which are greater than 25%. The relationship between F_1O_2 and P_aO_2 with various degrees of shunt (Benata *et al.*, 1973).

OXYGEN TOXICITY

Most of the apparatus available for continuous oxygen administration fails to increase inspired oxygen concentrations above 60%, but the increasing prevalence of intermittent positive pressure mechanical ventilation via a tracheal tube has made it possible to maintain concentrations approaching 100% for long periods.

It is now recognized that administration of high oxygen concentrations, particularly above 70%, may have deleterious effects when continued for more than 24 hours. Subjective symptoms may include paraesthesiae, nausea and vomiting, substernal distress and fatigue. Changes within the lung are probably caused by inactivation of surfactant and damage to pulmonary epithelium. There may be evidence of pulmonary capillary congestion, interstitial pulmonary oedema, atelectasis and bronchopneumonia, while 'hyaline membrane' formation may also occur. The resultant X-ray picture may be difficult to distinguish from that due to other causes of 'adult respiratory distress syndrome' and so the diagnosis may not be immediately apparent. It is probably that high F_1O_2 rather than a high resultant P_aO_2 is important, as a direct effect on pulmonary tissues occurs.

For these reasons there is now appreciation of the need to avoid unnecessarily high inspired concentrations of oxygen. Oxygen therapy should be monitored by repeated estimations of P_aO_2, and while there is seldom need for a value above 13 kPa, lower figures may be acceptable. F_1O_2 should therefore be adjusted to obtain an acceptable arterial oxygen tension. In the presence of shunts the F_1O_2, P_aO_2 and degree of shunt is important. Once values for F_1O_2 and P_aO_2 have been obtained, the shunt can be determined, and subsequent adjustment of F_1O_2 made without repeating P_aO_2 estimation.

OXYGEN ESTIMATION

The techniques of blood gas analysis will not be discussed here, but note should be taken of the various errors which may occur due to methods of sampling and storage (Adams *et al.*, 1967). Blood should be taken from an artery into a syringe, the deadspace of which has been filled with heparin. Care should be taken to exclude room air by avoiding the introduction of air bubbles and sealing the needle. The specimen once taken, the estimation should be carried out immediately as difficulties arise if the sample has to be stored. The oxygen consumption of the blood cells themselves cause a fall in PO_2 of the order of 0.4 kPa per min at body temperature (Nunn, 1962), though this can be minimized by cooling. It is now recognized that oxygen diffuses through the walls of plastic syringes, particularly when P_aO_2 values are high (Scott *et al.*, 1971). Significant changes can occur in minutes and it is important therefore to house the electrode close to the bedside and there is an advantage in the use of all glass syringes.

It is usual to estimate arterial oxygen tension and to calculate oxygen saturation. Although apparatus is available for direct measurement of saturation it is not in general hospital use in the United Kingdom.

F_1O_2 can be determined using the oxygen electrode, the paramagnetic oxygen analyzer (Nunn *et al.*, 1964), or using the fuel cell oxygen analyzer (Tordar and Grant, 1973).

PRINCIPLES OF OXYGEN ADMINISTRATION

Rational administration of oxygen requires an understanding of the principles of the various types of apparatus available. A classification into *fixed* and *variable* performance systems has been suggested (Leigh, 1970).

Fixed performance systems

Oxygen is inspired by the patient in such a manner that the concentration reaching the airways is unaffected by variations in ventilation. This can be achieved in various ways:

(1) The high air flow oxygen enrichment principle (HAFOE). Oxygen is supplied by a small tube and the Venturi principle used to obtain dilution with air. An oxygen flow of one litre per minute will entrain 10 litres of air, and an oxygen flow of four litres per minute, 40 litres of air. The use of a 4 l/min oxygen supply will therefore supply a flow of oxygen enriched air in excess of the usual inspiratory flowrate, the method will ensure a constant F_1O_2 if the air entrainment is suitably regulated, and the flow will be attained at an acceptable cost in terms of oxygen usage. This is the principle of the well-known Ventimask (see later).

(2) Low flow systems can be achieved using anaesthetic circuits; rebreathing is allowable if absorption of carbon dioxide by soda lime is used. The commonly used bag and mask (Mapleson circuit C) (Mapleson, 1954) is portable and can be used with piped oxygen or oxygen cylinders and with or without the soda lime canister. In a closed circuit system, however, the F_1O_2 may be well short of 100% due to the tension of nitrogen in expired air. Whereas it takes some two minutes to displace nitrogen from the lungs and about five minutes to remove nitrogen dissolved in the blood, it takes up to two hours to eliminate the gas from the body as a whole.

(3) Demand flow systems. These are not popular for use in the intensive care unit, but the use of pre-mixed nitrous oxide/oxygen (50:50) has been advocated for use in transport of critically ill patients (Baskett and Withnell, 1970). The Entonox apparatus allows inhalation of the gas mixture on a demand system and it can be argued the analgesia obtained from nitrous oxide is often valuable in the ambulance situation while high F_1O_2 is also supplied.

Variable performance systems

When these systems are used the percentage of oxygen in the gases reaching the lungs will vary from moment to moment with changes in the pattern of breathing. This occurs because the amount of dilution with air varies. The degree of air dilution can be minimized by the provision of some reservoir space.

Reservoirs

The commonest form of reservoir is a simple bag into which oxygen flows continuously and out of which the patient takes part or all of the inspiratory volume. Various systems can be considered:

(1) Reservoir bag without valves. Reservoir bags have been provided on various facemasks (e.g. the BLB mask). A higher F_1O_2 is obtained than if a bag is not incorporated, but there is a possibility of rebreathing with low oxygen flows.

(2) Reservoir bag with non-rebreathing valve. The use of a non-rebreathing valve eliminates the possibility of expired gases reaching the reservoir, but rebreathing can still occur if the deadspace of the mask and valve itself is significant.

(3) T-piece systems. A T-piece can be used in association with a facemask or tracheal tube (see Fig. 7.2). Oxygen is supplied to one limb of the T while the other is open to the atmosphere. The length of the open limb can be adjusted to provide variable reservoir volume. The T-piece system allows dilution with air when the oxygen flow is low and when the volume of the expiratory limb is less than the tidal volume, and rebreathing can occur with flows of less than two to three times the minute volume. Although the use of an actual T-connection is rare in oxygen therapy, the majority of commercial facemasks are in reality a modification of the T-principle; the deadspace of the mask is the equivalent of the expiratory limb of the T.

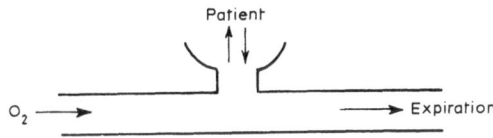

Fig. 7.2 T-piece system.

Other considerations. There are a number of other factors which affect the practical use of any oxygen device:

(1) Leaks: The F_1O_2 will fall where there is dilution due to leaks associated with poor facial fit. When the administration is purely nasal the degree of mouth breathing is important.

(2) Comfort: For continuous administration the patient must accept the oxygen device for long periods. Uncomfortable facemasks may be removed by the patient with consequent interruption of therapy which may be dangerous. Facemasks may also interfere with communication and nutrition.

TYPES OF APPARATUS

Facemasks

The rubber BLB mask (Boothby *et al.*, 1938; Bulbulian, 1938) was introduced in 1938 and was popular for many years in its nasal and oronasal designs. It delivered relatively high concentrations of oxygen and a small reservoir was incorporated. In recent years it has been superseded by the plastic disposable mask which has been available in a number of commercial designs. Some of these have been criticized on account of the relatively large deadspace in the mask, and masks such as the Polymask and Pneumask have lost popularity. A survey has shown that the MC mask, the Ventimask, the Harris mask and the Edinburgh mask are the most popular in present day use in Britain (Leigh, 1973).

The MC (Mary Catterall) mask (Catterall, 1960)

The mask takes the form of a transparent plastic cone with padded foam at the face to facilitate a good fit. Oxygen enters via a delivery tube at the apex of the cone and there are holes to allow inspiration of air for dilution and also expiration to the atmosphere. It is, therefore, a modified T-piece device. A flow of oxygen of six litres per minute should provide an F_1O_2 of about 60% with minimal rebreathing, though there is significant deadspace at low flows (Bethune and Collins, 1967).

Ventimasks

These masks utilize the HAFOE principle (see page 84). They provide a fixed performance system supplying known concentrations of oxygen with colour-code (24% blue, 28% clear, 35% yellow, 40% red). They are commonly used with an oxygen flow of four litres per minute and since this results in an air entrainment of about forty litres per minute carbon dioxide does not accumulate in the mask. These masks are used to provide step-like increases in F_1O_2 over a period of time in patients with obstructive airways disease. The small increases of P_aO_2 which result are associated with significant rises in S_aO_2 since changes occur on the steep portion of the haemoglobin oxygen dissociation curve. Tracheal oxygen concentrations are likely to be about 5% less than that supplied by the mask, probably due to addition of water vapour (Gilbert *et al.*, 1976).

Harris mask

This mask has a small deadspace volume. It is a stiff semi-translucent contoured mask with vent holes. Oxygen is supplied by feed tube and the concentrations supplied are of the order of 60% with six litre flow.

Edinburgh mask (Flenley *et al.*, 1963)

This plastic mask was designed to supply low concentrations of oxygen to patients with obstructive airways disease. A single mask provides a variable

$F_1 O_2$ according to the oxygen flowrate supplied. Less accurate than the Venti-mask, it supplies $F_1 O_2$ of 25 to 29% at one litre per minute, 31 to 35% at two litres per minute, and 33 to 39% at three litres per minute. It is claimed that this mask is sufficiently accurate for the treatment of patients with carbon dioxide retention but the authors have no personal experience.

Nasal catheters and cannulae

The anterior nares

Insufflation of the anterior nares with oxygen flows above three litres per minute is uncomfortable. Flow flows do provide a significant increase in $F_1 O_2$, though the system is patient dependent and variations occur according to tidal volume and the degree of mouth breathing. The method offers considerable advantages in that therapy is not interrupted by eating, drinking and talking. A catheter can be used with similar effect in the mouth of a pharyngeal airway or tracheal tube. In general, nasal catheters are more acceptable to patients than facemasks.

The nasopharynx

A catheter positioned in the nasopharynx is more efficient though less comfort-able. The technique is not entirely without risk since gastric distension and even rupture can occur (Walstead and Conklin, 1961), though this complication can be largely avoided by the use of a T-tube to a water blowoff 5 cm under water.

Choice of mask or catheter

Where high $F_1 O_2$ is desired

The MC and Harris masks are most popular for hospital ward use according to a survey. They can be expected to supply 60% inspired oxygen concentration at six litres per minute flow. Anaesthetic bag and mask (Mapleson circuit C) is convenient for acute resuscitation since concentrations approaching 100% can be obtained with flows of around ten litres per minute, and artificial respiration can be provided if required.

Where controlled $F_1 O_2$ is desired

The Ventimask or the Edinburgh mask are popular (see treatment of Obstructive Airways disease, page 93).

Where small increases in $F_1 O_2$ are required but the dosage is not critical

Nasal catheters have a place here since they are more comfortable than the facemask and are simple to operate with flows of two to three litres per minute.

For restless and unco-operative patients

Facemasks and catheters are not well tolerated. The head tent may be considered, but the restlessness may be due to hypoxia, at least in part, and it may be necessary to sedate the patient and administer oxygen enriched mixtures by IPPV via a tracheal tube.

Oxygen tents

Oxygen tents are rarely used in the intensive care unit. It is difficult to achieve high oxygen concentrations even with high flow rates. Tents are uncomfortable for the patient and interfere with nursing procedures and communication. The fire risk is significant due to the large volume of the tent.

There may be some place for the use of tents in paediatric practice and for the use of head tents for adults in whom lack of co-operation makes other techniques difficult and when controlled concentrations are not required. The Vickers Head Tent utilizes a Venturi producing concentrations up to 34% oxygen (Campbell and Gebbie, 1966). The degree of air entrainment is variable and for concentrations up to 30% the flow is large enough to prevent accumulation of carbon dioxide.

Incubators

Incubators are useful in the management of small babies. The Intensive Care Isolette Incubator (Air Sheilds (UK) Ltd.) provides oxygen concentrations from 26 to 44% with flow rates between 1 and 4.5 litres per minute (Simpson and Russel, 1967).

INTERMITTENT POSITIVE PRESSURE VENTILATION (IPPV)

When IPPV is applied via a tracheal tube it is possible to supply high concentrations of oxygen. The patient can be ventilated with room air or with oxygen enriched air and it is possible to supply oxygen concentrations approaching 100%. The techniques of IPPV are discussed in Chapter 6.

Positive end expiratory pressure (PEEP)

The use of positive pressure during the expiratory phase of mechanical ventilation may help to diminish the gradient between alveolar and arterial PO_2 in certain pathological situations. PEEP results in an increase in functional residual capacity (FRC), and in certain circumstances may bring the tidal volume range outside the closing volume (CV). PEEP may be considered when P_aO_2 remains low despite high F_1O_2 and when there is a significant degree of shunt suspected. The subject is considered more fully in Chapter 6.

HYPERBARIC OXYGEN

Hyperbaric oxygenation results in increased oxygen carriage in the blood by virtue of increased solubility of the gas in plasma. Solution of oxygen in plasma is directly proportional to PO_2. At atmospheric pressure breathing air only 0.3 ml oxygen is dissolved in 100 ml plasma, but as 2 atm. breathing pure oxygen this is increased to 4.2 ml/100 ml.

The technique of hyperbaric oxygenation is at present only available at special centres. In view of possible oxygen toxicity treatment can be maintained for relatively short periods only, and there are few indications for its use. Whereas it has been used over a wide clinical field there are few situations where it is accepted of proven benefit. The main value of the method would appear to be its use in carbon monoxide poisoning (Smith *et al.*, 1962) when high oxygen tension promotes displacement of carbon monoxide from combination with haemoglobin, but this condition is becoming rare as coal gas supplies are replaced by natural gas.

CLINICAL APPLICATIONS

Normal arterial oxygen tension approaches 13 kPa but it is now recognized that individuals in the older age groups live a normal life at tensions much lower than this figure (Nunn, 1965). The low 'normal' P_aO_2 with advancing age has been ascribed to the closure volume (CV) of the lungs increasing to encroach on the tidal volume (*Lancet*, 1972). Airways closure with airways trapping and resultant irregularities of ventilation-perfusion relationships ($\dot{V}/\dot{Q}$) in the lung occurs at higher lung volumes as age increases, in the recumbent posture, and in cigarette smokers. When the CV encroaches on tidal volume arterial hypoxaemia will result. The same end-effect will occur when FRC is reduced as in the patient with postoperative pain. The concept of airways closure, though not universally accepted, serves to explain the cause of arterial hypoxaemia in some clinical situations.

Clinical assessment of hypoxaemia is not possible and laboratory estimations are required. The clinician must have an objective in mind of what P_aO_2 is desirable. There is seldom need for P_aO_2 levels above normal and reference to the haemoglobin oxygen dissociation curve shows that oxygen tension can fall to low levels without a great effect on oxygen saturation. Even at P_aO_2 of 5.5 kPa, the S_aO_2 is 70%. Levels of oxygen tension above 6.5 kPa provide a reasonably high percentage saturation and are acceptable in the presence of major shunts.

Obstructive airways disease

It is well recognized that oxygen therapy may cause respiratory depression and hypercapnia, thus precipitating respiratory failure (Campbell, 1960). Controlled administration of oxygen is important in this context and the Ventimask is a useful device. A small rise in inspired oxygen concentration above that present in air may result in a small rise in P_aO_2 but a significant rise in S_aO_2. If the patient tolerates a low concentration Ventimask without deterioration, a change may be made to the model with next highest F_1O_2. Monitoring by blood gas measurements aids control. Intermittent oxygen therapy is however dangerous since if

89

P_aCO_2 has risen during oxygen administration P_aO_2 will fall to lower levels than prior to treatment (see the O_2-CO_2 diagram, page 80). In the absence of special masks, nasal oxygen at one litre per minute is allowable in incipient respiratory failure. Once frank respiratory failure, as evidenced by rising P_aCO_2 and exhaustion of the patient, has occurred it will be necessary to provide oxygenation by IPPV.

Oxygen in the neonate

Hyperoxia in the premature newborn has been shown to cause retrolental fibroplasia and it has been advocated that F_1O_2 should be restricted to 35% and PaO_2 not allowed to rise above 13 kPa. Intensive care of the neonate does, however, present complex problems (see Chapter 20) and there is no doubt that high inspired concentrations of oxygen should be used when indicated (Cross, 1973; Reynolds, 1974).

Shock

Diminished cardiac output leads to decreased oxygen availability to the tissues and a decreased coefficient of utilization (page 81). Abnormalities of gas exchange in the lungs are also likely in shock. There is also an increased workload associated with increased respiratory rate, dyspnoea, and possibly increased airway resistance. Oxygen therapy is necessary to ensure full saturation and in some cases controlled ventilation will be indicated. These considerations apply whatever the aetiology of the shock syndrome.

Postoperative patients (Nunn, 1965; Nunn and Payne, 1962; Alexander *et al.*, 1973)

Shunts of the order of 10% can develop during anaesthesia. In the immediate postoperative period arterial hypoxaemia may be aggravated by factors such as diminished FRC and significant airways closure, shivering and restlessness. Oxygen therapy in the postoperative ward is a rational routine and may be conveniently carried out by nasal catheter with flows of two to three litres per minute.

Resuscitation

Acute cardiorespiratory collapse from any cause is a major emergency and high inspired concentrations of oxygen should be used as soon as possible. Ventilation with air, as in the emergency treatment of cardiac arrest, should be replaced by ventilation with oxygen as soon as the latter is available. Apparatus such as the Ambu bag, even when the oxygen attachment is used, does not provide high F_1O_2 unless a reservoir attachment is used (Birt, 1965).

It is not possible to provide an exhaustive survey of the indications for oxygen therapy within the confines of this chapter. In general, high inspired concentrations of oxygen are indicated in the acute situation (e.g. cardiac arrest) or where reversal of an acute condition is anticipated (e.g. bronchial asthma). Oxygen is also indicated during transport of patients to the ICU and prior to technical manipulations (e.g. tracheal intubation, bronchoscopy and bronchial lavage). Rational oxygen therapy depends upon the education of medical and nursing staff, and hazards always exist when there is dependency on cylinders or where oxygen is fed into closed anaesthetic circuits. It should also be remembered that administration of dry gases is not desirable and proper humidification is important (see Chapter 6).

REFERENCES

Adams, A. P., Morgan-Hughes, J. O. and Sykes, M. K. (1967), pH and blood-gas analysis. *Anaesthesia*, 22, 575.

Alexander, J. I., Spence, A. A., Parikh, R. K. and Stuart, B. (1973), The Role of Airway Closure in Postoperative Hypoxaemia. *Brit. J. Anaesth.*, 45, 34.

Baskett, P. J. F. and Withnell, A. (1970), Use of Entonox in the Ambulance Service. *Brit. med. J.*, 2, 41.

Benata, S. R., Hewlett, A. M. and Nunn, J. F. (1973), The Use of iso-shunt lines for Control of Oxygen Therapy. *Brit. J. Anaesth.*, 45, 711.

Bethune, D. W. and Collis, J. M. (1967), An evaluation of oxygen therapy equipment—Experimental study of various devices on the human subject. *Thorax*, 22, 221.

Birt, R. C. (1965), The effects of addition of oxygen to various emergency inflating devices. *Anaesthesia*, 20, 323.

Boothby, W. M., Lovelace, W. R. and Bulbulian, A. H. (1930), Oxygen administration—the value of high concentration of oxygen for therapy. *Proc. Mayo Clinic*, 13, 641.

Bulbulian, A. H. (1938), Design and construction of masks for the oxygen inhalation apparatus. *Proc. Mayo Clinic*, 13, 654.

Campbell, E. J. M. (1960), The relation between oxygen concentrations of inspired air and arterial blood. *Lancet*, 2, 10.

Campbell, E. J. M. (1960), A method of controlled oxygen administration which reduces the risk of carbon dioxide retention. *Lancet*, 2, 12.

Campbell, E. J. M. and Gebbie, T. (1966), Masks and tent for providing controlled oxygen concentrations. *Lancet*, 1, 468.

Catterall, M. (1960), A new mask for delivering oxygen or other gases. *Brit. med. J.*, 1, 1940.

Comroe, J. H., Forster, R. E., Dubois, A. B., Briscoe, W. A. and Carlsen, E. (1962), *The Lung* 2nd Edn. Year Book Medical Publishers Inc., Chicago.

Cross, K. W. (1973), Cost of preventing retrolental fibroplasia? *Lancet*, 2, 954.

Editorial (1972), Closing Volume. *Lancet*, 2, 908.

Flenley, D. C., Hutchinson, D. C. S. and Donald, K. W. (1963), Behaviour of apparatus for oxygen administration. *Brit. med. J.*, 2, 1081.

Freeman, J. and Nunn, J. F. (1963), Ventilation-Perfusion Relationships after Haemorrhage. *Clin. Sci.*, 24, 135.

Gilbert, R. L., Comer, P. B., Beckham, R. W. and McGraw, C. P. (1976), Actual tracheal oxygen concentrations with commonly used oxygen equipment. *Anesthesiology*, 44, 71.

Leigh, J. M. (1970), Variation in performance of oxygen therapy devices. *Anaesthesia*, 25, 210.

Leigh, J. M. (1973), Present practice and current trends in oxygen therapy. *Anaesthesia*, 28, 164.

Mapleson, W. W. (1954), The elimination of rebreathing in various semiclosed anaesthetic systems. *Brit. J. Anaesth.*, 26, 323.

Nunn, J. F. (1962), Measurement of blood oxygen tension: Handling of sample. *Brit. J. Anaesth.*, 34, 621.

Nunn, J. F. (1965), Influence of age and other factors on hypoxaemia in the post-operative period. *Lancet*, 2, 466.

Nunn, J. F. and Payne, J. P. (1962), Hypoxaemia after general anaesthesia. *Lancet*, 2, 631.

Nunn, J. F., Bergman, N. A., Coleman, A. J. and Casselle, D. C. (1964), Evaluation of the Sergomex Paramagnetic Analyser. *Brit. J. Anaesth.*, 36, 666.

Nunn, J. F. (1969), In *Applied Respiratory Physiology*. Butterworths, London.

Reynolds, E. O. R. (1974), Methods of mechanical ventilation for hyaline membrane disease. *Proc. R. Soc. Med.*, 67, 248.

Scott, P. V., Horton, J. N. and Mapleson, W. W. (1971), Leakage of oxygen from blood and water samples stored in plastic and glass syringes. *Brit. med. J.*, 3, 512.

Simpson, H. and Russel, D. J. (1967), Oxygen concentrations in tents and incubators in paediatric practice. *Brit. med. J.*, 4, 201.

Smith, G., Ledingham, I. M., Sharp, G. R., Norman, J. N. and Bates, E. H. (1962), Treatment of coal-gas poisoning with oxygen at 2 atmospheres pressure. *Lancet*, 1, 816.

Sykes, M. K., McNicol, M. W. and Campbell, E. J. M. (1976), *Respiratory Failure*. 2nd ed. Blackwell, Oxford and Edinburgh.

Torda, T. A. and Grant, G. C. (1973), Test of a fuel cell oxygen analyser. *Brit. J. Anaesth.*, 45, 1108.

Walstead, P. M. and Conklin, W. S. (1961), Rupture of the normal stomach after therapeutic oxygen. *New Eng. J. Med.*, 264, 1201.

EIGHT

Specific respiratory problems

CHRONIC RESPIRATORY DISEASE (OBSTRUCTIVE AIRWAYS DISEASE)

The management of chronic obstructive airways disease, either as an elective post-operative procedure or as an emergency can pose many problems, not least of which is its recognition. Physicians, surgeons and anaesthetists should be on the alert for the apparently well compensated case where conditions can dramatically deteriorate in a dark corner of a medical ward or in the post-operative recovery room.

Clinical features

Two types of generalized airway obstruction are well recognized.

Type A or 'pink puffers'

These patients are generally lean smokers who, as the description implies, are not cyanosed. The story is of progressive dyspnoea but usually there is no history of recurrent bronchitis, i.e. cough and sputum. On examination the chest is overinflated and high pitched expiratory wheezes, if not present at rest, can often be induced by increasing the respiratory rate. Elevation of the JVP and ankle oedema are not present until the condition is very advanced. Cyanosis develops terminally and is a very grave sign. Lung function studies show a reduced forced expiratory volume, with a reduced vital capacity but the blood gases are usually normal at rest (the arterial oxygen saturation may fall after exercise). X-Rays show a normal size heart and emphysema with diminution of peripheral vascular markings.

Type B or 'blue bloaters'

These patients have a long history of recurrent bronchitis with expulsion of discoloured sputum. They are usually obese, pletheric and cyanosed. Oedema, elevation of the JVP, hepatomegaly are common. Pulmonary hypertension, due to chronic hypoxia with respiratory acidosis, is demonstrated both clinically and on the ECG and chest X-ray.

Severe reduction of the FEV occurs with a normal total lung capacity. The arterial oxygen saturation is reduced, P_aCO_2 is raised. A characteristic feature of

93

these patients is their inability to increase alveolar ventilation in response to an increased P_aCO_2.

Recognition of the patient at risk

Many patients with chronic obstructive airways disease are submitted to elective or emergency surgery. Pre-operative assessment should include a full history with particular emphasis on exercise tolerance, the quantity and nature of sputum and of course the smoking habits. Drug history is important, especially with respect to steroid therapy, the omission of which post-operatively could be catastrophic. Simple tests of respiratory function should be performed, at least the FEV_1, and Vital Capacity.

By definition failure exists when normal blood gas tensions cannot be maintained and if there is doubt as to the ventilatory status of the patient arterial blood gas estimations should be measured.

It should be remembered that the combination of anaesthesia, sedation, analgesia and diminished respiratory movement can cause rapid acceleration of respiratory insufficiency.

Clinical features that suggest respiratory failure

(1) exhaustion, irritability, drowsiness, insomnia
(2) coma
(3) rapid, shallow respiration
(4) sweating
(5) pallor/cyanosis
(6) inability to expectorate secretions

Management

Reversible components of chronic obstructive airways disease include infection, bronchospasm and heart failure.

(1) Infection—antibiotic therapy should always be undertaken if the sputum is purulent. Initially ampicillin is probably the drug of choice as it is effective against the common respiratory pathogens but bacteriological studies should always be carried out. It should be remembered that many patients with chronic disease will have had injudicious antibiotic therapy in the past leading to the emergence of resistant strains or opportunistic infection.
(2) Bronchodilator therapy—nearly always there is at least a small element of reversible airways obstruction which might respond to bronchodilators. Salbutamol, terbutaline or steroids should be given (see page 99).
(3) Diuretics—should be used if there is an element of heart failure. Generally frusemide (40–80 mg daily) is the drug of choice (with potassium supplements).

General management

Sedation

Sedation should always be used with the utmost caution, and only if facilities for artificial ventilation are immediately available. In general, sedation should be considered highly dangerous, particularly for restless patients in whom respiratory coma can only too readily be induced. It should be remembered that there are no 'safe' sedatives under these circumstances: even diazepam in low dosage depresses respiratory function.

Physiotherapy

Physiotherapy is of the utmost importance.
(1) to clear tracheobronchial secretion
(2) to preserve airway patency

Oxygen (see Chapter 7)

The dangers of oxygen therapy in chronic respiratory disease are well known and fully discussed elsewhere. A compromise needs to be met between the need for oxygen and the risks of respiratory depression. A modest increase in oxygen by use of a Ventimask (24 or 28%) should be the maximum allowed.

To ventilate or not?

Very often this is a difficult decision. It requires as full an assessment as is possible, often with limited time because once on a ventilator it is difficult to decide to abandon treatment.
(1) Is there a significant reversible component? Infection, heart failure and bronchospasm can all be treated. So can the effects of the injudicious use of sedation or uncontrolled oxygen therapy.
(2) Is the patient a respiratory cripple? Of vital importance is a history from relatives as to previous exercise tolerance. There is little point in treating end-stage respiratory failure in a patient in whom this is the latest in a sequence of hospital admissions and who is incapable of moving from a chair because of dyspnoea. It is relatively simple to restore blood gas levels to normal with mechanical ventilation, but this will be of little benefit to a patient who cannot ever be weaned off the instrument. Under these circumstances it would be kinder not to treat at all.
In summary therefore the management of acute respiratory failure in a patient with chronic obstructive airways disease will depend upon the presence of reversible factors taken into consideration in conjunction with the previous clinical state of the patient.

POSTOPERATIVE RESPIRATORY INSUFFICIENCY

IPPV may be carried out during the postoperative period as an elective or non-elective procedure. Respiratory function is depressed following abdominal surgery and this may be important after major procedures have been carried out in the elderly or critically ill patient. Arterial hypoxaemia occurs commonly following abdominal surgery and may not resolve for up to 5 days. The causes for this are probably multiple, but one aetiological factor is the changing relationship of functional residual capacity and closing volume when the patient suffers pain during the postoperative period. The patients lungs are held in a more expiratory position than formerly (lowered functional residual capacity) and the closing volume is likely to be increased. The closing volume, that volume of air remaining in the lungs when significant airways closure occurs during expiration, increases with advancing age, with adoption of the supine as opposed to the erect position, and in smokers. Postoperative patients are often elderly and are usually nursed in a horizontal position. If the tidal excursion encroaches on the closing volume, that is if functional residual capacity becomes less than the closing volume, ventilation and perfusion relationships are affected due to gas trapping. Shunts develop and arterial hypoxaemia occurs. Other causes of respiratory depression include the effect of anaesthetic drugs and postoperative narcotic analgesics, difficulty in expectoration and sometimes altered levels of consciousness.

It is common practice to administer oxygen to patients during the post-operative period to correct hypoxaemia. In selected patients this may be combined with IPPV which ensures adequate alveolar ventilation with an oxygen-rich mixture. Some workers have added nitrous oxide to the mixture for the first 12 hours to provide analgesia without cardiovascular depression. This can be achieved by dilution of Entonox (the commercially available mixture of 50% nitrous oxide in oxygen). 25% nitrous oxide is said to be equivalent to 10 mg morphine in analgesic effect. Long term administration of nitrous oxide is associated with bone marrow depression, but administration for up to 24 hours is considered safe.

Ventilation in management of head injury. See Chapter 10.

THE ADULT RESPIRATORY DISTRESS SYNDROME (ARDS)

Respiratory problems may arise in patients being treated in the intensive care unit for a variety of conditions. Where there is a progressive impairment of gas exchange P_aO_2 falls and $AaDO_2$ increases despite administration of high concentrations of oxygen. The patient becomes breathless with increased respiratory rate, accompanied by tachycardia and perhaps cyanosis. P_aCO_2 may fall as a result of hyperventilation in the early stages, but later it rises as lung function fails. Opacities develop in the chest X-ray, though not always immediately, and these later coalesce to produce the classical 'white-out' appearance, when only the major bronchi are filled with air. Histological changes include interstitial oedema, hyaline membrane, loss of surfactant and atelectasis.

The aetiology is not clearly understood. The syndrome is closely related to Shock Lung (see page 40) and resembles that of Fat Embolism (see page 168) in its effect on respiratory gas exchange. Oxygen toxicity can produce similar signs. The deposition of micro-aggregates in the lung capillaries as a result of blood transfusion are thought to be important and the use of blood filters when massive volumes of blood are given may aid prevention. Because of the multifactorial nature of the aetiology the syndrome has been described under a variety of labels but the term, adult respiratory distress syndrome, is now increasingly accepted, even though the condition can occur in children.

The mortality of this condition is high. Treatment is by controlled oxygen therapy, avoiding high $F_1 O_2$, and mechanical ventilation probably with PEEP. Fluid overload should be avoided and diuretics may be useful. Blood filters should be used if blood is transfused. The value of massive corticosteroid therapy is uncertain.

SEVERE ASTHMA—STATUS ASTHMATICUS

There is no clear-cut definition of status asthmaticus—it is unwise arbitrarily to define it as an attack of asthma that has defied ordinary treatment for so many hours; or to lay down a catalogue of abnormal blood gas studies which justify 'intensive therapy'. The decision to admit a patient to the ITU for treatment of severe asthma must depend upon informed clinical judgement, remembering that sudden death in asthmatic attacks is not always related to the duration of the attack, nor even to the severity as subjectively described by patients.

Warning signs

(1) *Cyanosis* is not common in asthmatics unless there is coexistent chronic bronchitis and emphysema. If present serious hypoxaemia will be present.

(2) *Tachycardia.* Pulse rates of over 130, similarly, are indicative of significant hypoxaemia. Pulsus paradoxicus is an important finding in severe asthma.

(3) *Level of consciousness.* Confusion or drowsiness will nearly always indicate serious blood gas disturbances.

(4) *Breathlessness* is often unreliable as an indication of severity, as sudden death may occur in patients who do not complain of undue dyspnoea but often have other ominous signs as described above. Unfortunately hyperventilation is a common finding in mild asthma.

(5) *Inability to expectorate*

(6) *Sleeplessness for over 24 hours*

Blood gas abnormalities

Hypoxaemia is the serious and significant abnormality in severe asthma. The P_aCO_2 is normal or reduced when the asthma is mild or moderate. A rise in P_aCO_2 is always a serious portent, and the effect of this is an acute fall of arterial pH because the situation is quite different to the chronic elevations of P_aCO_2 that occur in chronic bronchitis where buffering mechanisms in the blood prevent serious pH changes.

Assessment by blood gases is therefore important, particularly in respect of monitoring progress. A rise in P_aCO_2 and no improvement in arterial oxygen tension indicate that therapy is ineffective.

Respiratory function studies

These tests are often impracticable in severely ill patients, moreover there is not a clear relationship between them and functional severity of attacks. The simplest and most useful test, particularly in assessing progress is the FEV_1, which may be as little as 300–500 ml.

Pathology of fatal asthma

Autopsy findings in fatal asthma show mucous plugging of the small airways, the mucosa is oedematous and infiltrated with eosinophils. The mucous plugs are thick and tenacious.

Management of severe asthma

The mainstays of treatment are bronchodilating drugs, oxygen and steroids (Fig. 8.1).

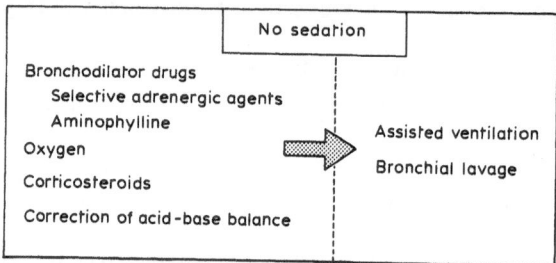

Fig. 8.1 Treatment of severe asthma.

Bronchodilating drugs

Most patients will already have been treated with adrenergic stimulators (often in inhalant form) but they remain an essential part of treatment. Emphasis should be on selective agents which are less likely to increase tachycardia or induce dysrhythmias.

Salbutamol (Ventolin) is administered by slow intravenous infusion. The rate is

3-20 mcg/min, the initial starting rate should be 5 mcg/min. (This preparation is available in 5 ml ampoules containing 5 mg of salbutamol. The contents of an ampoule should be added to 500 ml of dextrose saline giving a concentration of 10 mcg/ml. The infusion should be given using an infusion pump or paediatric giving set so that the dose can be given accurately. This drug can also be given by intramuscular or subcutaneous injection in a dose of 8 mcg/kg body weight repeated 4 hourly if necessary.

Terbutaline (Bricanyl); Orciprenaline (Alupent) are similar adrenergic agents more selective than adrenaline or isoprenaline.
    Terbutaline can be given by subcutaneous injection (0.25-0.5 mg 6 hourly in adults–0.005 mg/kg body wt in children). An intravenous preparation for infusion is also available.
    Selective adrenergic agents such as terbutaline and salbutamol can be very effectively administered as a nebulized solution. Both drugs are available as a respirator solution, which after dilution delivers a dose of 1-2 mg/hr using a suitable ventilator.

Fenoterol (Berotec) is a longer-acting bronchodilator which may be very useful especially in the form of an aerosol nebuliser.

Isoprenaline, Adrenaline should not be used, modern selective adrenergic agents are preferred.

Aminophylline remains a very useful drug in severe asthma, although it has a reputation of causing cardiac dysrhythmias. It is best given by slow infusion. The initial dose is 250-500 mg given over 10 minutes and followed by infusion of up to 2g in 24 hours.

Oxygen

There is less danger of affecting respiratory centre control in asthma than in chronic bronchitis, and therefore oxygen must be administered to all cases of severe asthma. High concentrations are not usually needed–35% Ventimask or nasal cannulae with a flow of 3-5 l/min are usually sufficient. But P_aCO_2 levels should be monitored.

Steroids

Steroids should be given to all cases. High doses are necessary, but tailing can be rapid with slight risk of hypoadrenalism afterwards. But remember that many severe asthmatics are on long-term oral steroids, and maintenance dose may be higher after the acute phase. The right time to give high dose steroids is at the beginning of treatment, it is a mistake to give too small a dose too late.

Dose–intravenous hydrocortisone–initial dose 250-500 mg followed by infusion 1 g-2 g/24 hours. The tailing off procedure should be over 24-48 h, but longer if the patient was on steroids before. Generally a de-crescendo course of oral prednisolone is commenced as i.v. steroid therapy is tailed off.

Correction of acid-base balance

When carbon dioxide retention occurs arterial pH falls (see above) and this acidosis may make the bronchial musculature less responsive to bronchodilators, and increase the risk of cardiac arrest. There may, therefore, be an argument for giving intravenous sodium bicarbonate, but a metabolic alkalosis may result if ventilatory function returns to normal.

Dehydration is common in severe asthma, and this will increase the viscosity of sputum plugs and careful fluid replacement is mandatory.

Monitoring therapy

The decision to pass an endotracheal tube and start mechanical ventilation will depend on several factors, the most important of which is observation of the patient. Physical exhaustion may occur without dramatic changes in blood gases. This therefore is the prime indication for proceeding to this form of treatment. A persistent tachycardia, cardiac arrythmia, increasing drowsiness are other important indicators of a deteriorating situation. Blood gas studies are valuable. Hypoxaemia, persistent or rising, despite adequate oxygen therapy; and most important—P_aCO_2 concentrations that fail to fall or rise should mean that IPPV will be indicated. In the context of asthma a P_aCO_2 of 6.6 KPa is a critical level.

However, it must be emphasized, important as blood gas estimations are, an exhausted patient must be ventilated regardless of blood gas levels that may be found.

Sedation

No sedative is safe in severe asthma unless the patient is on mechanical ventilation. Cough suppressants should not be used either.

Bronchial lavage

This technique may occasionally be justified if there is thick tenacious sputum with plugging of the bronchioles. It should never be undertaken unless mechanical ventilation has either been commenced or will be immediately after the prcoedure as there is a considerable risk of aggravating an already serious hypoxaemic state.

Mechanical ventilation

IPPV is particularly difficult in asthma. For details see page 6.

Antibiotics

Although severe asthma may be precipitated by bacterial infection this is not always so. As has been emphasized at many points in this book the decision to use antibiotics must be based on good evidence of bacterial infection. In this case, sputum culture is mandatory. A broad spectrum antibiotic is indicated in seriously ill patients pending bacteriology reports.

LUNG ABSCESS

Lung abscess will most commonly be seen in the ITU in association with prolonged respiratory infection and the best way of preventing such a complication is by meticulous attention to frequent and effective physiotherapy. All lung abscesses have their origin in an area of unresolved pneumonic consolidation. The possibility of an inhaled foreign body should, however, always be considered.

Table 8.1 Causes of lung abscess

Infection	Direct	especially staphylococcal infection
	Indirect	(1) haematogenous spread
		(2) by extension from a subphrenic abscess
		(3) following inhalation from an upper G.I. tract lesion
Distal to an obstructive lesion		Carcinoma of bronchus *Foreign body*
Traumatic		Infection of a lung haematoma
Pulmonary infarct		Infection following a pulmonary embolus

The diagnosis of lung abscess will usually be by observation of serial radiographs. The characteristic appearances of a cavity will appear and the exact location of the abscess must always be defined by means of X-rays in two planes, occasionally tomography will be necessary. Knowledge of the exact anatomical site is vital if effective physiotherapy is to be given.

Clinically, suspicion of abscess formation will occur with prolonged swinging fever, polymorph leucocytosis and possibly an increase in the quantity of sputum—which may become bloodstained. *Bacteriological* diagnosis can usually be made from sputum culture. However, a direct needle aspiration from the abscess cavity, the needle being inserted under X-ray control, may sometimes be necessary. If the abscess is complicated by empyema formation, pleural aspiration will be necessary. It is important to remember that all pathological material must be cultured for anaerobic organisms (Bartlett *et al.*, 1974).

Treatment

Physiotherapy. The physiotherapist must know in which lobe, or segment, of the lung the abscess is, so that effective drainage can be carried out. Prophylactic physiotherapy is particularly important, to prevent abscesses forming after small areas of atelectasis or consolidation have developed, especially in patients on

prolonged IPPV. Under these circumstances the attentions of a skilled physiotherapist are, at least, as important as a whole galaxy of (often inappropriate)
antibiotics.

Antibiotics. Bacteriological studies will dictate the choice of antibiotic. Particular
attention is drawn to the possibility of anaerobic organisms as aetiological agents,
when metronidazole may be the antibiotic of choice, alone or in combination
with drugs effective against aerobes.

Antibiotic therapy should be continued for at least a month.

Opportunistic infections may present as single or multiple lung cavities,
notably nocardia arteroides, cryptococcus neoformans and mucormycosis and
these organisms will require drugs other than conventional antibiotics (see
Chapter 25).

PNEUMOTHORAX

Pneumothorax in association with penetrating wounds of the chest is discussed
in Chapter 12. We are here concerned with the type of pneumothorax that
precipitates admission to the ITU, and also, importantly to pneumothorax
developing in cases in the unit, especially those on IPPV. Pneumothorax can be
defined as the presence of air in the pleural space, either from a breach of the
chest wall or, more commonly, from a leak of air from the lung.

Many pneumothoraces require no treatment, as a small amount of air within
the pleural space causes little or no respiratory embarassment, if lung function is
basically normal, and is rapidly absorbed. However, diagnostic and therapeutic
difficulties arise if pulmonary function is already impaired. Into this group fall
the following groups of patient:

(1) Chronic obstructive airway disease, bronchitis, asthma, pulmonary fibrosis

(2) The newborn

(3) Other chest diseases—bronchiectasis, fibrocystic disease, staphylococcal
pneumonia, bronchial carcinoma

(4) Patients on IPPV

In the ITU pneumothorax may also be caused by attempted cannulation of
the subclavian vein.

Diagnosis of pneumothorax

The classical physical signs are those of resonance with silence. To this can be
added the signs of mediastinal shift (away from the side of the lesion). However,
in patients with emphysema these physical signs may not be easy to elicit and
an X-ray must always be taken when a patient with chronic airways disease
becomes more dyspnoeic as the chronic over-inflation of the lungs may well
make the classical physical signs of pneumothorax impossible to elicit. It is, of
course, this group of patients who are not only vulnerable to pneumothorax,
but particularly at danger from its effects.

Types of pneumothorax

(1) Simple

A leak of air occurs, causing a greater or lower degree of lung collapse, but the amount of air stays constant, as the leak seals off, until absorption or therapeutic removal occurs, allowing the lung to re-expand.

(2) Open

The leak between lung and pleural space remains open, so that air continues to leak out replacing that which is removed or absorbed.

(3) Tension

A valve system at the leak occurs so that the amount of air in the pleural space increases with each inspiration. When this occurs intrapleural pressure becomes very high producing severe mediastinal shift, and this causes very severe symptoms of dyspnoea and collapse. When this occurs immediate needling of the chest might be life-saving.

The X-ray in pneumothorax

A chest film must always be taken. Inexperienced observers may easily miss the cap of air of an apical pneumothorax. It is always unwise to pass off a pneumothorax as insignificant wholly on the basis of X-ray findings—an X-ray may show pre-existing lung disease—and no pneumothorax is insignificant in chronic obstructive airway disease.

Another important reason for always X-raying the chest is to ascertain if fluid is present—usually indicating a haemo-pneumothorax.

Particular attention is drawn to the necessity for regular chest films of patients on IPPV, in whom the only clinical indications of pneumothorax may be changes in pulse rate.

Treatment of pneumothorax

In the ITU a pneumothorax will almost always need treatment—either because it is the reason for admission, such as in a patient with chronic airways disease who slides into respiratory failure, or because it is a consequence of treatment, e.g. IPPV, or as a complication of severe pneumonia, e.g. staphylococcal. Treatment is by use of an intercostal catheter attached to an underwater seal. The tube is best inserted, after local anaesthesia, into the axillary area. Caution should be used in large pneumothoraces to allow the initial escape of air to be slow (by means of a variable clip), because sudden changes in intrapleural pressure can produce acute pulmonary oedema, and rapid mediastinal shift can be dangerous. Serial X-rays will show that the lung is re-expanded and if the expansion is maintained after the catheter has been clamped off for some hours, it can be removed. Observation of the swing of fluid in the drainage system will indicate its patency.

103

If the pneumothorax remains despite simple drainage, apposition of the pleural surfaces, leading, hopefully, to a seal of the leak, can be achieved by using a low pressure suction unit attached to the underwater seal.

Tension pneumothorax. This is a grave emergency. If no time is available to set up an underwater system as above the air must be released by using a large bore intravenous cannula. Once the emergency is over a conventional intercostal catheter with underwater drain can be inserted. The intercostal catheter should always be removed as soon as the condition appears stable because of the risks of infection. If the pneumothorax is (a) bilateral, (b) remains open, (c) recurrent, a thoracic surgical opinion should be sought regarding definitive surgical treatment.

Haemopneumothorax—see Chapter 12.

EMPYEMA

An empyema is pus in the pleural space and will most commonly be encountered in the ITU as a complication of surgical or traumatic lesions of the oesophagus. In this respect the eclipse of the rigid oesophagoscope in favour of flexible fibre-optic endoscopic instruments may reduce the number of cases.

Extension from a subphrenic abscess is also an important cause. Broncho-pleural fistula after lung surgery is outside the scope of this book. Pneumonia, especially staphylococcal and lung abscess may be complicated by empyema formation.

Diagnosis

The diagnosis is made by identifying pus in the pleural cavity. Persistent pain with the X-ray appearances of a pleural effusion should always suggest the possibility of empyema, particularly if associated with fever, polymorph leuco-cytosis and anaemia. If there is suspicion of infection of pleural fluid a diagnostic tap is simple, but it should be remembered that very thick pus may require a wide bore needle for successful aspiration. Encysted or loculated empyema might also be difficult to aspirate.

Pleural pus should always be sent for bacteriological studies (including for anaerobic organisms such as actinomycosis).

Treatment

The use of systemic and intrapleural antibiotics with frequent chest aspiration will generally help with acute empyema secondary to lung infection. However, with underlying oesophageal pathology, or if the pus becomes loculated a surgical approach (decortication) will be necessary. This is probably better than attempting long periods of tube drainage.

When an empyema becomes chronic parenteral nutrition is an important aspect of therapy as these patients are often hypercatabolic.

'LEGIONNAIRES' DISEASE

First described in 1976, the onset is with malaise, fever, cough, chest pain and progressive dyspnoea. X-rays show patchy and then confluent consolidation either bilateral or unilateral. Several cases died despite full respiratory support and multiple antibiotics. Of the antibiotics erythromycin has been shown to be the most effective.

The diagnosis can be made using an indirect fluorescence antibody test. In post-mortem studies of the lungs the organisms can be demonstrated using a silver impregnation staining technique.

It should therefore be remembered that in patients with a severe pneumonia and blood gas abnormalities, where sputum is reported as showing 'commensals only', may be suffering from this disease and erythromycin prescribed.

DROWNING

By the time a case of near-drowning has reached hospital the critical period of immediate resuscitation will have been carried out by the ambulance crew. The immediate effect of near-drowning is asphyxia, and this occurs whether water has been aspirated into the lungs or not. Immediate resuscitation therefore is along the usual lines:

(1) clear the airway

(2) commence breathing, either by the mouth to mouth method, or by use of an airway such as the Brook airway, if available

(3) external cardiac massage, unless the femoral or carotid pulse is palpable

At this stage consideration should be given to the pathophysiology of near-drowning. With aspiration of either salt or fresh water into the lungs, pulmonary oedema occurs, probably due to direct chemical irritation and the blood changes are shown in Table 8.2.

Table 8.2 Pathophysiology of near drowning

Fresh water	Salt water
Hypervolaemia	Hypovolaemia
Haemodilution	Haemoconcentration
Haemolysis	
Na $\downarrow$	Na $\uparrow$
Cl $\downarrow$	Cl $\uparrow$
K $\uparrow$	K $\uparrow$

In hospital the immediate problem will be that common to all forms of circulatory arrest:

(1) Acidosis—treated with i.v. sodium bicarbonate 100–150 ml of 8.4% solution

105

(2) 100% oxygen, with endotracheal intubation and an Ambu bag until formal IPPV can be instituted.

(3) Correction of cardiac dysrhythmia. (In salt water drowning asystole is common and ventricular fibrillation more usual in fresh water drowning.)

When treating the cardiac component of near-drowning it should be remembered that these cases are frequently *hypothermic* and this should be considered when using drugs or D.C. cardioversion.

If the circulation is restored IPPV should be continued—and PEEP may be useful if pulmonary oedema is present (Golden and Rivers, 1975).

The management of the shock state is along the usual lines with cautious fluid and volume replacement and steroids are generally given in an attempt to prevent cerebral oedema (dexamethasone 4 mg 6-hourly).

HIGH ALTITUDE PULMONARY OEDEMA

This condition is unlikely to occur in the British Isles as it is described as developing at altitudes of over 9000 ft, usually at over 12 000 ft. It affects people who are not acclimatized to altitude, or who have spent weeks or months at sea-level after living at altitude and then return to high altitude. Young male adults are most likely to be affected. The clinical features are acute breathlessness with the physical signs of pulmonary oedema. The condition may be misdiagnosed as pneumonia because fever and leucocytosis occur and the X-ray may show changes suggestive of bronchopneumonia. Blood gas studies show severe hypoxaemia. Physical signs and catheter evidence of pulmonary hypertension are present. However the neck veins are not distended.

Pathophysiology

At post-mortem intravascular fibrin thrombi are seen in the lungs which suggests that disseminated intravascular coagulation (DIC) may occur. The degree of pulmonary hypertension is in excess of that normally found with similar degree of hypoxia. The arterial desaturation does not respond initially to 100% oxygen and this may be due to a functional right to left shunt produced by the opening of vessels that bypass the pulmonary arterioles and empty direct into pulmonary capillary beds. The X-ray appearances of diffuse bronchopneumonia could be explained by the non-uniform opening of these vessels.

Treatment

The patient should be removed from altitude and treated with bed rest and 100% oxygen, through a face mask at a flow of 6-8 l/min. Morphine may be helpful, as in other forms of pulmonary oedema, and frusemide 80 mg daily should be given. (It has been suggested that frusemide can be used prophylactically to prevent this condition.) High dose steroids have also been used.

FURTHER READING

Ambiavagar, M., Jones, E. S. (1967), Resuscitation of the moribund asthmatic. *Anaesthesia*, 22, 375

Bartlett, J. G., Gerbach, S. L., Tally, F. P. and Finegold, S. M. (1974), Bacteriology and treatment of primary lung abscess. *Am. Rev. resp. Dis.*, **109**, 510.

Blaisdell, F. N. and Schlobohm, R. M. (1973), The respiratory distress syndrome: a review. *Surgery*, **74**, 251.

Choo-Yang, Y. F., Parker, S. S., Grant, I. W. (1970), Response of asthmatics to isoprenaline and salbutamol aerosols administered by intermittent positive pressure ventilation. *Brit. med. J.*, **4**, 169.

Collins, J. V., Harris, P. W., Clark, T. J., Townsend, J. (1970), Intravenous corticosteroids in treatment of acute bronchial asthma. *Lancet*, **2**, 1047.

Editorial (1980). Lungs and Legionnaires Disease, *Brit. med. J.*, **281**, 339.

Golden, F. St. C. and Rivers, J. F. (1975), The Immersion Incident. *Anaesthesia*, **30**, 364.

Grimwood, K., Johnson-Barrett, J. J. and Brent Taylor (1981), Salbutamol: tablets, inhalation powder or nebuliser? *Brit. med. J.*, **282**, 105.

Houston, C. S. (1960), Acute Pulmonary Oedema of high altitude. *New Eng. J. Med.*, **263**, 478.

Kliner, J. P., Nelson, W. P. (1975), High altitude pulmonary oedema—a rare disease? *J.A.M.A.*, **234**, 491.

Knowles, G. K., Clark, T. J. H. (1973), Pulses paradoxus as a valuable sign indicating severity of asthma. *Lancet*, ii, 1356.

Rees, H. A., Millar, J. S., Donald, K. W. (1968), A study of the clinical course and arterial blood gas tensions of patients in status asthmaticus. *Q. J. Med.*, **37**, 541.

Singh, I. (1965), High altitude pulmonary oedema. *Am. Heart J.*, **70**, 435.

NINE

Coronary care

The management of the complications of myocardial infarction will often require the full resources of a cardiac care unit, but it should be remembered that there is a continuing controversy over the indiscriminate admission of all patients with myocardial infarction to hospital (Mather *et al.*, 1976). There can be no doubt that the life-threatening dysrhythmias and cardiogenic shock require intensive monitoring facilities. However coronary care has most to offer if the patient can be admitted during the first four hours, when the risk of serious dysrhythmia is at its greatest. If the patient is in a stable haemodynamic state 24–48 h after an infarction the advantages of coronary care in hospital are less easily demonstrated. In general, patients over the age of 65 who have survived the first eight hours after infarction without cardiac failure or significant dysrhythmia are often better treated at home. The principal role of the coronary care unit is the recognition and treatment of dysrhythmias by continuous monitoring and in this respect, therefore, management in general wards offers little advantages over home care. The psychological hazards of coronary care are very real (Hackett *et al.*, 1968 and see Chapter 22) and may contribute to mortality. Coronary care units should, if possible, be adjacent to the medical wards and separate from Intensive Therapy Units concerned with the management of the other conditions discussed in this book. Although possibly extravagant with limited resources and opposed by administrative staff, in our view it is inappropriate to manage myocardial infarction in a multi-disciplinary ITU.

CARDIAC ARREST—CARDIO-PULMONARY RESUSCITATION

Whilst the definitive treatment depends on observation of the ECG and electrical and drug therapy, if successful resuscitation is to be achieved, it is the early recognition and resuscitating measures that are vital. Basic cardio-pulmonary resuscitation must immediately be instituted.

(1) The patient must be laid flat on a hard surface, often the floor is best. A springy bed is no place for successful cardiac massage.

(2) The legs should be elevated.

(3) The airway should be established by extending the head.

(4) External cardiac massage commenced.

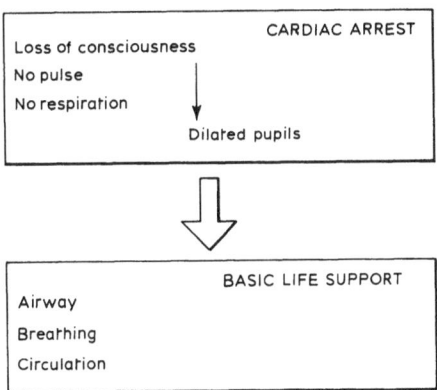

Fig. 9.1 Cardiac arrest and cardio-pulmonary resuscitation.

(5) Ventilation commenced, either by mouth to mouth breathing or by use of an airway, such as the Brook airway.

Ventilation

The tendency to leap on the chest before airway and ventilation is secured must be resisted. Maintenance of oxygenation is equally important and there is no point in applying circulatory support to a hypoxic patient.

In hospital an airway will usually be available and mouth to mouth breathing will not be necessary as a Brook Airway or Ambu bag should be available on all resuscitation trolleys. Endotracheal intubation will be required in cases where the circulation is not rapidly restored.

The ventilation rate should be 12/min and obviously the lungs should not be inflated at the same time as the compression phase of cardiac massage. One inflation every 5 cycles of cardiac compression is required. In the hospital environment it will be possible to administer high concentrations of oxygen during cardio-respiratory resuscitation.

External cardiac massage

The technique of external cardiac massage which can effectively maintain the circulation until definitive therapy is commenced, depends upon producing a cardiac output by compressing the heart between the sternum and the thoracic vertebrae.

The object of external massage is not to break the ribs and induce a pneumothorax or worse. Pressure from the broad heel of the palm should be applied to the lower sternum, the second hand placed over the first gives extra pressure and the sternum moved about 1½ inches 60–70 times a minute (Kouwenhoven *et al.*, 1960).

Specific therapy

By the simple manoeuvres of ventilation and external massage it is possible to maintain vital functions for many minutes. Observation of pupil size is a useful gauge of the efficiency of these measures.

(1) Correction of acidosis

Acidosis occurs rapidly and inevitably in all cases of circulatory arrest. If not corrected successful resuscitation is unlikely.

Intravenous bicarbonate should always be given. Hopefully, in the CCU, access via an intravenous line will already be available; if not an i.v. line must be set up immediately and 100–150 mmol sodium bicarbonate given quickly. In order to avoid overloading an already compromised circulation this is best given as 100–150 ml of 8.4% sodium bicarbonate. It is however important not to exceed this figure. More bicarbonate may be necessary, especially if VF proves intractable, but in general further doses should be calculated after blood pH estimations have become available.

(2) Correction of dysrhythmia

The technique of defibrillation and drug therapy is described on page 122.

(3) Other measures

(1) *Mannitol* may be helpful in protecting the kidneys if prolonged hypotension has occurred. 200 ml of 20% solution is given over 20 minutes.

(2) *Dexamethasone* may also be given to reduce cerebral oedema. The dose is 4 mg 4 hourly for 24 hours.

(4) Cardiogenic shock

Treatment of this is described on page 126.

ACUTE MYOCARDIAL INFARCTION

The principal reason for admission to the CCU is acute myocardial infarction, but there will inevitably be a proportion of patients with a suggestive history who are being observed with serial ECGs and enzyme studies, and it is this group who may well suffer adverse psychiatric effects, especially if the tests are negative. However, it is probably wiser that such cases should be treated in the CCU as initial cardiograms may be unreliable and the possibility of serious dysrhythmia is always present.

Where haemodynamic disturbance or dysrhythmia is present there is no doubt that prognosis is better in the CCU. It should however be recalled that the principal mortality in myocardial infarction occurs within the first hour and unless a coronary ambulance is available such cases are unlikely to be admitted to a unit with monitoring facilities within that time. The population of a CCU is therefore selected by virtue of having survived the lethal early stage of infarction. Moreover only a relatively small proportion of patients in the CCU develop significant complications to justify the huge expense and psychological hazards that are an inevitable part of coronary care.

Symptoms

The principal symptom of acute myocardial infarction is chest pain. However although the classic description is of constricting pain radiating across the chest to the arms, and accompanied by collapse, pallor, sweating and vomiting, it is important to remember that the pain may be felt entirely in the abdomen, throat or arms. 'Silent' infarction without pain is well recognized. Many patients have had preceding angina and will differentiate the pain from agina because of severity, systemic symptoms and lack of response to TNT.

Physical findings

There are no specific physical signs. The pulse rate is increased and the blood pressure usually reduced (occasionally a hypertensive response is seen). Vaso-constriction and sweating may in part be due to pain. A triple rhythm indicates left ventricular failure, a fourth heart sound is more common in cases uncompli-cated by failure. The jugular venous pressure is not usually raised in the early stages, in the presence of shock a raised JVP can indicate tamponade due to rupture of the heart. Pericardial friction rubs do not usually appear in the first 24 h. Fever develops during the first 24 h and often persists for up to a week particularly if there is a large area of muscle necrosis.

Diagnosis

(1) ECG

The principal pathological findings in the ECG of acute myocardial infarction are:
  (a) Q waves
  (b) ST elevation
  (c) T wave inversion
For details of the electrocardiography of cardiac infarction the reader is referred to a textbook of cardiology. It should, however, be remembered that the ECG may not show any abnormality for 2-3 days and serial observations are therefore essential. Also it is important to try and identify the site of the infarct because of the different types of dysrhythmia that may be anticipated with lesions at different sites (see below).
  (a) Anterior infarction—changes in I, II AVL and the chest leads
  (b) Inferior infarction—changes in II, III AVF
  (c) A lesion on the posterior aspect of the heart may only be identified by a tall R wave and an upright T wave in V_1

(2) Enzyme studies

Cardiac enzyme studies play little part in the acute diagnosis of myocardial

111

infarction. The earliest rise (3–6 h with peak at 16–20 h) is in the creatine kinase (CK), the glutamic oxalo-acetic transaminase (SGOT) follows this. Lactic dehydrogenase (LDH) levels start rising some hours later reaching their peak at 72 hours (Sobel and Shell, 1972).

(3) Chest X-ray

There are no pathognomonic findings in the chest film. It is difficult to obtain technically satisfactory film on portable machines in the CCU, and the principal reason for performing such X-rays is to detect early signs of pulmonary congestion and left ventricular failure. These signs may appear on the chest X-ray before there are physical signs of heart failure.

Differential diagnosis

The diagnosis of acute cardiovascular collapse is not always easy and there are many causes other than myocardial infarction. We are particularly concerned here with the patient who collapses in hospital, often in the course of investigation or treatment of other conditions. In the context of an ITU, often the most difficult differential diagnosis is *massive pulmonary embolism*. This condition is described in Chapter 11. The ECG may be equally normal in both conditions. A raised JVP and breathlessness *without* orthopnoea is more suggestive of pulmonary embolism. If ECG changes are present they may be confused with inferior infarction, but the presence of a S wave in lead I and no Q in AVF help to differentiate. Changes in III in inferior infarction are not accompanied by the T wave changes in right chest leads that may be seen in pulmonary embolism.

It should be remembered that the circulatory failure of *endotoxic shock* can develop quite suddenly (see Chapter 3).

Admission to the CCU

An intravenous line, preferably with a long catheter, should be introduced as soon as the patient is comfortably placed in bed. A slow drip of 5% dextrose is started so that access to the venous system is available should complications develop. In general, patients should not be placed flat in bed even if the blood pressure is low. Unless shock or dysrhythmias occur he should be allowed to use the commode rather than be strictly confined to bed. The legs should be kept uncrossed and movement encouraged as this might reduce the risk of venous thrombosis.

Management

(1) Relief of pain

This is of the utmost importance and is probably the most neglected aspect of coronary care. Either morphine or heroin should be used in sufficient doses to relieve symptoms and repeated as necessary. Vomiting can be controlled with cyclizine. Synthetic drugs such as pethidine or pentazocine (Fortral) are not suitable for use in this context because of possible cardiovascular ill-effects (tachycardia, hypotension or rise in pulmonary arterial pressure).

(2) Relief of anxiety

This is almost as important. Opiates will help in this respect in the early stages when pain is a predominant feature. However adequate sedation is essential, Diazepam is the drug of choice, and large doses may be beneficial (Melsom *et al.*, 1976).

(3) Oxygen

Invariably given because hypoxaemia is a constant finding after myocardial infarction. The best mode of administration is by nasal cannulae, but it is not clear whether the outlook is in any way influenced.

(4) Diuretics

A small dose of a thiazide diuretic (e.g. Navidrex K) is nearly always justified because some degree of failure is common. But often the diuretic can be discontinued if heart size remains normal and X-rays confirm the absence of heart failure in the convalenscent stage.

(5) General mangement

In the absence of severe complications such as left ventricular failure or serious dysrhythmia bed rest is unnecessary after the pain has subsided, or after 2-3 days.

(6) Controversial drugs

(a) *Anticoagulants.* The controversy with regard to the use of anticoagulants has now somewhat settled in that it is generally accepted that the course of the infarct is not affected by their use. However the risks of thrombo-embolism are such that in many units heparin is given for 5-7 days in all cases. If Q waves are present, with transmural infarction and risk of mural thrombus, or prolonged immobilization has been necessary the case for anticoagulants is stronger. Routine anticoagulation is probably best avoided, but they should seriously be considered in the situations mentioned above (Ebert, 1972).

(b) *Firbinolytic therapy.* A series of studies have produced conflicting results. A controlled trial in the UK has shown no significant decrease in mortality by the administration of streptokinase for 24 hours to patients admitted to a CCU within a presumptive 12 hours of infarction. However the incidence of deep vein thrombosis and pulmonary embolus was reduced. There is probably no place for the routine use of fibrinolytic agents in myocardial infarction (Aber *et al.*, 1976.)

COMPLICATIONS OF MYOCARDIAL INFARCTION

Dysrhythmias

The incidence of dysrhythmia after acute myocardial infarction is high (90–95%), fortunately the majority do not produce haemodynamic consequences, but the principal function of the CCU is the early recognition and treatment of significant disturbances of rhythm (Lown *et al.*, 1969).

Bradycardia

Sinus bradycardia is very common in the early stages (first 3–4 h) of myocardial infarction especially with inferior lesions. A rate below 50 will often be associated with hypotension and there is an increased risk of ventricular dysrhythmias at this level. The mechanism of the bradycardia is either due to damage to the sino-atrial node or as a complication of increased vagal tone (in this respect control of pain is very important) (Webb *et al.*, 1972).

The indications for the treatment of sinus bradycardia are as follows:
(1) Heart rate less than 50
(2) Associated ventricular extrasystoles or atrio-ventricular junctional rhythm
(3) Clinical evidence of falling cardiac output.

Treatment

(1) *Atropine* is usually effective. 0.6 mg is given i.v. The injection should be given slowly. The dose can be repeated to a total of 2.0 mg. It should be remembered that there is a risk of inducing ventricular dysrhythmias when atropine is given for sinus bradycardia.

(2) *Isoprenaline* is potentially dangerous under these circumstances because there already is a risk of ventricular extrasystoles and the drug itself will increase this risk. The dose must, therefore, be carefully titrated and should not exceed 1–2 microgram/minute by slow infusion.

(3) *Pacing* should not be delayed if the above measures are unsuccessful.

Heart block. Heart block occurs in 5–10% of patients with myocardial infarction. Its significance depends on the site of the infarction. In *anterior* infarction the prognosis is poor; in *inferior* infarction the outlook is considerably better and pacing often not necessary. This difference in mortality is because the occurrence of complete heart block in anterior infarction implies an extensive area of muscle necrosis, whereas in an inferior lesion a much smaller infarct can have the same effect (Rotman *et al.*, 1972).

First degree heart block is common and does not usually progress. There are no haemodynamic consequences and no treatment is necessary.

Second degree heart block. Two types are observed and the significance depends on both the type of block and the site of infarction.

(a) Mobitz Type II where a fixed P-R interval is present but occasionally an atrial contraction is not followed by a ventricular contraction and so on the cardiogram a P wave is not followed by a QRS complex and a beat is dropped. This can occur in a 2:1, or 3:1 regular rhythm. Mobitz type II heart block is of significance because of a frequent progression to complete heart block and its association with anterior infarction.

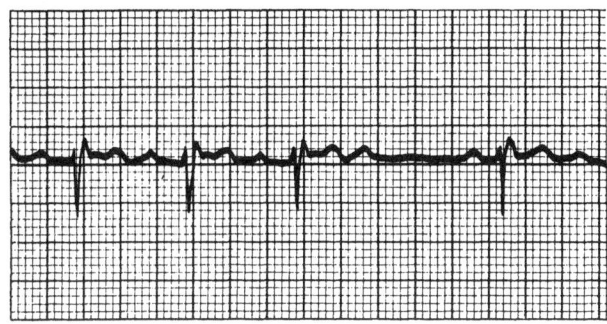

Fig. 9.2 ECG Mobitz type II.

(b)*Wenkebach phenomenon.* The P-R interval progressively lengthens until a beat is dropped, the next cycle commencing with a short P-R interval which again lengthens and the cycle is repeated. This is most often seen with inferior infarction and does not carry the same grave implications of Mobitz Type II with anterior infarction.

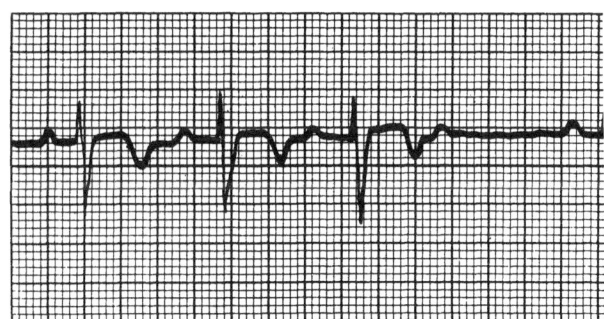

Fig. 9.3 ECG Wenkebach phenomenon.

Treatment

Pacing is mandatory in the presence of anterior infarction. In inferior lesions treatment with atropine or isoprenaline should be tried (as above)—but pacing will be indicated if there is evidence of haemodynamic disturbance.

Third degree heart block. In this condition the atria contract normally (regular P waves on the ECG) but the impulse is not conducted to the ventricles and ventricular contraction is initiated within the ventricular muscle, producing a slow (30–45 beats per minute) often bizarre QRS complex on the ECG. These slow escape rhythms are associated with serious clinical consequences—Stokes-Adams attacks, asystole and congestive cardiac failure.

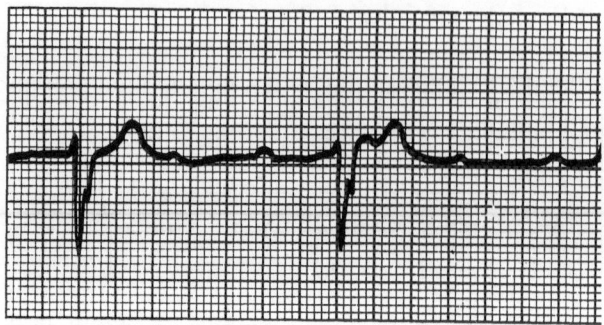

Fig. 9.4 ECG Complete heart block.

Treatment

As with second degree block the treatment and prognosis is related to the site of the infarct. Drug treatment may be effective in inferior lesions but hypotension, failure or asystole are indications for pacing wherever the lesion is. If there is any doubt it is usually wiser to pace than use drugs.

Tachycardia

Sinus tachycardia. This is very common after myocardial infarction. It may be aggravated by apprehension, so that relief of pain and anxiety is an important component of treatment. It should however be remembered that a persistent sinus tachycardia may be the first manifestation of a failing heart. The indiscriminate use of beta adrenergic blocking drugs in this situation can aggravate the situation. The drug of choice, if indicated by reason of failure or low output state, is digoxin.

Supraventricular tachycardia
   (i) *Atrial tachycardia*
   (ii) *Junctional tachycardia* (nodal)
These supraventricular tachycardias occur frequently, and interpretation of the cardiogram may be difficult. Often the QRS complex appears normal, and under these circumstances the supraventricular origin of the dysrhythmia is clear. However difficulty may occur if ventricular conduction is aberrant. If V_1 shows an RSR (i.e. RBBB type pattern) there is an approximate 85% chance of the tachycardia being supraventricular. Often atrial tachycardias imply pump

failure and are probably induced by atrial distension secondary to a rise in left ventricular end-diastolic pressure.

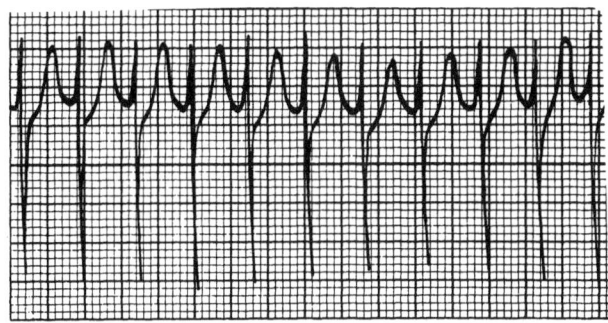

Fig. 9.5 Nodal tachycardia.

Treatment

(1) Carotid sinus pressure should always be tried, but caution is necessary because of the risk of inducing serious ventricular dysrhythmias, especially if the patient has been digitalized.

(2) DC shock will be indicated if the cardiac output is low and peripheral perfusion poor.

Drug therapy

(a) *Verapamil (Cordilox)* 5 mg i.v. repeated every 5 min to a total of 20 mg is usually effective.

(b) *Beta-adrenergic blocking agents.* Practolol (Eraldin) given i.v. in a dose of 5-20 mg. Not to be given in association with Verapamil.

(c) *Disopyramide (Rythmodan).* This drug is useful in the control of supraventricular dysrhythmias. The dose is between 300-800 mg daily, given orally in divided doses. To prevent recurrence, disopyramide should be continued in a dosage of 300 mg daily.

(d) *Digoxin* may sometimes be helpful. If the patient has not previously been on the drug, the dose schedule on page 127 is used. Digoxin and disopyramide can be given together. Many cardiologists would be opposed to the use of digoxin in these circumstances and advise that it should only be used if there is no response to disopyramide, beta blockers, or DC shock.

Ventricular tachycardia: ventricular extrasystoles. These important complications of myocardial infarction are described together as the methods of treatment are essentially similar. Moreover the presence of ventricular ectopic beats may be a warning of the development of ventricular tachycardia, or ventricular fibrillation.

Ventricular extrasystoles

The majority of patients after an infarct will develop some ventricular ectopics and often they are of no haemodynamic, clinical or prognostic significance. There is no need to try and suppress ectopics except under the following circumstances

(1) Over 10/min.

(2) Occur in pairs or runs (ventricular tachycardia).

(3) Are multiform (implying origin from different foci).

(4) Show the R on T phenomenon, i.e. the R wave of the ectopic impulse occurs near the peak of the T wave of the preceding beat.

(5) The patient has had preceding VT or VF.

Under these circumstances there is a considerable risk of ventricular tachycardia or fibrillation. However both VT and VF are not necessarily preceded by evidence of ventricular dysrhythmias.

Treatment

(1) *Lignocaine* is the treatment of choice (Mogensen, 1970). It is safe and effective without serious side effects. Occasional CNS depression and hypotension may be seen. The drug is given intravenously. 50–100 mg is given over 1–2 minutes; followed by an intravenous infusion at a rate of 1–4 mg/minute. An infusion pump is desirable but not essential.

An intramuscular injection is available. 200–300 mg is given into the deltoid muscle. Blood levels may be variable using this route which has its primary use as 'coronary first-aid' outside hospital.

Generally i.v. treatment is continued for 2–4 days and oral therapy (see below) continued for 3–6 weeks because of the risk of recurrence.

(2) *Other drugs*

(a) *Practolol*—i.v. doses of 5 mg to a total of 25 mg can be used if lignocaine is ineffective, either alone or in combination with lignocaine. *Propanolol* and *Metoprolol* can also be given intravenously, but should be avoided if cardiac failure is present.

(b) *Procainamide*—25–50 mg per minute is given i.v. to a total of 1 g. Oral treatment is best achieved with the longer acting durule form of the drug, 3–4.5 g daily. Prolonged exposure to this drug may produce agranulocytosis and an LE type syndrome (Koch-Weser *et al.*, 1969).

(c) *Mexiletine*—this drug has anticonvulsant properties and CNS side effects may be troublesome, including drowsiness, dysarthria and ataxia. It has the advantage of being available both in an oral and intravenous preparation (Talbot *et al.*, 1975).

i.v. dose schedule

(a) 100–250 mg over 10 min.

(b) followed by 250 mg in 1 h.

(c) 250 mg in the next 2 h.

(d) followed by an infusion rate of 1 mg/min.

Oral therapy

(i) rapid blood levels can be achieved by giving a loading dose orally of 400 mg with a slow (5-10 min) i.v. injection of 200 mg and continuing 200-250 mg tds or qds after 2 h.

(ii) A loading oral dose of 400-600 mg followed 2 hours later by 200-250 mg tds/qds orally.

Mexiletine is a useful alternative to lignocaine and is free of the potentially serious side effects of procainamide. Careful administration is necessary to achieve therapeutic levels and avoid toxic side effects.

(d) *Phenytoin* in doses of 50 mg i.v. to a total of 300 mg.

(e) *Bretylium tosylate* i.m. 5 mg/kg (may cause severe hypotension). Bretylium should always be given slowly over 10 min (Romhilt *et al.*, 1972).

(f) *Disopyramide* 100 mg 6-hourly is useful oral therapy for prophylaxis of extrasystoles and can be used after i.v. lignocaine has been discontinued.

It should be noted that despite this formidable array of drugs, a course of i.v. lignocaine for 24-72 h during the acute phase of infarction is satisfactory treatment for the majority of patients. The temptation to indulge in polypharmacy for ectopic beats of no haemodynamic significance must be resisted.

Ventricular tachycardia

Ventricular tachycardia occurs when a run of extrasystoles occurs to produce a rate of over 100. The dysrhythmia is usually accompanied by hypotension and may precede ventricular fibrillation.

Treatment is essentially as for significant ventricular extrasystoles, but if a bolus of lignocaine and/or practolol is ineffective within a few minutes DC shock is necessary (50-300 J). If VT recurs acidosis or hypoxia should be suspected.

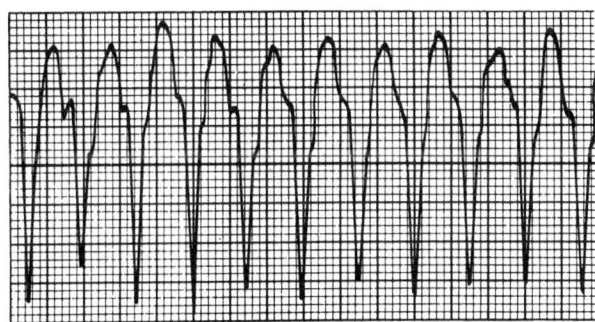

Fig. 9.6 ECG ventricular tachycardia.

(4) *Atrial flutter/fibrillation.* As with atrial tachycardia, atrial flutter or fibrillation is associated with failure and digitalization will almost always be indicated. It should be noted that atrial flutter does not respond to carotid sinus pressure.

However if the ventricular rate is less than 100 digitalization can be deferred. With very rapid ventricular rates and clinical evidence of low output DC shock (followed by digitalization) should not be delayed. Practolol can be used to control the ventricular rate, but this should always be used with caution because of the risk of inducing or aggravating cardiac failure. *Verapamil* has been suggested for use in refractory cases, but there is a considerable risk of asystole if this drug is used in conjunction with beta-adrenergic blocking agents.

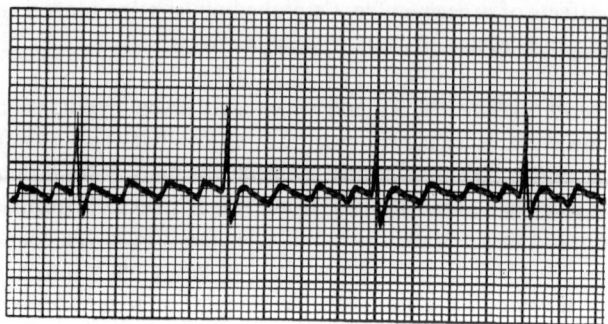

Fig. 9.7 ECG atrial flutter.

(5) *Conduction defects.* Bundle branch blocks are not uncommon as transient occurrences after infarction. If persistent, a progression to complete heart block may occur. A particularly dangerous finding is left axis deviation with right bundle branch block. This carries a very high risk of asystole and a pacing catheter should always be inserted.

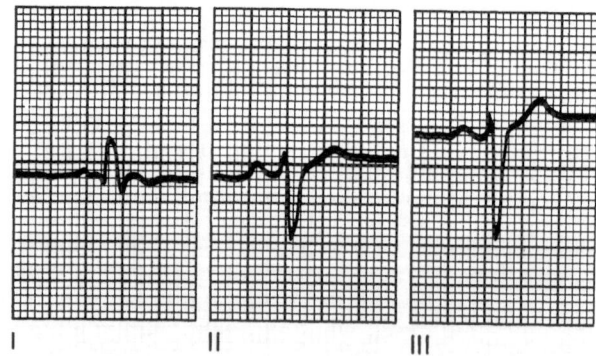

I   II   III

Fig. 9.8 ECG left axis deviation (LAD) with right bundle branch block (RBBB).

(6) *Ventricular fibrillation.* There may be no warning of this lethal condition, although often there are indicators of ventricular dysrhythmias with significant ventricular extrasystoles and ventricular tachycardia. Ventricular fibrillation can

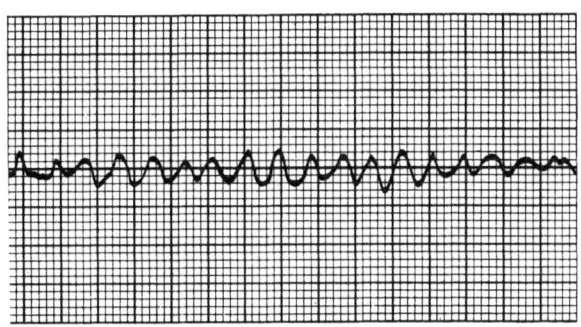

Fig. 9.9 ECG ventricular fibrillation (VF).

occur in any patient who has sustained an infarction and does not always occur in patients with extensive myocardial damage who already have a poor prognosis. There must be a straightforward procedure laid down so that there is minimum delay in instituting resuscitation.

Ventricular fibrillation causes cardiac arrest, and unless permanent cerebral damage is to ensue the circulation must be restored within 2–3 minutes. The longer cardiac standstill has been present the less likely effective restoration of the circulation.

When VF occurs in the CCU (or ITU) defibrillation should be commenced within seconds. However when it happens outside a unit with monitoring facilities there is inevitably some delay in recognition of the syndrome and as a defibrillator is unlikely to be at hand the procedure for cardiac arrest (see above) must be carried out until the resuscitation team arrives.

Technique

Note: The management of cardiac arrest is described on page 108

A defibrillator should be portable and preferably independent of the mains supply. However a short charging time is essential, to avoid delay, and the best models are powered by nickel-cadmium rechargeable batteries, and the machine is on permanent charge when not in use so that there is no possibility of the batteries being flat when needed. It must be the responsibility of one of the resuscitation team to check the defibrillators daily in order to avoid an un-serviceable machine being produced for the treatment of cardiac arrest. A very useful facility is the provision of a small oscilloscope on the defibrillator, the tracing being obtained from the electrode paddles. In this way, outside a monitored area, VF can be recognized instantly without the necessity (and delay) of attaching limb leads.

The paddles, liberally coated with electrode jelly, should be applied to the praecordial area and laterally to the left of the apex. It is important that the jelly should not be so liberally applied as to conduct the current across the skin, there must be a clear area between the paddles.

Defibrillation is potentially dangerous for the operator and onlookers. The procedure should be treated with respect and no-one must be touching the patient when the shock is applied. Again, indiscriminate use of electrode jelly must be avoided so that there is no possibility of the current being conducted to the operator's hands.

The usual current is 200–300 Joules, but higher currents may be necessary if there has been any delay, in particular if acidosis has developed.

Repeated shocks may be necessary if a normal QRS complex does not appear within a few seconds. If there is no return of both electrical and mechanical activity of the heart the full cardiac arrest procedure—airway attention, ventilation, external massage and treatment of acidosis must be continued.

Failure to defibrillate is most likely to occur when there has been a long delay producing acidosis and a large infarct has produced cardiogenic shock.

If the fibrillation pattern on the oscilloscope is fine i.v. adrenaline 10 ml of 1 : 10 000 may be given to coarsen the fibrillation, which may then be more responsive to electrical defibrillation.

Other drug therapy is likely to be disappointing, but lignocaine 100 mg, phenytoin 200 mg or bretylium 300 mg, given slowly, may be tried.

It is, of course, essential that while this electrical therapy is proceeding i.v. bicarbonate has been given, as described under cardiac arrest procedure.

At this stage 10 ml of 10% calcium chloride may occasionally help. If an electrical pattern is restored without mechanical activity the use of isoprenaline, as in the treatment of cardiogenic shock (see below) may be tried, but at this stage the chances of successful resuscitation are remote. External massage and ventilation should be continued until it is evident that further electrical or drug therapy is ineffective.

After successful resuscitation from VF a drug regime to prevent recurrence should be started, using lignocaine, procainamide or mexilitine as described on page 118.

(7) *Cardiac asystole.* Resuscitation from asystole is less likely to be successful than with VF, it usually implies massive cardiac damage. In some cases there will have been some warning and a cardiac pacemaker may be inserted. Transient asystole may respond to light blows on the praecordium. Emergency pacing is rarely practicable. Drug therapy is often ineffective.

(1) Calcium chloride 10 ml of 10% soln i.v. as a bolus
(2) Adrenaline 10–20 ml of 1 . 10 000 soln i.v.
(3) High dose isoprenaline infusion

External massage must, of course, be continued together with attention to the treatment of acidosis and hypoxia.

HEART FAILURE

Some degree of pulmonary venous congestion occurs in most cases of infarction and modest diurectic therapy is indicated. Several of the dysrhythmias described in the preceding section either imply failure or may themselves reduce cardiac

Table 9.1 Dysrhythmias after acute mycoardial infarction

Tachycardia			Bradycardia			Ventricular extrasystoles	Atrial fibrillation	Ventricular fibrillation
Sinus	Supraventricular	Ventricular	Sinus	A.V. block (2nd or 3rd degree)				
				Anterior infarction	Inferior infarction			
Relief of pain (Watch for failure) ↓ Digoxin and diuretics.	Carotid Sinus Pressure ↓ (Disopyramide Verapamil − β-blockers ↓ ? Digoxin ↓ D.C. shock	Lignocaine + − Practolol ↓ D.C. shock	Relief of pain Atropine Isoprenaline Pacing		Watch closely ↓ Atropine ↓ Isoprenaline	Lignocaine → Mexilitene → Disopyramide → Procainamide Beta-blockers Phenytoin Bretylium	Digoxin + − Practolol + D.C. shock if fast ventricular rate.	D.C. shock
				Mobitz Type II LAD + RBBB Complete Block → PACING		Maintenance Disopyramide Beta-blockers Procainamide Mexilitene		

efficiency. It should be remembered that beta-blocking drugs may also be implicated in depressing cardiac function.

Assessment of cardiac function depends upon observation of the JVP and serial X-rays of the chest. Obvious pulmonary oedema can readily be diagnosed clinically, but severe X-ray changes may be accompanied by dyspnoea and a minimum of physical findings, although a gallop rhythm will usually be audible.

If powerful diuretics such as frusemide are used careful watch on serum potassium levels must be maintained. Digoxin may be indicated if there is a supraventricular dysrhythmia, but should not be given routinely.

Acute deterioration of cardiac function may occur if structural abnormalities develop

(1) *Rupture of papillary muscle*—dysfunction of the papillary muscle producing a variable apical systolic murmur is frequent in the early stages, probably functional in origin rather than structural, and this normally improves as cardiac function improves. Rupture usually precipitates acute left ventricular failure and a loud apical pansystolic murmur appears. Surgical repair is the only effective treatment.

(2) *Acquired septal defect* occurs less frequently. Acute right and left heart failure develops with a loud pansystolic murmur at the left sternal edge. Surgery is again the only effective treatment.

Ventricular aneurysms occur in about 10–15% of patients but do not always produce haemodynamic consequences. However in some cases persistent dysrhythmias and refractory failure may be due to aneurysms. The diagnosis is suggested by ST elevation persisting after about 6 weeks, and clinically, by paradoxical pulsation in the anterior chest wall. The diagnosis is confirmed by angiography—routine screening of the heart can miss aneurysms, especially if the lesion is inferior. Aneurysms carry an increased risk of embolic problems.

Pericardial effusions are rarely large enough to embarrass cardiac function, unless the patient is on anticoagulants, when haemorrhage into the pericardium can occur. Pericarditis occurs commonly within a few days of an infarct. If it occurs later, in the convalescent phase it is usually due to Dresslers syndrome, when it is often accompanied by fever, leucocytosis, a raised ESR, arthralgia and occasionally pleurisy. This, probably auto-immune, condition responds to steroids, but often it is self-limiting and usually analgesics only are necessary.

Shock associated with myocardial infarction

When shock develops after myocardial infarction the prognosis is always extremely poor. However a potentially treatable cause should always be searched for. Some of the aetiological mechanisms are given in Table 9.2 with specific therapies that may be indicated.

Cardiogenic shock

Many patients are hypotensive, pale and sweaty after myocardial infarction. Cardiogenic shock is difficult to define and a decision to embark upon potentially

Table 9.2 Shock after myocardial infarction

Aetiology	Treatment
Primary pump failure – related to size of infarct	Treatment of cardiogenic shock Mechanical circulatory support
Dysrhythmias	Drug therapy Cardioversion Pacemaker

Mechanical complications
– acquired septal defect
    papillary muscle rupture
    ventricular aneurysms
	Surgery

Other cardio-pulmonary causes
– cardiac tamponade
    pulmonary embolism
    pneumothorax
    dissecting aneurysms
	As for the complication

dangerous treatment should rest upon objective observations. If hypotension and signs of poor peripheral perfusion do not improve following general measures as described above, of which relief of pain is most important, observations of urinary output and altered consciousness are important indicators of primary pump failure. These patients will usually have obvious clinical indications of pulmonary oedema due to left ventricular failure.

A decision to use vaso-active drugs or mechanical support for the circulation should be made after other treatable causes for shock have been excluded (see Table 9.2 above).

Cardiogenic shock is likely to occur if over 40% of the myocardium is infarcted. When considering this figure it should be remembered that muscle damage from previous infarction produces an additive total of non-functioning myocardium.

Pathophysiology

(1) *Central venous pressure* (mean right atrial pressure) is increased due to sympathetic activity. Under these circumstances a rise in CVP does not indicate an increase in total blood volume. It can be assumed that if the CVP is elevated the pulmonary artery wedge pressure will be at least the same or even higher, resulting in pulmonary congestion.

Rarely the CVP is low and a haemodynamic disturbance similar to hypovolaemic shock is present, which may require fluid and volume replacement measures, but this must only be attempted cautiously and with frequent monitoring of right atrial pressures. Indirect left atrial pressures can be measured using a Swan-Ganz catheter floated into the pulmonary artery (see Chapter 10).

(2) *Effects on left ventricular function*. Myocardial infarction principally involves the left ventricle and impaired contractions lead to a reduction in stroke

volume with an increase in end-diastolic pressure due to a larger diastolic volume. Because of this mean left atrial pressure is increased. Pulmonary congestion therefore invariably occurs.

(3) *Effects on coronary circulation.* Coronary artery perfusion diminishes as the cardiac output drops. If peripheral vasodilatation is induced in an attempt to improve tissue perfusion, coronary artery flow will further be diminished unless the cardiac output can be increased. If this is to be achieved by the use of inotropic agents it should be remembered that myocardial oxygen requirements may be increased.

The therapy of cardiogenic shock depends on an appreciation of the effects of extensive infarction on cardiac function. If logical therapy is to be applied haemodynamic monitoring is necessary. Generally a central venous line giving mean right atrial pressure is practicable, and this measurement can be supplemented with a pulmonary artery wedge pressure if the Swan-Ganz catheter is available.

Treatment of cardiogenic shock

Table 9.3 Treatment of cardiogenic shock

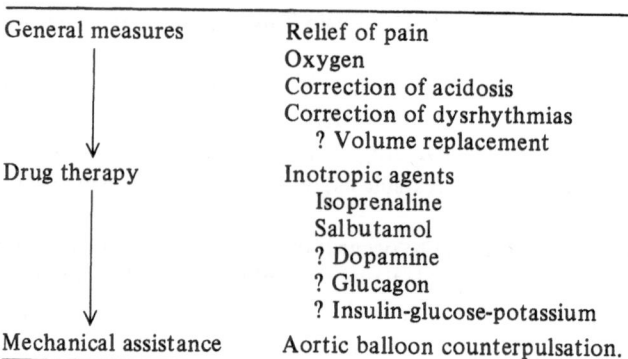

General measures	Relief of pain
	Oxygen
	Correction of acidosis
	Correction of dysrhythmias
	? Volume replacement
Drug therapy	Inotropic agents
	Isoprenaline
	Salbutamol
	? Dopamine
	? Glucagon
	? Insulin-glucose-potassium
Mechanical assistance	Aortic balloon counterpulsation.

General measures

(1) *Relief of pain* is of paramount importance. Diamorphine is the drug of choice. 5 mg is given by slow i.v. injection and a further 2.5 mg may be given if pain persists.

(2) *Oxygen* should be given by an effective delivery system. High flow rates are necessary.

(3) *Correction of acidosis.* Blood gas estimations should be carried out and appropriate bicarbonate therapy given (page 9).

(4) *Dysrhythmias* should be treated as described above.

(5) *Volume replacement* may cautiously be indicated if the CVP is low. This syndrome of hypovolaemic shock is due to venous pooling. The right atrial pressure is normal or reduced and the left atrial pressure is less than 15 mm Hg.

100 ml of 5% dextrose is infused rapidly and if there is no rise in the CVP repeat 100 ml boluses are given over 5-10 min.

This procedure must only be adopted if the CVP can be monitored or if a balloon catheter has been floated to the pulmonary artery to measure indirect left atrial pressure.

If the clinical condition deteriorates with falling blood pressure, oliguria and alterations in consciousness a decision to use vasoactive drugs may be necessary. In general, a urine flow falling to 0.3 ml/min indicates both a very grave prognosis and the need for inotropic agents.

(A) *Drug therapy.* Drug therapy of cardiogenic shock is fraught with great dangers. Inappropriate therapy may further damage already compromised myocardial function by increasing myocardial oxygen requirements, inducing tachydysrhythmias or diverting blood from the coronary arteries. No ideal drug exists which increases cardiac output, raises blood pressure and improves tissue perfusion without risks (Shubin and Weil, 1970).

(1) *Isoprenaline* is a pure beta-receptor stimulator. It therefore has a positive inotropic effect. Its peripheral vasodilatory action is achieved without a fall in blood pressure. However myocardial oxygen requirements are increased and a considerable increase in heart rate may occur. Isoprenaline is however the drug most commonly used in cardiogenic shock.

Dose. Isoprenaline is given by slow intravenous infusion, preferably using an infusion pump. The initial dose is 1 pg/min and this can cautiously be increased to 5 pg/min if necessary. The infusion should be prepared with 5 mg isoprenaline in 500 ml dextrose 5%. Careful monitoring of heart rate and rhythm must be continued while isoprenaline is being infused and the drip stopped or slowed if tachycardia or dysrhythmias occur. The infusion should always be freshly prepared. If no clinical improvement occurs continuation of isoprenaline may increase the size of an infarct. If the blood pressure falls during isoprenaline infusion cautious volume replacement with low molecular weight dextran may be indicated. Isoprenaline should be given into a large vein as extravasation from an inadequate superficial vein may cause severe tissue necrosis.

(2) *Digoxin* increases cardiac output, reduces end-diastolic left ventricular pressure, and slows the heart. However its pharmacological activity in the acutely infarcted heart is less predictable. Little or no effect on cardiac output is seen when more than 25% of the myocardium has been destroyed. Supraventricular tachycardias may be an indication for its use. Caution is necessary if ventricular dysrhythmias are present (these are common in cardiogenic shock) and it should be remembered that serum potassium levels must always be monitored as hypokalaemia increases the risk of digoxin toxicity. Before administering intravenous digoxin it is essential to check that the patient is not already receiving the drug.

Dose. Digoxin is given intravenously. Intravenous digitalization can best be achieved by a slow infusion: 1.5 mg in 2 hours, the first 0.5 mg dose in 30 minutes. The drug is diluted in 5% dextrose and given through a drip.

In general digoxin is not indicated in acute cardiogenic shock.

(3) *Glucagon* has a positive inotropic effect on the heart, but its clinical effects have been disappointing.

Dose. It has a short action and must be given intravenously. 2–4 mg is given intravenously over 2–3 min and repeated hourly if improvement occurs. Blood glucose levels must be monitored and a fall in serum potassium may occur if the glucose rises, this could be dangerous if the patient is digitalized (Luoff and Witchen, 1972). Vomiting is a common side effect.

(4) *Dopamine* is a biochemical precursor of noradrenaline. It has similar actions to isoprenaline but it is claimed that there is less increase in oxygen demand and a considerably reduced risk of dysrhythmias. It is too early to assess its use in cardiogenic shock but preliminary reports are encouraging. This agent should not be used in the presence of uncorrected tachydysrhythmias or ventricular fibrillation. Infusion should be into a large vein to reduce the risk of tissue necrosis from extravasation. (If extravasation occurs the area should be infiltrated with 10–15 ml of saline containing 5–10 mg of phentolamine (Holyer *et al.*, 1973).)

Dosage and administration. Dopamine must not be added to bicarbonate or other alkaline solution, as it is inactivated in alkaline solutions. Suitable dilution is with normal saline or 5% dextrose. 200 mg dopamine diluted in 500 ml gives a concentration of 400 μg/ml. The initial infusion rate should be 2 μg/kg/min. This can be increased slowly to 50 μg/kg/min, but at this level very careful monitoring of urine flow is necessary, and if urine output falls, even in the presence of hypotension, the dose of dopamine should be reduced. Increments in the dose administered will depend on monitoring of systemic blood pressure, urine flow and pulmonary wedge pressure, if available.

(5) *Salbutamol*, a beta$_2$-specific adrenergic agonist has recently been used in the treatment of cardiogenic shock (Timmis *et al.*, 1981). Its effects are peripheral rather than central, by reduction of systemic vascular resistance, cardiac output improves, with much less risk of increasing myocardial oxygen consumption than dopamine. The dose used in this study was 10–40 μg/min.

(6) *Glucose-Insulin-Potassium mixture* has been claimed to increase efficiency of the failing heart without depleting myocardial energy reserves. A beneficial effect on dysrhythmias is also claimed. The rationale for this treatment is as follows. Normally the myocardium is dependent on aerobic metabolism, but at the cellular level, after infarction, metabolism is anaerobic and glucose is necessary as a ready energy source. However insulin suppression is part of the sympathetic activity that occurs in cardiogenic shock, and glucose can only get to the cells in the presence of adequate levels of insulin (Majid *et al.*, 1972).

Dose. 1 litre 50% glucose + 60 units Soluble Insulin, or 1 litre 18% glucose +

40 units Soluble Insulin, or 1 litre 10% glucose + 20 units Soluble Insulin. The amount of KCl per litre will depend on the serum potassium level

$$> 5.6 \text{ mmol/l} \quad -\text{none}$$
$$5.0\text{-}5.6 \text{ mmol/l} - 20 \text{ mmol/l}$$
$$4\text{-}5 \text{ mmol/l} \quad -40 \text{ mmol/l}$$
$$< 4 \text{ mmol/l} \quad -60 \text{ mmol/l}$$

The infusion is given over 8 hours. Blood sugar levels should be monitored to remain between 120-150 mg%. The insulin can be increased by 5-10 units if these levels rise.

(7) *Steroids* have been enthusiastically advocated in cardiogenic shock (as in other forms of shock). Their possible actions are reviewed on page 27. No convincing evidence of therapeutic effect has been produced but in short term use, even in very high dosage, serious side effects are not likely to occur. They are, therefore, often used with hope rather than expectation of clinical improvement, with the knowledge that ill-effects should not result from short term use.

Dose. (As on page 28.)

(8) *Alpha-Blocking agents* are described on page 26. Their use in cardiogenic shock is not recommended. Peripheral tissue perfusion will be achieved at the price of reduced cardiac perfusion if the cardiac output remains static.

(B) *Mechanical circulatory support.* If the above measures have failed to improve cardiac infarction facilities are available in some centres for mechanical support. The condition of the patient will usually preclude transfer to a special unit.

Aortic balloon counter-pulsation depends upon the introduction of a balloon into the aorta which is deflated immediately before systole and then inflated during diastole. The circulation is thus artificially boosted and the work of the heart diminished.

The most useful application of this technique is to 'buy time' pending evaluation of possible surgical treatment of an acquired lesion. In primary cardiogenic shock the mortality rate remains extremely high (Michels *et al.*, 1980).

CONVALESCENCE AFTER MYOCARDIAL INFARCTION

Most patients are moved from the CCU to a general ward when their condition appears stable—usually after 3-4 days. There remains a risk of late dysrhythmias, notably ventricular fibrillation, and the nurses of the ward where post-infarction patients are kept should be fully trained in the techniques of cardiorespiratory resuscitation. The aim should be to have the patients fully ambulant by the time they are discharged home—usually about 10-12 days in uncomplicated cases. Patients who have survived major dysrhythmias should be retained under in-patient observation for a longer period, this should also apply to diabetics (Gilson *et al.*, 1976).

The psychological aspects of rehabilitation will not be discussed in detail. It should be remembered that the patients so often afflicted with myocardial infarction are young men, to whose morale the condition is a shattering blow. Although it would be a grave mistake to minimize the importance of a cardiac infarct, a reassuring positive attitude from medical and nursing staff is essential to prevent cardiac necrosis (Delipiani et al., 1976). The majority of patients who have sustained an infarct should be back at their normal work within 8-10 weeks.

REFERENCES

Aber, C., Bass, N., Berry, C., Cardon, P., Dobbs, R., Fox, K., Hamblin, J., Haydu, S., Howitt, G., Maciver, J., Portal, R., Raftery, E., Rousell, R. and Stock, J. (1976), Streptokinase in acute myocardial infarction: a controlled multicentre study in the United Kingdom. Brit. med. J., 2, 1100.

Delipiani, A. W., Cay, E. L., Philip, A. E., Vetter, N. J., Colling, W. A., Donaldson, R. J. and McCormack, P. (1976), Anxiety after a heart attack. Brit. Heart J., 38, 752.

Ebert, R. V. (1972), Use of anticoagulants in myocardial infarction. Circulation, 45, 903.

Gilson, A. D., Carson, P. H., Tucker, H. H., Phillips, R., Clarke, M. and Oakley, G. D. (1976), Course of patients discharged early after myocardial infarction. Brit. med. J., 1, 1555.

Hackett, T. P., Cassem, N. H. and Wishnie, H. A. (1968), The Coronary Care Unit. An appraisal of its psychologic hazards. New Eng. J. Med., 279, 1369.

Holyer, J., Karliner, J. S., O'Rourke, R., Pitt, W. and Ross, J. (1973), Effectiveness of Dopamine in patients with Cardiogenic Shock. Am. J. Cardiol., 32, 79.

Koch-Weser, J., Kelin, S., Foo-Canto, L., Kaster, G. A. and De Sanctis, R. (1969), Anti-arrythmic prophylaxis with procainamide in acute myocardial infarction. New Eng. J. Med., 281, 1253.

Kouwenhoven, W. B. et al. (1960), Closed chest cardiac massage. J.A.M.A., 173, 1-64.

Lown, B., Klein, M. D. and Hershberg, P. I. (1969), Coronary and pre-coronary care. Am. J. Medicine, 46, 705.

Lvoff, R. and Witchen, D. E. L. (1972). Glucagon in heart failure and cardiogenic shock. Circulation, 45, 1972.

Majid, P., Sharma, B., Meeran, M. and Taylor, S. (1972), Insulin and glucose in the treatment of heart failure. Lancet, ii, 937.

Mather, H. G., Morgan, D. C., Pearson, N. G., Read, K. L., Shaw, D. B., Steed, G. R., Thorne, M. G., Laurence, C. J. and Riley, I. S. (1976). Myocardial infarction: a comparison between home and hospital care for patients. Brit. med. J., 1, 925.

Melsom, M., Andreassen, P., Melsom, H., Hansen, T., Grendahl, H. and Hillestad, L. (1976), Diazepam in acute myocardial infarction. Brit. Heart J., 38, 804.

Michels, R., Haalebos, M., Kint, P. (1980), Intra-aortic balloon pumping in myocardial infarction and unstable angina. Europ. Heart J., 1, 31.

Mogensen, L. (1970), Ventricular Tachyarrhythmias and lignocaine prophylaxis in acute myocardial infarction. Acta med. scand. Suppl., 513.

Romhilt, D. W., Bloomfield, S. S. and Lipicky, R. J. (1972), Evaluation of bretylium tosylate for the treatment of premature ventricular contractions. *Circulation*, **45**, 800.

Rotman, M., Wagner, G. S. and Wallace, A. G. (1972), Bradyarrhythmias in acute myocardial infarction. *Circulation*, **45**, 703.

Shubin, H. and Weil, M. H. (1970), Practical considerations in the management of shock complicating acute myocardial infarction. *Am. J. Cardiol.*, **26**, 603.

Sobel, B. E. and Shell, W. E. (1972), Serum enzyme determination in the diagnosis and assessment of myocardial infarction. *Circulation*, **45**, 903.

Talbot, R. G., Nimmo, J., Julian, D. G., Clark, R. A., Neilson, J. M. and Prescott, L. F. (1975), Treatment of ventricular arrhythmias with Mexiletine. *Lancet*, ii, 399.

Timmis, A. D., Fowler, M. B. and Chamberlain, D. A. (1981), Comparison of haemodynamic responses to dopamine and salbutamol in severe cardiogenic shock complicating acute myocardial infarction. *Brit. med. J.*, **282**, 7.

Webb, S. W., Adgey, A. A. and Pantridge, J. (1972), Autonomic disturbance at onset of acute myocardial infarction. *Brit. med. J.*, **3**, 89.

TEN

Monitoring of the cardiovascular system

OBJECTIVES

The main purpose of haemodynamic monitoring in intensive care is the maintenance of an optimal cardiac output and the detection of early signs of a fall allowing the rapid initiation of treatment to prevent or reverse such an event. The haemodynamic variables and cardiac output can be measured either directly or assessed indirectly by observing other signs. The decision as to which method is appropriate in any particular case will depend on the clinical state of the patient and the nature of the underlying disease. For example in the immediate post-operative phase after open heart surgery direct measurement of several variables is essential whereas in many other conditions not primarily affecting the cardiovascular system the indirect techniques are more appropriate.

HEART RATE

The heart rate may be continuously monitored from the electrocardiogram, the direct arterial pressure recording or an indirect pulse wave recording from a transducer placed over an accessible artery. When using the electrocardiogram it must be remembered that the electrical rate and the mechanical heart rate may differ, as for example, in rapid atrial fibrillation in which many electrical beats fail to result in opening of the aortic valve and there is therefore no left ventricular ejection.

An unexpected increase in cardiac rate is frequently an early sign of impending left ventricular failure which may be easily treated before overt pulmonary oedema develops.

ELECTROCARDIOGRAM

The principles of electrocardiographic monitoring are fundamentally the same as those applied to acute coronary care and are described in Chapter 9. Any of the dysrhythmias associated with myocardial infarction can occur in the intensive care unit and are treated in the same way. The importance of maintaining normal serum potassium levels is especially great in post-operative patients whose fluid balance, electrolyte balance and renal function are often deranged. Maintenance of normal serum potassium levels and close attention to acid/base balance will result in the incidence of dysrhythmias being minimized and will help also in the control of such dysrhythmias as do occur.

ARTERIAL BLOOD PRESSURE

Monitoring of the arterial pressure is essential in the management of all patients. In the absence of severe cardiac disease adequate pressure monitoring can be obtained in most patients by indirect measurement using a sphygmomanometer in the conventional way. This however is inaccurate and therefore not advisable in patients with a low cardiac output or shock. In such cases, and in all patients with primary cardiac disease likely to develop hypotension, direct arterial pressure monitoring is advisable. This is most easily and safely accomplished by percutaneous cannulation of the radial artery. Use of the brachial or femoral artery is also possible but carries a higher complication rate and is not recommended. Radial artery cannulation can be performed, with experience, even in the presence of profound hypotension and vasoconstriction.

Changes in arterial pressure are generally late signs of a change in cardiovascular dynamics. A serious fall in cardiac output may be masked in terms of its effects on arterial pressure by increasing vasoconstriction so that hypotension occurs only when a drastic reduction in cardiac output has already happened. When interpreting changes in arterial pressure therefore it is advisable to consider these in conjunction with changes in the heart rate, cardiac filling pressures and cardiac output.

The maintenance of arterial pressure should not be regarded as an end in itself. In patients with reduced cardiac output the arterial pressure can often be maintained by vasopressors but without any improvement in organ perfusion and often at the expense of a further reduction in cardiac output by increasing cardiac work (Franciosa *et al.*, 1974).

An unexpected rise in arterial pressure may be due to the inappropriate use of vasoconstricting drugs or the unopposed effect of the release of endogenous catecholamines. Control of such hypertension may be important to reduce the demands on the left ventricle and the possible development of arrhythmias due to catecholamine stimulation of the heart.

Occasionally, hypertension will be a reflection of an underlying increase in intracranial pressure.

CENTRAL VENOUS PRESSURE

Central venous pressure recording requires the placement of a cannula either in the right atrium, superior vena cava or internal jugular vein. The percutaneous approach to either the subclavian or internal jugular veins is recommended (Craig *et al.*, 1968). Great care must be taken to ensure that all connections are securely made because the risk of air embolism is very great should the catheter become disconnected from the flushing system. The subclavian vein can be approached from either above or below the clavicle. Care must be taken in angling the introducing needle to avoid puncturing the pleura and inducing a pneumothorax. Inadvertent puncture of the subclavian artery can also be avoided by maintaining close contact between the needle and the clavicle. Should arterial puncture occur the needle must be withdrawn. It is rare for

133

any harmful consequence to result other than the formation of a large haematoma.

When measuring the central venous pressure the zero reference point may be taken as either the mid-chest level or the sternal angle. The former is preferred as it is more easily located irrespective of the patient's posture. Having chosen the reference point, all subsequent measurements should utilize this same point to avoid confusion.

A rise in venous pressure particularly when coupled with a rise in heart rate and fall in cardiac output is a sign of right ventricular failure. When due to disease of the left side of the heart the rise in venous pressure may be a late sign since the left heart failure must be reflected through the pulmonary circulation in the form of right heart failure before the rise in venous pressure occurs.

A fall in central venous pressure associated with a rise in heart rate, fall in cardiac output and fall in arterial pressure reflects underhydration or inappropriate vasodilation, usually due to drug treatment, for example with opiates. This condition can be reversed by the infusion of fluid (preferably plasma or a synthetic substitute) until the central venous pressure is restored to normal.

LEFT ATRIAL PRESSURE

The direct measurement of left atrial pressure is only practicable in patients who have undergone cardiac surgery. A direct left atrial line may be left in position and brought through the chest wall. Subsequently the line may be removed by simple traction.

In other cases, assessment of the left atrial pressure is possible either by monitoring the pulmonary artery pressure or pulmonary arterial wedge pressure. In the absence of pulmonary vascular disease the diastolic pressure in the pulmonary artery is equal to the left atrial pressure. Measurement of pulmonary artery or wedge pressure can be obtained by use of balloon-tipped flow-directed catheters. These can be passed percutaneously into the subclavian vein and advanced about 15 cm into the right atrium. The balloon is then inflated and the catheter advanced smoothly while monitoring pressure. The inflation of the balloon ensures that the direction of blood flow carries the catheter through the right ventricle to the pulmonary artery, recognized by their characteristic pressure waveforms. When a wedge pressure is recorded the balloon is deflated and pulmonary artery pressure can then be measured. Further wedge recordings can be obtained by re-inflating the balloon.

Fluoroscopy is not required for catheter insertion but the final position must be checked by a penetrated chest X-ray. The balloon must never be left continuously inflated or pulmonary infarction will occur. Clumsy passage of the catheter through the heart may result in the formation of loops or knots. The catheter tip may tend to displace into small pulmonary artery branches with time. When the balloon is then inflated pressure on the catheter lumen occurs giving spuriously high readings of wedge pressure. This is avoided by slow inflation of the balloon, stopping as soon as a wedge pressure waveform is seen. The design of the balloon tip ensures that there is minimal disturbance of rhythm during passage through the right ventricle.

Measurement of left atrial pressure in this way has advantages over central venous pressure recording in that left ventricular failure is reflected more quickly in changes in left atrial pressure. The time lag between rise in left atrial and right atrial pressure is avoided. Particularly, when infusing fluid to correct hypovolaemia and raise a low venous pressure the risk of inducing pulmonary oedema before the central venous pressure has risen is averted.

In the interpretation of left atrial pressure recordings the same principles apply as for central venous pressure measurement.

It is essential to prevent thrombosis within the catheter. This is best achieved by the use of a continuous flushing device which enables simultaneous pressure measurement and flushing of the catheter at a very low flow rate. Commercially available systems provide a flow rate of between 2 and 4 ml/h of heparinized saline. Care of the catheter connection is again extremely important to avoid the possibility of disconnection and air embolism. With care of the catheter entry site and prevention of thrombosis pressure monitoring with this type of catheter can be maintained for several days.

TEMPERATURE MEASUREMENT

Indirect measurement of the systemic vascular resistance is obtained from measurement of skin temperature and its relation to central, or core, temperature. Skin temperature is measured with a transducer taped to one of the toes. Central temperature can be measured rectally. An increase in the temperature difference between core and skin indicates increasing vascular resistance and reduced peripheral perfusion. This may be an early sign of a fall in the cardiac output and is often followed by hypotension if the fall in output continues. Hypotension associated with a normal skin temperature is one of the few indications for the use of a vasopressor and often results from the excessive use of vasodilating drugs in patients with hypovolaemia or a fixed cardiac output.

URINE OUTPUT

In the absence of primary renal disease or the use of drugs directly affecting urine flow such as diuretics the rate of urine production is a function of cardiac output, systemic vascular resistance and local regulation of renal blood flow. Changes in urine flow reflect the interplay between these factors. In patients with a poor haemodynamic state or those in whom the haemodynamic state is expected to be labile accurate continuous monitoring of urine flow is essential and can only be reliably performed by bladder catheterization with continuous drainage into a measuring burette. Output should be measured at least hourly in such cases. Changes in the rate of urine production will generally closely reflect changes in skin temperature. However, under certain circumstances this is not the case, for example, when urine flow is being maintained by the use of potent diuretics or when drugs preferentially increasing renal blood flow are used.

In patients with shock a resumption of urine flow will occur as the cardiac output is restored to near normal levels unless acute tubular necrosis has resulted from a prolonged period of hypotension.

CARDIAC OUTPUT

Since a primary objective of monitoring of the cardiovascular system is the maintenance of a normal cardiac output it is clearly desirable that this should be measured directly when possible. However, accurate measurement of the output, particularly when it is low, is difficult and because of the reliability of the other methods of assessing the haemodynamic state such as urine output, skin temperature, arterial pressure and ventricular filling pressures direct measurement of the cardiac output is not required in most patients.

Two methods are potentially suitable for use in the intensive care unit. The direct Fick technique relies on the measurement of the oxygen content of mixed venous and arterial blood and calculation of the oxygen consumption from the oxygen difference between inspired and expired air. The cardiac output is calculated as oxygen uptake divided by arteriovenous oxygen difference. The mixed venous blood sample can be taken from the pulmonary artery if a flow-directed catheter has been placed or from the right atrium through a central venous pressure line although this is less reliable as a true mixed venous sample. The risk of bacteraemia due to the presence of central cannulae is increased if blood is either withdrawn or infused through them. The arterial sample can be obtained from the arterial pressure monitoring line with the same risks. Because of the need to collect expired air over a fixed period of time, and the requirement that ventilation during the collection period should be stable, this technique is not the most convenient for patients who are critically ill.

Indicator dilution techniques are more suitable. Dye dilution using indocyanine green has been largely superceded by thermal dilution which has the advantage of no recirculation of the indicator and an easily available reagent. Multiple measurements can be performed over a short period of time and cannulae already in place for other monitoring purposes can be used (Forrester *et al.*, 1972). In most cases, the thermal dilution technique is easily applied by using a balloon-tipped flow-directed catheter carrying an additional thermistor mounted close to the tip in the pulmonary artery and a side lumen at the level of the right atrium. Ice-cold dextrose (10 ml) is rapidly infused into the right atrium and the temperature change in the pulmonary artery recorded continuously by the thermistor. The resulting temperature curve is integrated either by manual planimetry or preferably electronically and the cardiac output calculated from the known volume of the injectate. Since the dextrose is rapidly warmed to body temperature on its passage through the circulation no recirculation occurs and further measurements may be made within a few seconds. This technique is accurate, reliable and reproducible.

INTERPRETATION OF HAEMODYNAMIC DATA

In patients with established derangement of the haemodynamic state various combinations of abnormal haemodynamic information will be available from the monitored sources. Some examples are shown in Table 10.1. It must be remembered that the early detection of impending deterioration in cardio-vascular function is important to prevent serious impairment. In these early phases many of the abnormal findings listed will not yet have become manifest. It cannot be assumed that the presence of only one or two abnormal findings excludes serious haemodynamic disturbance. It is at this stage that early treat-ment should be initiated to restore normality.

The common feature of the conditions listed in the table is a fall in cardiac output. This is reflected by a fall in skin temperature except when vasodilatation, due to drugs or certain types of shock such as that associated with septicaemia, occurs. The suggested lines of management differ considerably depending on the relative state of the ventricular filling pressures, arterial blood pressure, heart rate and urine output. Patients with a gross haemodynamic derangement cannot therefore be satisfactorily managed unless all of these variables are being monitored.

BLOOD VOLUME

Derangements of blood volume in the intensive care unit may result from bleed-ing, failure to ensure adequate hydration or excessive fluid administration. The overenthusiastic use of potent diuretics can result in serious hypovolaemia. Measurement of the circulating volume is rarely if ever necessary. Acute changes will be apparent by their effects on heart rate, arterial and venous pressures and cardiac output. Administration of excess fluid can result in severe pulmonary oedema particularly if oliguria is present. Diuretics administered at this stage may be ineffective and the pulmonary oedema extremely difficult to treat. Hydration of the patient should therefore be carried out whilst observing the effects of the increasing fluid load on the venous pressure and the cardiac output.

MYOCARDIAL OXYGEN SUPPLY AND DEMAND

The left ventricle depends on a critical balance between oxygen requirement and availability. Availability is governed by coronary blood flow which may be affected by coronary atherosclerosis. It is also largely determined by the level of the diastolic arterial pressure and the duration of diastole. Relatively little coronary flow occurs during systole because the high tension in the left ventricu-lar wall tends to obstruct flow in the intramyocardial branches of the coronary arteries. The major component of flow is diastolic. The oxygen requirement is governed by the heart rate, systolic left ventricular pressure and duration of systole (Sarnoff,*et al.*, 1958). Myocardial oxygen availability can be maximized by maintaining a high diastolic arterial pressure and avoiding tachycardia. At the same time, the oxygen requirement can be reduced by a controlled reduction in

Table 10.1 Sample findings showing various abnormal haemodynamic states

Skin temp.	Venous pressure	Arterial pressure	Urine flow	Heart rate	Cause	Action
Low	High	Normal	Low	Fast	Heart failure	Diuretic, vasodilator
Low	High	Low	Low	Fast	Cardiogenic shock	Inotropic drugs, diuretic, intra-aortic balloon pump
Low	Low	Low	Low	Fast	Hypovolaemia	Infuse fluid
Low	High	Low	Low	Slow	Dysrhythmia and heart failure	Pacing, inotropic and chronotropic drugs, diuretic
Normal	Low	Low	Low	Fast	Inappropriate vaso-dilatation	Infuse fluid, vasopressor, inotropic drug
Normal	High	Low	Low	Fast	Vasodilatation and heart failure	Diuretic, inotropic drugs

left ventricular systolic pressure, chiefly by preventing undue increases in systemic vascular resistance. Myocardial oxygen availability together with the oxygen availability to all other tissues will also be affected by changes in the oxygen-carrying capacity of the blood resulting from severe anaemia or disturbed acid/base state. Frequent estimation of blood gases is required in all patients with shock.

CLINICAL ASSESSMENT

Regular clinical examination of the patient is a vital aspect of monitoring of the cardiovascular system. Certain physical signs of cardiac dysfunction can confirm or precede abnormalities in haemodynamic measurements. A third heart sound or gallop rhythm indicate cardiac failure except in children or young adults in whom they may be normal findings. Reversed splitting of the second heart sound during spontaneous respiration is due to prolongation of left ventricular systole and results from left ventricular dysfunction. Fixed splitting of the second sound is a sign of fixed stroke volume due to biventricular failure except in patients with atrial septal defect.

The appearance of a late systolic or pansystolic murmur indicates mitral regurgitation (or less commonly tricuspid regurgitation) due to ventricular dilatation or rupture of the subvalve apparatus. In the former case the murmur ofen disappears after treatment of the underlying heart failure.

A pericardial rub may be a clue to the subsequent development of cardiac tamponade. This will be associated with a rise in venous pressure and arterial pulsus paradoxus. Severe airways obstruction can however also cause this abnormal arterial pulse variation.

In the absence of a central venous pressure line the jugular venous pulse can be used to estimate venous pressure. It is essential that the patient be able to sit up if this method is to be used. The presence of a large systolic wave in the jugular pulse indicates tricuspid regurgitation due to right ventricular dilatation. This need not be associated with a pansystolic murmur.

PATIENT CARE AFTER CARDIAC SURGERY

Following open heart surgery arterial blood pressure, venous pressure, skin and core temperature and urine output should be measured. In some units direct left atrial pressure measurement is used, particularly after mitral valve replacement. Measurement of the cardiac output is not routinely performed in most centres. The necessary monitoring lines will have been inserted at the time of induction of anaesthesia and the initial post-operative recordings should be made before the patient leaves the operating theatre.

Acid/base and potassium balance are particularly important in these patients and are liable to considerable fluctuation. Close control is required if dysrhythmias are to be avoided and the cardiac output maintained. If any difficulty has been experienced in discontinuing cardiopulmonary bypass the patient may be receiving inotropic support with intravenous dopamine, dobutamine, isoprenaline, noradrenaline, adrenaline or salbutamol. In exceptional cases more than one of these may be given simultaneously and, if an adequate cardiac output has not been restored, intra-aortic balloon counterpulsation may have been started.

Positive pressure ventilation is normally continued for several hours until the haemodynamic state is quite stable and the patient conscious and co-operative. If the cardiac output is low, or the patient was assessed pre-operatively as being at special risk, a more prolonged period of ventilation may be advisable.

The principles outlined in Table 10.1 are applied in the treatment of any haemodynamic disturbance. It is particularly important to ensure that adequate blood replacement is given and the output from drainage tubes accurately and frequently measured. Hypovolaemia is one of the commonest causes of a low cardiac output in the post-operative period.

A chest X-ray should be performed immediately on return to the intensive care unit and daily there after. Routine antibiotic cover is preferred by most cardiac surgeons. The precise schedule varies depending on the local experience of likely pathogens. The combination of a penicillinase-resistant penicillin and an aminoglycoside is commonly chosen.

THE CARDIAC PATIENT SUBMITTED TO SURGERY

Careful pre-operative assessment of patients with heart disease is essential before considering any surgical procedure and in patients with severe heart disease only essential surgery should be undertaken. In the presence of coronary artery disease periods of hypotension must be avoided. These can cause myocardial infarction. Hypoxia can similarly affect patients with ischaemic heart disease but can also be particularly dangerous in those with intracardiac shunts, in whom the consequent increase in pulmonary vascular resistance may cause reversal of the shunt with serious arterial desaturation. Patients with a history of heart failure require attention to fluid balance to avoid overhydration. Pulmonary oedema can be controlled by diuretics and positive pressure ventilation if excessive fluid replacement has been given.

Continuous electrocardiographic monitoring is advisable and mandatory if any previous rhythm disturbance has been noted. Care is required in managing patients with normal rhythm but the combination of right bundle branch block and extreme left or right axis deviation. These findings indicate bifascicular block affecting the left anterior or posterior divisions of the bundle of His respectively. There is conflicting evidence as to the risk of higher degrees of block developing during anaesthesia in these patients but caution is advised.

Patients with first degree atrioventricular block also require careful monitoring. Second degree or complete heart block, even in the absence of any previous symptoms or evidence of instability of rhythm, require the insertion of a temporary demand pacing system to cover the period of induction, surgery and the immediate post-operative phase. This will avoid the risk of Stokes–Adams attacks due either to asystole or ventricular tachyarrhythmias.

Many patients with cardiovascular disease receive long-term treatment with a variety of drugs such as diuretics, antihypertensives, beta-adrenergic blocking drugs and digitalis preparations. Patients with heart failure controlled by maintenance diuretic therapy may develop severe pulmonary oedema as a result of omitting a dose of diuretic while being fasted awaiting anaesthesia. This can be avoided by giving the diuretic by intramuscular injection at the normal time. Beta-adrenergic blocking drugs can cause problems of hypotension and masking of the tachycardia normally associated with hypovolaemia during surgery. However in patients with coronary disease there is thought to be an increased risk of myocardial infarction and unstable angina if beta-blocking drugs are withdrawn abruptly. If it is thought essential that such treatment be discontinued it should be done gradually over a period of weeks. It is likely that the patient's symptom level will deteriorate as a result and other drugs such as vasodilators should be given over this time to counter the effects of withdrawal.

NEW TECHNIQUES AND FUTURE TRENDS

The increasing interest in non-invasive investigation of the cardiovascular system is spilling over into the field of intensive care and can be expected to continue to do so. Two techniques which are currently being applied in some centres and are likely to become more widely available are echocardiography and nuclear methods.

(1) Echocardiography

Echocardiography enables visualization of the cardiac chambers, pericardial space and heart valves without trauma to the patients. A transducer emitting sound at a frequency of 2.25 MHz in pulses 1000 times a second is placed over the precordium and the resulting echoes from cardiac structures recorded in two-dimensional form. Changes in left ventricular function can be detected by serial measurement of the dimensions of the ventricular chamber at end-systole and end-diastole. Pericardial effusion is immediately apparent as an echo-free space outside the epicardium (Horowitz *et al.*, 1974). Certain deductions can be made about cardiac function from an analysis of valve movement. More detailed evaluation of left ventricular function can be made using computer analysis of the echocardiogram and can be particularly useful in conjunction with other non-invasive techniques such as apexcardiography.

Further evaluation of cardiac function is possible using the method of ultrasonic sector scanning in which the transducer rapidly and continuously scans through an arc of 90 degrees, thereby adding a third dimension to the resulting images. These can then be displayed as video pictures showing details of the movement of the various chambers and valves allowing examination of cardiac structure and function.

(2) Nuclear methods

Radioisotopes can be used to image the left ventricular wall, myocardial infarcts and ventricular cavities. Normal myocardium takes up [201]thallium in proportion to regional myocardial blood flow. Areas of active ischaemia and both fresh or old infarcts appear as defects on [201]thallium scintigrams (Bailey *et al.*, 1977). Areas of infarction preferentially take up [99m]technetium stannous pyrophosphate whilst normal myocardium does not. Imaging with this isotope therefore identifies areas of recent infarction as hot spots. Interpretation of pyrophosphate scans can be confusing because of the high avidity of bone for this radionuclide (Botvinick *et al.*, 1975).

Ventricular cavity size and regional wall motion can be assessed using either the first-pass technique or gated scanning. In the former [99m]technetium as pertechnetate is injected intravenously and the precordial activity continuously recorded from the time of injection for about two minutes. A computer analysis of the time/activity display permits measurement of the ejection fraction, defined as ventricular diastolic counts minus systolic counts divided by diastolic counts, and observation directly of wall motion. In the gated technique, [99m]technetium labelled to human serum albumin is injected and the counts collected in frames related to the electrocardiogram. Each cardiac cycle is divided into 16 to 32 frames. The counts obtained from about 350 beats are then summed, frame by frame, so as to produce an isotope 'angiogram' (Rigo *et al.*, 1974). Computation of ejection fraction and wall motion abnormalities are performed as before. These methods require a mobile gamma camera which can be brought to the patient's bedside and suitable computing facilities for storage and processing of the data.

REFERENCES

Bailey, I. K., Griffith, L. S. C., Rouleau, J., Strauss, H. W. and Pitt, B. (1977), Thallium-201 myocardial perfusion imaging at rest and during exercise. *Circulation*, **55**, 79–87.

Botvinick, E. H., Shames, D., Lappin, H., Tyberg, J. V., Townsend, R. and Parmley, W. W. (1975), Non-invasive quantitation of myocardial infarction with technetium-99m pyrophosphate. *Circulation*, **53**, 390–396.

Craig, R. G., Jones, R. A., Sproul, G. J. and Kinyon, G. E. (1968), The alternate methods of central venous system catheterization. *Am. Surg.*, **34**, 131–134.

Forrester, J. S., Ganz, W., Diamond, G., McHugh, T., Chonette, D. W. and Swan, H. J. C. (1972), Thermodilution cardiac output determination with a single flow-directed catheter. *Am. Heart J.*, **83**, 306–311.

Franciosa, J. A., Guiha, N. H., Limas, C. J., Paz, S. and Cohn, J. N. (1974), Arterial pressure as a determinant of left ventricular filling pressure after acute myocardial infarction. *Am. J. Cardiol.*, **34**, 506–512.

Horowitz, M. S., Schultz, C. S., Stinson, E. B., Harrison, D. C. and Popp, R. L. (1974), Sensitivity and specificity of echocardiographic diagnosis of pericardial effusion. *Circulation*, **50**, 239–247.

Rigo, P., Murray, M., Strauss, H. W., Taylor, D., Kelly, D., Weisfeldt, M. and

Pitt, B. (1974), Left ventricular function in acute myocardial infarction evaluated by gated scintigraphy. *Circulation*, **50**, 678–684.

Sarnoff, S. J., Braunwald, E., Welch, C. H., Jr., Case, R. B., Stainsby, W. N. and Macruz, R. (1958), Haemodynamic determination of oxygen consumption of the heart with special reference to the tension-time index. *J. Physiol.*, **192**, 148–156.

ELEVEN

Pulmonary embolism

Massive pulmonary embolism occurs when 50% of the pulmonary arterial circulation is occluded by thrombus. The origin of such emboli will usually be in the deep veins of the leg or pelvis, particularly in the ileo-femoral area. Many patients will have had no preceeding symptoms and the presence of distal venous thrombosis will have been unsuspected. Death from massive pulmonary embolism may occur within minutes and, of fatal cases, 50% die within 2 hours (Gerham, 1961; Turnier *et al.*, 1973). Such cases present with predominantly cardiac or neurological symptoms—the diagnosis must be made rapidly and treatment initiated within minutes. Treatment of massive pulmonary embolism may be considered as

    (1) immediate resuscitation measures

    (2) definitive therapy.

It is also appropriate to consider the prophylaxis of pulmonary embolism.

Diagnosis of massive pulmonary embolism

The features of massive pulmonary embolism are predominately due to cardiovascular dysfunction consequent upon acute obstruction of the right ventricular outflow (Miller and Sutton, 1970a).

    (1) Acute reduction of cardiac output

    (2) Acute right ventricular failure

    (3) Disturbance of pulmonary perfusion and ventilation.

SYMPTOMS AND SIGNS OF ACUTE MASSIVE PULMONARY EMBOLISM

(1) *Cerebral.* Loss of consciousness, confusion, agitation

(2) *Dyspnoea.* Hyperventilation and tachypnoea. It should be noted that patients with acute massive pulmonary embolism often prefer to lie flat and do *not* complain, therefore of orthopnoea. This is an important consideration in the differential diagnosis—patients with pulmonary venous hypertension due to, for example, left ventricular failure after a myocardial infarction prefer to sit upright.

(3) *Chest pain.* An anginal type of central chest pain may occur. This may

represent acute right ventricular ischaemia associated with diminished coronary perfusion.

The characteristic pleuritic pain (and hemoptysis) of minor pulmonary embolism (see below) does not occur commonly when massive occlusion of the pulmonary arteries occurs.

(4) *Tachycardia.* This is usually sinus in type. Dysrhythmias do not occur frequently unless there is pre-existing cardiac disease.

(5) *Acute right ventricular failure*
    (a) elevation of JVP
    (b) gallop rhythm at left sternal edge
    (c) normal second heart sound (unless pre-existing pulmonary hypertension).
The previously normal right ventricle cannot generate sufficient pressure to overcome the obstruction and therefore the physical signs of pulmonary hypertension are absent.

(6) *Signs of acute drop in cardiac output*
    (a) hypotension
    (b) small volume pulse with sharp upstroke
    (c) peripheral vasoconstriction.

(7) *Cyanosis*

Minor pulmonary embolism

No cardiac or haemodynamic complications usually occur when small thrombi lodge in the peripheral pulmonary arteries but 'minor' pulmonary emboli are of importance as 30% of patients who sustain massive pulmonary emboli have premonitory small emboli which may easily be overlooked or misdiagnosed as post-operative chest infections. Also, repeated small pulmonary emboli may eventually lead to irrecoverable chronic thromba embolic pulmonary hypertension. A 'minor' pulmonary embolism indicates the presence of peripheral venous thrombosis which may, later, be the cause of massive embolism.

Features of 'minor' pulmonary embolism

    (a) chest pain—classically pleuritic in nature
    (b) pleural friction rub with signs of consolidation or crepitations (abnormal signs in the lungs may be delayed for 24 h).
    (c) cough
    (d) hemoptysis.

Investigations

(1) *Chest X-ray.* A massive pulmonary embolism may not produce any gross radiographic changes, especially when the films are taken supine on critically ill

patients. The cardinal feature of the chest film is oligaemia of affected areas, i.e. there is a diminution of normal vascular markings. A fullness of hilar shadow is often seen. There may also be evidence of preceding minor emboli:

(a) Wedge-shaped, often indistinct peripheral shadows,

(b) Pleural fluid,

(c) Elevation of lobe of diaphragm.

However, these appearances are not to be expected invariably and their absence does not imply that no embolism has occurred (Kerr *et al.*, 1971).

(2) *ECG*. The ECG almost invariably show changes, but these are variable and may be quite transitory. Minor pulmonary emboli do not cause ECG abnormalities (Cutforth and Oram, 1958).

(3) *Blood gases*. The combination of low PO_2 with low PCO_2 is very suggestive of massive pulmonary embolism but can also occur in pulmonary oedema with hyperventilation (Oakley, 1970). A chest X-ray will usually demonstrate the presence of pulmonary oedema.

The above investigations are simple to carry out, give a rapid result and do not involve much movement of the patient. They are, therefore, suitable for critically ill patients. Further information on the pulmonary circulation can be obtained from lung scanning and pulmonary angiography, but these investigations are relatively slow to perform and although they are valuable aids to accurate diagnosis they should not be considered as routine first-line investigations.

(4) *Lung scan*. An area of low uptake on a lung scan (using labelled 1^{131} or ^{99m}Tc macro-aggregated human albumin) indicates an area of poor perfusion and therefore may be due to causes other than pulmonary embolism. But an area of low uptake in association with a normal chest X-ray is very suggestive of embolism. If it is considered justifiable to submit a patient with acute cardiovascular collapse to lung scanning, a normal uptake excludes massive pulmonary embolism. If a gamma camera is available a lung scan can be obtained in about 10 minutes; this is considerably faster than routine scintillation scanning. A combined ventilation perfusion scan will help to eliminate false positive results (Williams *et al.*, 1974).

(5) *Pulmonary angiography*. This technique provides the means of definitive diagnosis, and has the advantages that the haemodynamic consequences of massive pulmonary embolism can be studied while the cardiac catheters are *in situ*. However it is not without risk and the vasodilation effect of radio-opaque media may produce further hypotension in the patient who is already in a state of shock. It should not be carried out casually in the X-ray department but only in a fully equipped cardiac catheter laboratory (Miller and Sutton, 1970b). The haemodynamic findings may be summarized as follows

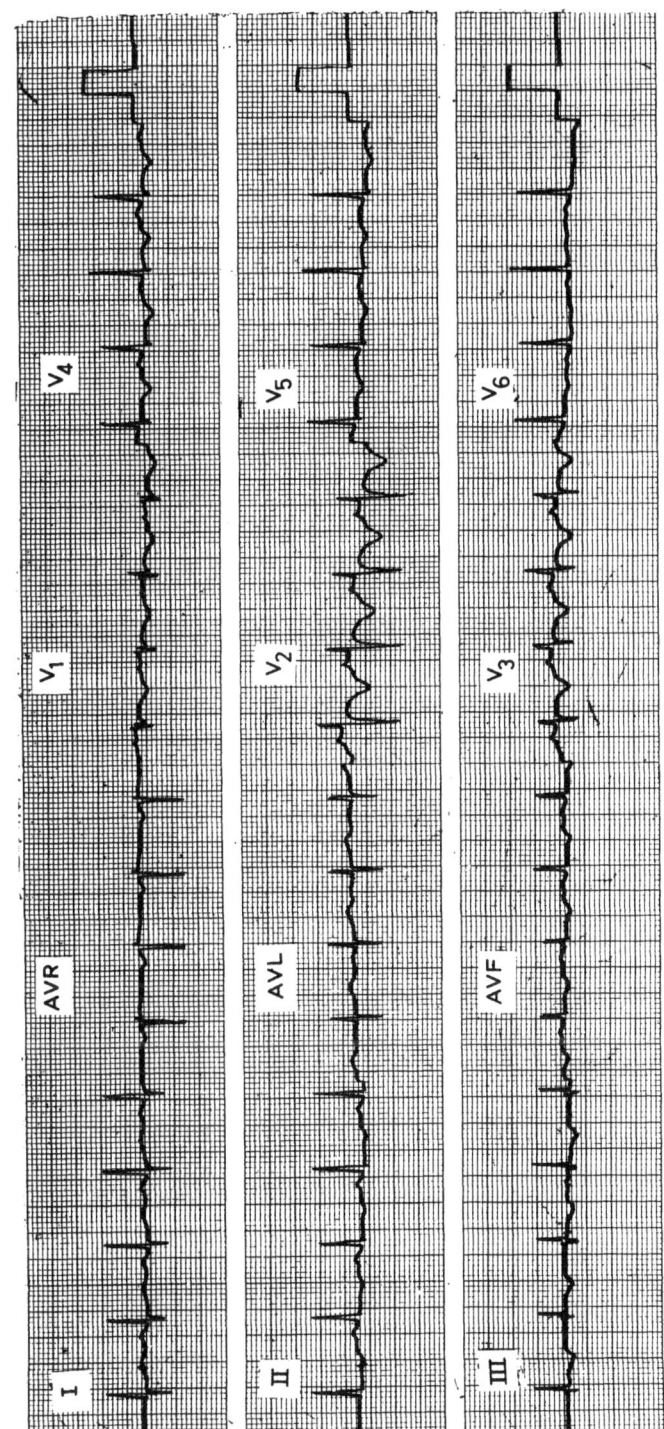

Fig. 11.1 ECG patterns (1) $S_1 Q_3 T_3$ pattern-S wave in lead I, Q wave in lead III with I wave inversion; (2) $S_1 Q_3 T_3$ with I wave inversion in V compare with ECG (1); (3) Right bundle branch block compare with ECG (2); (4) Left side changes with ST-T changes in V_{5-6}.

147

(1) moderate elevation of pulmonary artery systolic pressure (average 38 mmHg, range 26–57 mmHg)

(2) wide pulmonary arterio-venous oxygen difference

(3) lowered arterial PO_2

(4) elevation of right ventricular end-diastolic pressure with a commensurate rise in right atrial pressure ($\equiv$ RVF) (Miller and Sutton, 1970)

(6) *Enzyme changes.* The value of abnormalities in the serum enzymes (LDH. SGOT) in pulmonary embolism is not clear. It is unlikely that they will be of any value in the management of massive embolism.

Treatment

Table 11.1 Treatment of acute massive pulmonary embolism

Immediate	Definitive
External cardiac massage	Anticoagulants
Oxygen	Fibrinolytic therapy
i.v. Heparin	Surgery
Reversal of acidosis	

Immediate resuscitary measures

(1) *External cardiac massage.* Death occurs in massive pulmonary embolism because of a gross fall in stroke volume consequent upon a fall in venous return because of outflow obstruction of the right ventricle. The object of external massage is to propel the thrombus towards the periphery of the pulmonary artery where it will produce less haemodynamic disturbance.

(2) *Oxygen.* This must be administered via an efficient delivery system and many patients will require intubation and IPPV (see Chapters 5, 6).

(3) *Heparin.* It has been demonstrated that serotonin released from platelets involved in the thrombus may cause a broncho-constriction and a vaso-constriction effect. This observation may not be applicable in all cases, but the administration of 15 000 units of heparin i.v. will block this effect and cannot prejudice other more definitive therapeutic manoeuvres.

(4) *Reversal of acidosis.* With 100 ml 8.4% sodium bicarbonate.

Definite therapy

Anticoagulants

Anticoagulants have no thrombolytic activity and cannot influence the status of an existing pulmonary embolus or the deep vein thrombus that caused it.

However mortality is reduced with anticoagulant therapy. The beneficial effects of anticoagulant therapy may be due to the following factors

(1) inhibiting effect on serotonin release as discussed above. In order to achieve this on a longer term basis large doses of heparin have to be given, about 100 000 units/24 h; and with this dosage haemorrhagic complications are likely.

(2) prevention of extension of clot *in situ*

(3) prevention of further emboli from underlying DVT (Barritt and Jordan, 1970)

Fibrinolytic therapy

The prospect of drug therapy which will actually dissolve clots is immediately attractive. It has been shown that treatment with streptokinase is effective in lysing thrombus but evidence that mortality is improved is less well defined (Tibbutt *et al.*, 1974). The natural history of thrombus is for lysis to occur eventually, although full lysis may take several months. There seems no doubt that the haemodynamic consequences of pulmonary embolism can at least be improved by the use of thrombolytic agents and most clinicians now accept that this form of therapy is indicated in serious pulmonary embolism. The difficulty arises in deciding which patients need fibrinolytic agents and which require surgical treatment with embolectomy.

Treatment with fibrinolytic agents may also have a beneficial effect on the underlying deep vein thrombosis, although thrombus which has been present for some days is unlikely to be lysed. However free-floating ileo-femoral thrombus, which is so often the cause of severe pulmonary embolus, might be expected to respond favourably.

The two agents in general use are streptokinase and urokinase. Details of the hazards and contra-indications to fibrinolytic therapy are given below.

Surgical treatment

Pulmonary embolectomy, first described in 1907 (Trendelenberg, 1908) still carries a high mortality, even when carried out with cardio-pulmonary bypass. However if the patient has survived 2 hours and remains in a critical state, and it is evident that any improvement in the haemodynamics that could be expected with fibrinolytic agents is going to be too slow, pulmonary embolectomy must be considered. It should also be employed where the clinical situation is deteriorating despite the use of anticoagulant or fibrinolytic therapy. An angiographic score system has been suggested for selection of patients for embolectomy, but this requires the facilities of a full cardiac catheter laboratory (Tibbutt *et al.*, 1974; Miller *et al.*, 1971).

The mortality from embolectomy without bypass (where the clinical situation is too severe to allow bypass) even with modification of the original Trendelenberg procedure is 87%. With bypass mortality rates between 25% and 57% are reported. 100% mortality occurs if embolectomy is attempted with the wrong diagnosis (e.g. cardiac infarction) (Cross and Mowlem, 1967; Miller, 1972).

149

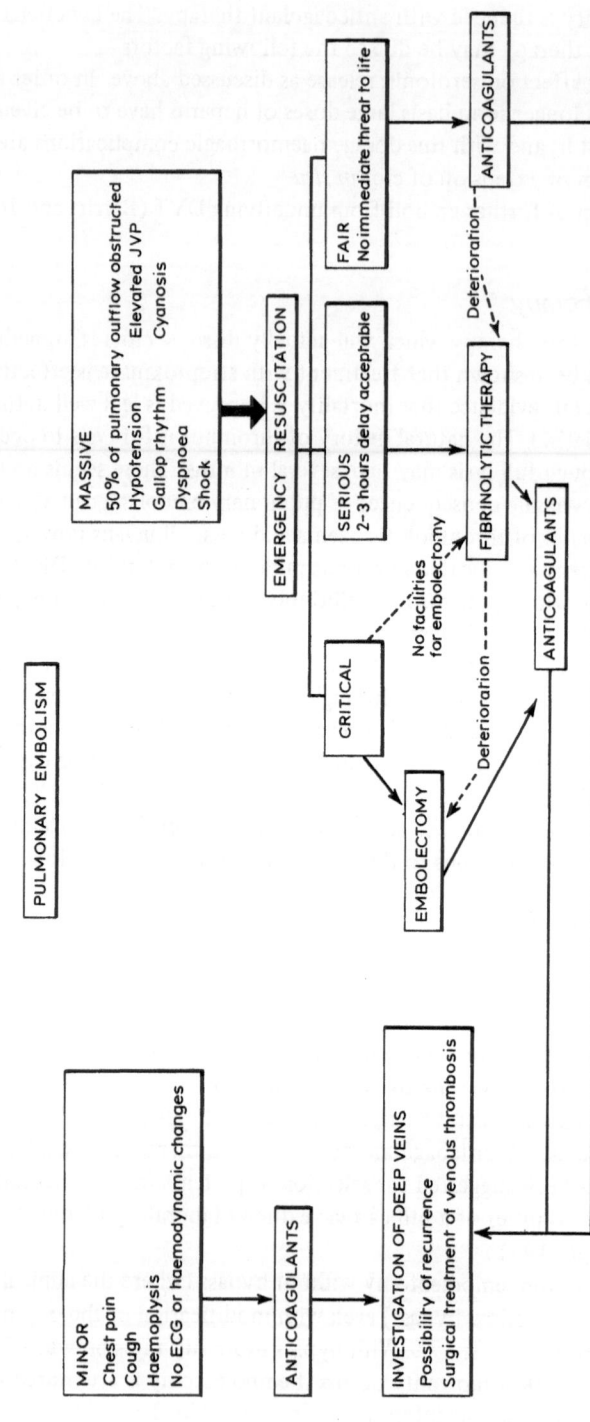

Fig. 11.2 A therapeutic approach to the management of pulmonary embolism.

150

The management of pulmonary embolism

The management of a patient will depend upon the clinical condition and the facilities available. A therapeutic approach is suggested in Fig. 11.2.

Anticoagulant therapy

Heparin 10 000 units 6 hourly, followed by Nicoumalone (Sinthrome) 8 mg on the first day; 6 mg on the second day and thereafter the dose is controlled by the prothrombin time.

If anticoagulation with heparin is to be followed by oral anticoagulants the first dose of Nicoumalone is given 24 h before the heparin is discontinued as its therapeutic effect is delayed for this period of time.

Fibrinolytic therapy

The principle of fibrinolytic therapy is to enhance the normal fibrinolytic process which occurs when plasminogen (present in tissue extracts and plasma) is converted into plasmin. This proteolytic enzyme converts fibrin into fibrin degradation products. The whole process of fibrinolysis is normally in equilibrium with the coagulation system (see Chapter 19). The conversion of plasminogen into plasmin can be accelerated by the intravascular administration of plasminogen activators of which streptokinase and urokinase are commercially available.

Dosage of streptokinase

250 000 units in 100 ml N/saline over 30 minutes.
100 000 units hourly maintenance (in 500 ml N/saline over 8 hours.
Continued for 36–48 h.

Control of streptokinase therapy. The main hazard of fibrinolytic therapy is haemorrhage. Although the dose schedule above will be effective and safe in the majority of patients (but see list of contra-indications below) laboratory control with thrombin clotting-time (TCT) should be done before the infusion is started, 6 hours later and then twice daily while therapy continues. The aim is to increase the TCT to 2-3 times the control time.

Complications.
(1) *Fever* is frequent but can usually be suppressed by intravenous hydrocortisone 100 mg.
(2) *Bleeding.* Haemorrhage may be minor or severe. If minor and from an easily accessible source such as a venepuncture site, pressure bandages and occasionally pressure with a swab soaked in epsikon amino-caproic acid (EACA) will usually control the situation and the infusion can be continued.
Major haemorrhage, often from the gastro-intestinal tract, is an indication for discontinuing fibrinolytic therapy. Fresh blood should be given if available, if not fresh frozen plasma or fibrinogen may be used. If these measures are not

effective the antifibrinolytic agent tranexamic acid can be given. But this should be avoided unless necessary because of the risk of re-thrombosis.

The dose of tranexamic acid (Cyklokapron) is 1.0 g by slow infusion over 6-8 hours.

Contra-indications to streptokinase

Absolute contra-indications
Active peptic ulcer
Haemorrhagic diathesis
Severe hypertension
Haemorrhagic retinopathy (hypertensive or diabetic)
Recent surgery or trauma (5-10 days)
Preceding streptokinase therapy within 3-6 months

Relative contra-indications
Elderly patients
History of asthma or other severe allergic disease
? long-standing atrial fibrillation

(3) *Transfer between anticoagulant and streptokinase.*
(a) If it is decided to undertake streptokinase treatment it will be necessary to reverse heparin first. This is done with protamine sulphate, given i.v. with a concentration of 10 mg/ml. 1 mg protamine will neutralize 110 units of heparin.
(b) Anticoagulant therapy will always follow the streptokinase infusion. Generally heparin can be commenced immediately; 7500 units in the first 12 hours followed by 10 000 units in the next 12 hours. The heparin infusion continues for 5-6 days and is followed by oral anticoagulants.

Aetiology of pulmonary embolism
Emphasis has been placed upon the emergency treatment of pulmonary embolism. It is now appropriate to discuss its aetiology and prophylaxis.

Pulmonary embolism is secondary to distal thrombosis in the venous system: 70-80% in the leg veins and 10-15% in the pelvic veins; a small number originate in the right side of the heart and are associated with dysrythmias, myocardial infarction, ventricular aneurysms, congenital heart disease and cardiomyopathies. Very often the venous thrombosis is unsuspected clinically and produces neither clinical signs nor symptoms. It is estimated that 30% of patients undergoing surgery or confined to bed in a Coronary Care Unit develop deep vein thrombosis. Many patients who develop acute massive pulmonary emboli have had premonitory small emboli. Predisposing factors towards venous thrombosis and therefore pulmonary embolism are shown in Table 11.2.

The diagnosis of deep vein thrombosis
(1) *Clinical.* The clinical physical signs of deep vein thrombosis are of little value

Table 11.2 *Predisposing factors towards venous thrombosis and pulmonary embolism*

Bed rest – lower limb venous stasis
Trauma – particularly fractures of the legs
Surgery – particularly pelvic and abdominal
Malignant disease (may be presenting symptom)
Treatment with oral contraceptives
Congestive cardiac failure
Obesity
Age and general immobility
Previous deep vein thrombosis
Pregnancy

in the diagnosis of the condition as up to 80% of patients do not demonstrate them (Browse, 1969). Moreover the classical signs of calf pain, tenderness and swelling may be present in patients in whom more sophisticated investigations show no venous thrombosis to be present. It is free-floating thrombus in the ileo-femoral area which carries the maximum risk of pulmonary embolism, and although this can be associated with calf pain, it is not invariably so and routine negative calf palpitation may well induce a false sense of security. It must be emphasized however that the acutely painful swollen leg that clinically indicates acute thrombophlebitis, whether deep or superficial, does carry a risk of pulmonary embolism.

(2) *Isotope examination.* ^{125}I-labelled fibrinogen is incorporated into thrombus as it is formed, and by use of a scanning technique a rise in count will indicate thrombus formation. The advantage of this technique is that it is simple and non-invasive, without risk. However it is ineffective for the diagnosis of ileo-femoral thrombosis because of high background count: it requires blocking of the thyroid first to prevent uptake of the isotope and it is of limited value in the detection of established thrombus as no fibrinogen is being incorporated at this stage. This technique permits very early diagnosis of subclinical calf thrombosis, but the correlation between this type of venous thrombosis and serious morbidity is not great (Kline *et al.*, 1975). It has been suggested that radio-active labelled streptokinase will help in the diagnosis of established thrombus (Kempi *et al.*, 1974).

(3) *Ultrasound.* By use of the Doppler effect when the calf is compressed manually a characteristic disturbance in blood flow can be obtained and this method correlates well with radiography and Isotope investigation. This method is rapid and does not require administration of diagnostic agents or blocking drugs. It is very useful as a screening method in patients who are particularly at risk. However it is not reliable in the detection of minor calf thrombosis or pelvic vein lesions. Partial occlusion of a major vein may be missed. A good

collateral circulation around an occlusion will produce a negative result (Evans and Cockett, 1969).

(4) *Radiology*. Demonstration of the leg and pelvic veins by the use of radio-opaque dye—ascending venography—is the only diagnostic method which provides full anatomical diagnosis of both location and nature of the thrombus. It is the latter observation that is of particular importance because, by this technique free-floating thrombus with only partial attachment to the vein, especially in the ileo-femoral area, can be demonstrated.

It is time-consuming and may be difficult, especially in patients with oedematous legs and is therefore unsuitable for routine screening, but it must be performed in all patients with suspected or proven pulmonary embolism when the clinical situation allows it (Lea-Thomas, 1971).

Prophylaxis of deep vein thrombosis

It has been estimated that 5% or more of hospital deaths are due to pulmonary embolism and of those dying 60% would have returned home to near normal life but for the fatal incident (Evans, 1970). As the majority of these deaths occur in patients who have no preceding symptoms in the legs or chest a programme of prophylaxis of deep vein thrombosis is essential.

There are two approaches to the problem:

(1) *Mechanical.* To prevent venous stasis, especially through the operation, various devices have been described to flex the foot—either by a mechanical foot mover or by electrical stimulation of the calf muscles. More recently pre-operative intermittent calf compression has been used successfully—reducing the incidence of post operative DVT by 82%. This technique appears to be particularly helpful in patients with malignant disease (Roberts and Cotton, 1975).

(2) *Chemical.* Many drugs have been used including aspirin, dextran 70, dipyridamole, hydroxychloroquine and heparin. Of these agents low-dose subcutaneous heparin (5000 units 2 hours before surgery, and 8 hourly afterwards for 7-10 days) appears to be most likely to provide effective prophylaxis. With this regime haemorrhagic complications are unusual. The role of dextran 70 remains uncertain, but some trials have demonstrated a satisfactory reduction in the incidence of pulmonary emboli (Carter and Eban, 1974; Kakkar, 1975; Kline *et al.*, 1975).

REFERENCES

Barritt, D. W. and Jordan, S. C. (1970), Anticoagulant Drugs in the treatment of pulmonary embolism: controlled trial. *Lancet*, i, 1309.

Browse, N. L. (1969), Deep Vein Thrombosis. *Brit. med. J.*, 4, 676.

Carter, A. E. and Eban, R. (1974), Prevention of Post-operative DVT in the legs by orally administered Hydroxychloroquine Sulphate. *Brit. med. J.*, 3, 94.

Cross, F. S. and Mowlem, A. (1967), A survey of the current status of pulmonary embolectomy for massive pulmonary embolism. *Circulation*, 35, Suppl 1, 86.

Cutforth, R. H. and Oram, S. (1958), The E.C.G. in pulmonary embolism. *Brit. Heart J.*, 20, 41.

Evans, D. S. (1970), The early diagnosis of deep vein thrombosis by ultrasound. *Brit. J. Surg.*, 57, 726.

Evans, D. S. and Cockett, F. B. (1969), Diagnosis of deep vein thrombosis with an ultrasonic Doppler technique. *Brit. med. J.*, 2, 802.

Gerham, L. W. (1961), A Study of Pulmonary Embolism. *Intern. Medicine*, 108, 8.

Kakkar, V. V. (1975), Prophylaxis of venous Thrombo-embolism. *Proc. Roy. Soc. Med.*, 68, 263.

Kempi, V., Van Der Linden, W. and Von Scheete, C. (1974), Diagnosis of deep vein thrombosis with 99 m Tc-streptokinase: a clinical comparison with Phlebography. *Brit. med. J.*, 4, 748.

Kerr, I. H., Simon, G. and Sutton, G. C. (1971), The value of the plain radiograph in acute massive pulmonary embolism. *Brit. J. Radiol.*, 44, 751.

Kline, A., Hughes, L. E., Campbell, H., Williams, A., Zlosnick, J. and Leach, K. J. (1975), Dextran 70 in Prophylaxis of Thromboembolic disease after surgery. *Brit. med. J.*, 2, 109.

Lea-Thomas, M. (1971), Radiology of Deep Vein Thrombosis. *Brit. J. Hosp. Med.*, 6, 735.

Miller, G. A. (1972), The diagnosis and management of massive pulmonary embolism. *Brit. J. Surg.*, 59, 837.

Miller, G. A. and Sutton, G. C. (1970a), Acute massive pulmonary embolism. Clinical and Haemodynamic findings in 23 patients studied by cardiac catheterisation and pulmonary angiography. *Brit. Heart J.*, 32, 518.

Miller, G. A. and Sutton, G. C. (1970b), Massive Pulmonary Embolism. *Brit. J. Hosp. Med.*, 3, 847.

Miller, G. A., Sutton, G. C., Kerr, I. H., Gibson, R. V. and Honey, M. (1971), Comparison of Streptokinase and Heparin in treatment of Isolated Acute Massive Pulmonary Embolism. *Brit. med. J.*, 2, 681.

Oakley, C. M. (1970), The diagnosis of pulmonary embolisms. *Brit. med. J.*, 2, 773.

Roberts, V. C. and Cotton, L. T. (1975), Blood flow and prophylaxis of deep vein thrombosis. *Proc. Roy. Soc. Med.*, 68, 262.

Tibbutt, D. A., Davies, J. A., Anderson, J. A., Fletcher, E. W., Hamill, J., Holt, J. M., Lea-Thomas, M., De J. Lee, G., Miller, G. A., Sharp, A. A. and Sutton, G. C. (1974). Comparison by controlled trial of Streptokinase and Heparin in Treatment of life-threatening Pulmonary Embolism. *Brit. med. J.*, i, 343.

Trendelenberg, F. (1908), Uber die operative behandlung der embolie der lungenarterie. *Arch. Klin. Chir.*, 86, 686.

Turnier, E., Kerth, W. J. and Gestrode, F. (1973), Massive Pulmonary Embolism. *Am. J. Surg.*, 125, 611.

Williams, O., Lyall, J., Vernon, M. and Croft, D. (1974), Ventilation Perfusion scanning for pulmonary emboli. *Brit. med. J.*, 1, 600.

TWELVE

Trauma

HEAD INJURIES

The Registrar General's Statistical Review for the year 1973 (1975) found that some 18 000 deaths in England and Wales were attributable to trauma. Between the ages of 15 and 29 years injuries accounted for 48% of all deaths and mortality was also significant in the young and the elderly. Head injuries are the cause of about 35% of all deaths due to trauma and the mortality is increased when there is associated chest injury (Campbell, 1977). The value of improved immediate care services remains unproven (Norman and Moles, 1977; Campbell, 1979), but improvements in ambulance services continue (Snook, 1977). On arrival in hospital about half the deaths occur in the first 24 hours (Hoffman, 1976) and it is in the Accident Centre and ITU that intensive treatment must be instituted.

The patient with a severe head injury is commonly admitted to the intensive care unit of a general hospital. This patient is usually unconscious and is likely to require support to the airway, continuous observation of vital signs, special investigations and skilled nursing management. Sometimes the decision has to be made that brain death has occurred so that life support systems can be discontinued. In other circumstances, head injury is only one facet of the management of the patient with multiple trauma. The clinical picture may vary from that of mild concussion to deep coma and the management must take into account the overall interests of the patient.

The effects of injury to the brain

Primary impact damage
Results from acceleration/deceleration forces applied to the skull contents. There may be contusions of the cortex both beneath the site of impact and contracoup while microscopic lesions may affect nerve fibres in the white matter, the long tracts, and the reticular formation.

Secondary damage
Results from haemorrhage and oedema. Intracerebral and subdural bleeding usually relates to the time of injury. Extradural haemorrhage is a complication

of fractured skull. Haematoma within the rigid skull gives rise to *increased intracranial pressure* and perhaps *brain shift*. *Infection* can also occur.

Skull fractures

These cause problems when segments of bone form a *depressed fracture* which requires elevation or when they are compound and therefore infection may be introduced. *Fractures of the base of the skull* may be associated with bleeding into the nasopharynx with the consequent danger of inhalation of clots. Fractures may also involve the nasal sinuses causing rhinorrhoea with danger of ascending infection.

Extradural haematoma

This is an important condition since the blood clot can often be evacuated via a burr hole with resulting dramatic improvement in the clinical condition of the patient. The classical clinical picture is one of a blow to the temple region with loss of consciousness; there is a stage of recovery before the patient again deteriorates with increasing drowsiness, dilatation of the pupil on the side of the lesion, hemiparesis of the contralateral side; the condition progresses until apnoea develops and the other pupil dilates and death occurs. This classical picture is, however, by no means always present (Jamieson and Yelland, 1968) and the classic lucid interval is only present in a minority of patients. Successful treatment depends on careful observation and accurate diagnosis so that surgery can be instituted to arrest the natural progression of the condition at an early stage.

Cerebral oedema

This is present whenever there is a significant head injury. It increases gradually, following trauma, to reach a maximum within the first week. It is associated with increased intracranial tension, increasing coma, and ultimately to fixed dilatation of the pupils and respiratory failure. Cerebral oedema does not of itself produce localizing signs. Steroids are commonly used to diminish its effect, for example dexamethasone 4 mg 4 to 6 hourly.

'Steal' and 'inverse steal'

Localized damage to the brain produces local tissue acidosis and maximal dilatation of blood vessels (Lassen, 1966). These vessels do not then respond to changes in arterial PCO_2 as do those in normal areas of the brain. The effect of a rise in $PaCO_2$ is therefore to cause vasodilation in unaffected regions of the brain and divert blood from the traumatized regions which have a *luxury perfusion*. The overall result is harmful because the damaged areas are denuded of blood supply while overall the intracranial pressure rises. Treatment by IPPV results in hypocapnia and the reverse situation develops. Intracranial pressure is reduced and blood is diverted to perfuse the traumatized brain substance. This is the theoretical basis by which IPPV may be of benefit in head injury. It also

157

ensures that the arterial blood is well-oxygenated, and also, because tracheal intubation is necessary, it ensures a clear airway and reduces body oxygen consumption as the work of the respiratory muscles is diminished.

Prevention of harm

Harm is caused as a result of hypoxia, hypercapnia, respiratory straining and coughing. All these are causes of a rise in intracranial pressure, which, in the presence of a pre-existing high level due to haemorrhage or oedema, may be critical. They are to be avoided by tracheal intubation and if necessary IPPV. Tracheal intubation may itself provoke some rise in intracranial pressure, particularly if suxamethonium is used to facilitate laryngoscopy, but this is short-lived and is preferable to allowing a continued state of partial obstruction over a long period. Blind nasal intubation may obviate the need for suxamethonium in suitable cases as may topical analgesia.

Patients may need general anaesthesia to allow carotid arteriography, the use of the CAT scanner, or for surgical exploration. It should be remembered that anaesthetic agents can themselves cause a rise in intracranial tension. The problems of anaesthesia have been reviewed by various authors (Hunter, 1975; McDowell, 1976; Greenbaum, 1976).

First aid management

The first priority is to secure the airway of the unconscious patient. The prone position with suction to clear the mouth and pharynx of blood and debris affords immediate protection, but passage of an orotracheal tube is preferable whenever the patients reflexes are sufficiently depressed to allow this to be done without trauma. The stomach should also be emptied using a wide-bore tube to prevent possible vomiting or regurgitation with subsequent soiling of the bronchial tree. When masseteric spasm prevents laryngoscopy for tracheal intubation the blind nasal technique should be considered or else the trachea intubated after the use of a muscle relaxant. Pre-oxygenation should be carried out prior to intubation. Care must be taken when the patient is turned or moved, and particularly when manoeuvres such as tracheal intubation are carried out, because fractures of the cervical spine may be present and manipulation might cause trauma to the spinal cord.

Once the trachea is intubated, an assessment should be made of respiratory function. Whenever there is doubt about the adequacy of gas exchange, respiration should be assisted or controlled using an oxygen rich mixture, until the neurological evaluation has been completed.

The next priority is to control haemorrhage and maintain an adequate circulation. Blood loss from scalp wounds (Illingworth and Jannett, 1965) and associated with other injuries can be considerable and may need to be replaced. An intravenous line should be set up and appropriate fluids infused.

Routine examination of the patient should then be carried out and basic observations commenced. These should include: level of consciousness, presence or absence of localizing signs on neurological examination, pupil size equality and reaction to light, systolic and diastolic arterial pressure, pulse rate, respiratory rate and pattern. Associated injuries should also be sought, for example fractured ribs and pneumothorax, intra-abdominal injuries, major bone fractures.

The *signs of rising intracranial pressure* must be observed if present. They include: deteriorating level of consciousness, bradycardia, rise of arterial blood pressure, dilating pupils which may become unequal and non-reacting to light, a change in the respiratory pattern leading eventually to apnoea.

Assessment of level of consciousness

A rough assessment can be made (Horton, 1975):

(1) Is the patient alert and orientated?
(2) Is the patient drowsy but rousable?
(3) Does he obey simple commands?
(4) Does he react to a painful stimulus?

A more sophisticated assessment can be made using the Glasgow Coma Scale (Teasdale and Jennett, 1974). Three separate scales are used:

(1) The stimulus required to induce eye opening
  (a) Spontaneous
  (b) Response to verbal command
  (c) Response to painful stimulation
  (d) No response
(2) Best Verbal Response
  (a) Orientated
  (b) Confused
  (c) Intelligible articulation used in exclamatory random way
  (d) Incomprehensive sounds (e.g. groaning)
  (e) No response
(3) Best motor response
  (a) Obeying commands
  (b) Localized response
  (c) Flexion responses
  (d) Extension responses
  (e) No response

The scoring system can be charted and observations made several times a day to indicate an improving or deteriorating clinical picture.

Eye signs

Examination of the size and reactivity of the pupils is an integral part of evaluation of the central nervous system function following head injury. *Unilateral dilatation of one pupil which does not react to light* suggests involvement of the third cranial nerve, the dilated pupil being on the same side as the lesion. Light shone in the eye gives rise to consensual constriction of the opposite pupil, distinguishing a third nerve lesion from an optic nerve injury.

Small pupils suggest hypothalamic involvement.

Deviation of the eyeballs may be seen towards the affected side in frontal lesions. When epileptic fits occur the eyes are usually deviated to the side opposite to the focus.

Hemiplegia and unilateral facial weakness are signs of supratentorial damage.

Respiratory pattern

Observation of the pattern of spontaneous respiration in the patient with a head injury is very important. Raised intracranial pressure may result in a depression of respiratory function so that breathing becomes shallow, irregular or of Cheyne-Stokes character. Apnoea may then supervene, and no drugs should be administered which depress the activity of the respiratory centre unless the administrator is prepared to proceed to IPPV.

Another abnormal respiratory sign is one of hyperventilation, often associated with extensor muscle spasms. This pattern may occur after brain stem injury. The prognosis is often good in the absence of localizing signs, but the oxygen consumption is increased by the muscle work involved while at the same time chest wall rigidity may interfere with respiratory movement. The overall result may well be arterial hypoxaemia and IPPV has been recommended (Hunter, 1975).

Fits

Epileptic seizures may occur in either localized or generalized form. The former may aid in diagnosis of the site of a lesion. If fits continue they represent a danger to the patient; the muscle effort increases oxygen consumption and hypoxia may develop as a result of masseter or laryngeal spasm. Muscle relaxants and IPPV prevent the harmful effects of muscle spasms.

Monitoring

Standard charts should be kept of systolic and diastolic arterial pressure, heart rate and respiratory rate. Neurological notes should be kept of changes in the level of consciousness and of the eye signs.

Monitoring of intracranial pressure is possible in units equipped for this. A catheter can be placed in one lateral ventricle though this introduces an infection hazard. A transducer can also be implanted in the extradural space (Turner and McDowall, 1976). Monitoring of intracranial pressure is available at present only in some neurosurgical centres, but its value seems clear as marked increases (above 40 mmHg) may indicate the need for further investigation and surgery. Also the beneficial effects of IPPV on intracranial tension can be demonstrated directly.

Radiology

Skull X-rays should be obtained in lateral, antero-posterior and Towne's view. The presence of a fracture may act as a guide to the site of an extradural haematoma. Depressed fractures may be seen. Fluid levels in the paranasal sinuses suggest base of skull fractures. The calcified pineal gland, if seen, may be a guide to possible intracranial shifts.

Further investigations may be required should the clinical picture deteriorate and localizing signs develop. A *brain scan* may suggest a localized lesion but more accurate information can be obtained by *carotid angiography* or the use of the *CAT scanner*. These often require general anaesthesia to ensure that the patient remains motionless for the duration of the investigation. The place for *echo-encephalography* remains doubtful (Klinger *et al.*, 1975). The electro-encephalogram has a place in patient care, though its place in the diagnosis of brain death is limited (see below).

Active treatment

Steroids

Steroids significantly diminish the degree of brain oedema in patients and experimental models. The response is, however, less apparent in the case of severe head injuries than in the presence of tumour. Dexamethone has become the most commonly used steroid in the treatment of cerebral oedema (French and Galichich, 1964). It is often prescribed in a dose of 4 mg 4 to 6 hourly, perhaps with an initial intravenous dose of 10 mg (Horton, 1975).

IPPV

Moderate hypocapnia (3.3 to 4.0 kPa) has been shown to reduce intracranial pressure (Lundberg *et al.*, 1959). It also produces a redistribution of blood within the brain, diverting blood to the damaged brain tissue. IPPV also reduces respiratory work and oxygen consumption, which may be considerably raised in the hyperventilating subject. The following indications for IPPV have been stated (Horton, 1975):

(1) Intracranial pressure above 30 mmHg without adequate response to other measures

(2) Presence of uncontrolled convulsions and decerebrate spasms

(3) PaO_2 below 10 kPa not responding to increase of FIO_2

(4) Hyperventilating patients with $PaCO_2$ below 3 kPa

When the patient does not accept the mechanical ventilator drugs may have to be used. Muscle relaxants (Horton, 1975) have the advantage that central neurological depression does not occur, but agents such as diazepam (Rossanda *et al.*, 1973) and phenoperidine have also been advocated. The $PaCO_2$ should not be allowed to become too low (below 3 kPa) in case tissue hypoxia should occur as a result of vasoconstriction. Monitoring of neurological status during IPPV may depend upon observations of arterial pressure, pupil reaction, pulse rate and direct intracranial pressure measurement. It is also possible to allow spontaneous respiration from time to time (Horton, 1976). There is evidence that treatment by hyperventilation does reduce mortality (Gordon, 1971).

Control of body temperature

Active hypothermia is not now thought to be desirable (Potter, 1967), and cooling measures are nowadays restricted to the use of fans with removal of coverings to prevent rises in body temperature.

Brain death

The brain is the most important organ which can suffer irreversible damage, tantamount to brain death, while other body systems continue to function with mechanical support. Since this state of affairs can continue for long periods of time to the distress of relatives and without benefit to the patient it has become important to define the criteria by which brain death may be diagnosed so that mechanical support can be withdrawn.

This subject has been considered in depth by the Conference of Medical Royal Colleges and their Faculties in the United Kingdom and this has resulted in publication of a statement summarizing current opinion (1976). The aim is to distinguish between patients who have a chance of even partial recovery and those who do not. The main factors may be summarized as follows:

(1) *Coma.* The patient must be deeply comatose and the drug history carefully reviewed to exclude any possibility of their continued action. Likewise primary hypothermia must be excluded as a cause of coma (temperature must be at least 35°C) as must metabolic and endocrine disturbances that can contribute to coma. There should be no profound disturbance of serum electrolytes, acid base balance or blood sugar concentration.

(2) *Apnoea.* Spontaneous respiration must have ceased, the implication being that the patient is maintained by artificial ventilation. It is clear that muscle relaxants and other drugs must be excluded as a cause of respiratory failure. No respiratory movements must occur when the $PaCO_2$ is allowed to rise to 6 kPa as measured by arterial sampling. In practice the patient is ventilated with 100% oxygen for 10 minutes, followed by 5% carbon dioxide in oxygen for 5 minutes. The ventilator is then disconnected for 10 minutes while oxygen is insufflated to the trachea at 6 l/min. This ensures that hypoxia does not occur while the test is being made. Even if facilities for blood gas measurement are not available this regime should ensure that the respiratory centre (if viable) receives sufficient stimulus to initiate respiration. Care in assessment is necessary, however, in patients with chronic respiratory disease who normally depend on hypoxic drive to stimulate respiration.

(3) *Brain-stem reflexes.* These must be absent. It is necessary to ensure that the following observations have been made.

162

(a) The pupils should be fixed in diameter and non-reacting to light stimuli.

(b) There should be no corneal reflex.

(c) The vestibulo-ocular reflexes must be absent. They are tested by slowly instilling 20 ml of ice cold water into each external auditory meatus in turn. Eye movements occur during or following this procedure if the reflex arc is intact. It is necessary to inspect the ear drum beforehand to ensure that the meatus is not blocked. Local trauma may interfere with performance of the test.

(d) There should be no motor responses to skin stimulation anywhere within the cranial nerve distribution.

(e) There must be no pharyngeal reflexes or responses to the stimulus of tracheal suction.

(4) *Repetition of testing.* It is usual to repeat the above tests after a suitable interval. No time can be fixed to this interval which will depend on a variety of factors, but it may be up to 24 hours.

(5) *Spinal reflexes.* It is accepted that spinal reflexes can be present even when brain death has occurred.

(6) *Confirmatory investigations.* It is now accepted that electroencephalography is not essential in the diagnosis of brain death, though it may be valuable at an earlier stage in patient care. Likewise there is no place for cerebral angiography or measurements of cerebral blood flow in the diagnosis of brain death.

(7) *Specialist opinions.* It is accepted that there is no need to request specialist opinions (e.g. neurologist) unless the primary diagnosis is in doubt.

(8) *Status of doctors concerned.* It is recommended that the diagnosis of brain death should be made by either;

(a) a consultant in charge of the case and one other doctor, or

(b) the consultant's deputy, who should have been registered for 5 years or more and who should have had adequate experience in the care of such cases, and one other doctor.

It should be emphasized that the diagnosis of brain death has no connection with transplant surgery, nor with euthanasia (Editorial, 1976). The decision should be made when the patent is dead, but respiration and circulation are maintained. There is no advantage, and every disadvantage, to continued therapy in these circumstances.

CHEST INJURIES

Trauma to the chest may result in injury to one or several intrathoracic organs. Many of these injuries will be managed best on an intensive care unit.

Patients with a recent severe chest injury will inevitably be in a state of shock which demands immediate treatment. This is likely to be due to loss of blood

163

and abnormal cardiorespiratory dynamics. The two immediate questions to be answered are: does the patient need a transfusion and has he respiratory distress? The management of shock has been described in Chapter 3. Respiratory distress must be evaluated. The breathing may be noisy due to obstruction of the airway and there may be a sucking wound. Tachypnoea may be due to chest wall pain or pneumothorax. The patient must be examined carefully and the cause for respiratory distress found. It should be remembered (Keen, 1974) that there may be no obvious external abnormality and a chest X-ray should be part of the assessment of any patient with multiple injuries.

Blunt trauma to the chest

Fractured ribs without damage to other structures seldom can pose serious problems especially in the elderly or bronchitic subject. The resultant pain may result in shallow respiration and an aversion to coughing. This can lead to retained secretions, atelectasis, bronchitis, bronchopneumonia and even lung abscess, especially in elderly patients and those with chronic respiratory disease. Adequate physiotherapy and pain relief should prevent these complications. 'Wet lung' syndrome which has been described (Burford and Burbanks, 1945) and investigated (Daniel and Cate, 1948) can be prevented by the use of analgesics which allow adequate coughing. Retained secretions which cannot be removed by such means will require tracheal suction and even bronchoscopy. Good pain relief can be obtained in selected cases by the establishment of an extradural block (Dittman *et al.*, 1978). It is claimed that not only does this allow expectoration and mobilization of the patient but it produces improvements in lung volumes. Of course the catheter must be placed in the extradural space at an appropriate level and small doses of analgesic solution used in order to avoid side effects such as hypotension. The technique is comparable to that used for pain relief in obstetrics by extradural catheter injections though the segmental level required to be blocked is rather higher. The thoracic approach is needed and due to the overlapping of the spinous processes in this region the direction of the needle has to be modified during insertion; in fact the mid-thoracic spaces are best avoided if possible. Pain relief can also be obtained by intercostal block of individual nerves but this is often less satisfactory except in simple fractures as a number of injections have to be given. The insertion of catheters in the paravertebral space has, however, been investigated recently; this allows repeated top ups and solution injected at one point will usually spread to involve several segmental levels (Eason and Wyatt, 1979).

Where the damage to the rib cage is more serious, and particularly when a flail segment is present, other measures must be taken. Mechanical ventilation of the lungs avoids paradoxical respiration and allows the chest wall to stabilize in an optimal position. It is the treatment of choice when paradoxical respiration is present, when there is contusion to the lung itself and when there are major associated injuries in other parts of the body. Mechanical ventilation carries a risk of pneumothorax and chest drains should usually be inserted on the side where the ribs are fractured. The flail chest problem is discussed on page 166.

Pneumothorax

Air in the pleural cavity nearly always originates from damaged lung. Occasionally it follows a penetrating injury through the chest wall, and rarely it results from rupture of the oesophagus or damage to a bronchus or the trachea.

When large, the diagnosis of pneumothorax is easily made on clinical grounds (see Chapter 8).

A small pneumothorax may not require drainage. A space 1 cm or less in depth between chest wall and lung can often be managed conservatively unless there is surgical emphysema in the tissues or unless IPPV is to be instituted.

The best and simplest site to insert the drain is in the mid-clavicular line at the 2nd intercostal space. The tube should be at least 6 mm in diameter and connected to a water seal drain. No suction is necessary provided X-ray shows full expansion of the lung. When negative pressure is applied the type of suction used is important. Three types are available: the small piston type, the larger type based on the vacuum cleaner principle and 'wall' suction which is connected to a central high-powered suction pump. The piston type works at a high suction pressure but can only remove small volumes and should never be used in the presence of an air leak. 'Wall' suction can remove large volumes but needs careful regulation as it tends to be too powerful. The vacuum cleaner type is best since it can remove a large volume due to air leak and is easily adjusted.

The chest drain may be removed once air bubbling has stopped provided the lung is fully expanded. A clamp may be placed on the tube for 24 hours before removal to make sure that the lung remains expanded without drainage.

When the lung fails to expand despite adequate suction, and furious bubbling occurs in the under water seal drainage bottle a diagnosis of ruptured bronchus may be entertained and bronchoscopy carried out to exclude this.

Haemothorax

Unless massive, a haemothorax may be difficult to diagnose clinically. Chest X-ray is mandatory if haemothorax is suspected. A film taken in the erect posture shows an obvious opacity, but when the patient is recumbent the blood may be distributed throughout the pleural cavity giving a ground glass appearance on the X-ray film. A fluid level may be seen when blood and air have escaped from a contused lung.

Blood replacement is indicated if shock is present. A drain should be inserted to remove the blood from the pleural cavity. Otherwise loculation may occur with difficulty in subsequent removal and in the long term fibrous reaction may result in the need for cortication. Removal of the blood allows measurement of the quantity, which if large may prevent expansion of the lung.

Needle aspiration of blood is unsatisfactory and carries a risk of the introduction of sepsis. The drainage tube should normally be inserted in the 8th intercostal space 10 cm from the vertebral column. This allows drainage from the lowest part of the pleural cavity. Use of a clear plastic tube allows inspection of the material leaving the chest. It should be connected to a water seal drain by tubing with walls thick enough to allow suction if necessary without the wall collapsing. Rubber tubing is advantageous in that it can be 'milked' if clots block the lumen. If pneumothorax is also present an apical drain should also be inserted. Should negative pressure be necessary it should be applied simultaneously to both drains.

Following insertion of the chest drain and removal of collected blood, subsequent measurements given an indication of continued blood loss, though false recordings can occur if the tubing becomes blocked with clot. Contused lung usually stops bleeding once it expands and continued haemorrhage suggests damage to an intercostal or pulmonary vessel. Loss of more than 200 ml per hour for more than 3 hours suggests the need for exploratory thoracotomy though massive haemorrhage may indicate this earlier.

Thoracotomy should be performed through a standard incision in the 6th space regardless of the site of the penetrating injury. This allows access to any intrathoracic organ as well as the site of perforation. Haemorrhage from the lung should be controlled, but only extensively damaged lobes should be removed.

Intrapleural haemorrhage provides one of the rare opportunities in surgery for autotransfusion. Such a technique may be life-saving occasionally. The simplest technique is to connect an intrapleural cannula directly to an ACD blood bag and milk the pleural contents into it. The contents of the bag can then be transfused into a vein, the clot being held back by the filter of the transfusion set. A bold early decision to heparinise the patient (20 000 units) prevents clot formation and facilitates autotransfusion.

Flail chest

The term is used to indicate fracture of the anterior and posterior ends of several ribs, producing a mobile segment of chest wall which is sucked in during inspiration and blows out during expiration. The result is, in effect, an increase in dead space which when more than 3 or 4 ribs are affected may exceed tidal volume. The patient compensates by taking deeper, laboured and more rapid respirations and this leads to greater movement of the flail segment. Hypoxia, hypercarbia and exhaustion are the end result though these factors may not be apparent clinically for some hours. There is often associated damage to the underlying lung and perhaps a haemo-pneumothorax. Flail segments can occur on both sides or may be central if the sternum is depressed and separated from its anchoring ribs.

Treatment is almost always necessary when flail chest has been diagnosed. As a first aid measure the flail segment may be supported manually or by rolling the patient onto the affected side, but a decision must be made regarding treatment policy.

Tracheal intubation and IPPV is the method favoured in most units. Paradoxical respiration is abolished and gas exchange in the lungs improved. Preoxygenation is an important procedure in association with tracheal intubation which is not without hazard in the hypoxic patient. Atropine may be administered in small doses to discourage salivary and bronchial secretions during instrumentation and reduce the possibility of reflex vagus effects on the heart. General anaesthesia should be used if the patients condition allows and when awake intubation is considered more stressful. An intercostal drain is also indicated because of the danger of pneumothorax.

Once initiated IPPV may have to be continued for several weeks before the flail segment becomes fixed. The ultimate position is likely to be good since with IPPV it fixes in the expiratory position, whereas with spontaneous respiration it may become fixed in the inspiratory position.

Another method of treatment in selected cases is the use of Rush nails to unite the fractures. This method is only applicable where the patients condition is relatively good and in the absence of associated injuries, since it involves surgical exploration under general anaesthesia.

Thoracic extradural block maintained by serial injections of local analgesic solution through an indwelling catheter has also been advocated (Dittman *et al.*, 1979). This relieves pain, allows coughing and expectoration and may improve lung volumes. It is a useful technique in selected patients without associated injuries.

Traumatic rupture of the diaphragm

This injury is produced by compression of the abdomen. The right diaphragm is protected by the liver and is ruptured less commonly than the left. Most lesions are radial in the long axis of muscle fibres. The edges of the hole may therefore trap and incarcerate any viscera that enter the chest. Commonly the stomach enters the chest, less often the small and large intestine. The injury is usually diagnosed from a chest X-ray which shows gas shadows in the chest. Occasionally the diagnosis is not made until obstruction occurs. The treatment is early operation through a standard thoracotomy incision in the 8th interspace. The viscera are reduced and the tear repaired with unabsorbable sutures.

Wounds of the heart

80% of patients with penetrating cardiac wounds do not survive long enough to reach hospital alive (Sugg *et al.*, 1968). In most patients who do blood pressure is likely to be unobtainable or at least below normal as a result of shock due to tamponade. This condition can be diagnosed readily by observation of a paradoxical pulse and recording the venous pressure which can reach very high levels, ranging from 12 to 60 cm H_2O in one series (Sugg *et al.*, 1968).

Chest X-ray may show an enlarged cardiac outline. Aspiration of blood from the pericardium confirms the diagnosis, but failure to do so does not exclude it. There may be technical problems with the tap and it may be that blood in the pericardium has clotted. Until the 1960's pericardiocentesis was the only treatment, with an associated mortality of 36 per cent, but the use of early exploration has reduced this to 14% (Sugg *et al.*, 1968). The approach should be through a median sternotomy, unless associated chest trauma indicates thoracotomy.

Injury to the great vessels

When a major vessel is lacerated survival until admission to hospital is unlikely. Occasionally, injury is manifest later as aneurysmal dilatation of a large vessel such as the aorta. Widening of the mediastinal shadow on serial chest X-rays gives rise to suspicion and special investigations such as injection of contrast medium may clinch the diagnosis. Operative measures will include the facility of cardiopulmonary bypass. (See also Keen, 1975.) For consideration of *Shock Lung* see Chapter 3.

FAT EMBOLISM

This important complication of trauma requires early diagnosis and prompt treatment. It is most commonly associated with fractures of the long bones of the legs, but has also been described with fractures of the pelvis. This group of patients are those who are particularly vulnerable to develop the full life-threatening syndrome, but fat emboli, particularly in the lungs, have been demonstrated histologically in many other conditions including burns, cardiac massage, liver injury, cardio-pulmonary bypass and pancreatitis. In traumatic cases, with a fatal outcome, the histological incidence has been claimed to be as high as 93% (Scully, 1956).

Clinical picture

The classical picture is that of petechial haemorrhages appearing in the skin, conjunctivae and fundi. This is associated with cerebral and pulmonary signs. Neurologically the picture is variable—coma with or without focal signs, epileptic fits or episodic confusion with restlessness. Respiratory symptoms are almost invariably present. Tachypnoea, hyperventilation, bronchospasm, cyanosis and severe blood gas abnormalities are associated with radiological changes varying from extensive bilateral consolidation to minor variants from normal. Generally the features of fat embolism appear within 48 hours of the injury.

However, the diagnosis must be made early, and it is very unwise to wait until petechiae appear—the pulmonary and cerebral changes may frequently antedate any cutaneous lesions, and these are by no means an invariable finding even in fatal cases. Beware, therefore, of patients with skeletal injuries who become confused or comatose—under these circumstances a chest X-ray and blood gas estimations will often be more valuable than either sedatives or neuro-radiology.

Blood gas changes in fat embolism

The cardinal finding is marked reduction in arterial oxygen tension, the $PaCO_2$ is, too, often reduced. The degree of hypoxia is often far in excess of that suspected clinically, and is not always accompanied by cyanosis. The overall picture is that of a severe disturbance of the ventilation/perfusion relationship.

Differential diagnosis

The problem of diagnosis is often complex, particularly with reference to the neurological picture because most of the cases will have been involved in major trauma, with its concomitant risks of head injury. The pulmonary events are unlikely to be confused with either chest infection or pulmonary emboli because of the time-relationship to the injury, i.e. fat embolism tends to occur early, rather sooner than would anticipate other pulmonary complications.

If there is any doubt about the neurological status appropriate investigations to exclude, e.g. subdural haematoma must be carried out. But, as has been suggested above, the respiratory component may well be revealed by chest X-ray and, particularly, blood gas estimations, at a time when *clinical* indications of lung problems are not present, or insignificant.

The picture of '*shock-lung*' is described in Chapter 3 page 40, and that syndrome is probably due to a combination of factors including micro-embolization by a variety of aggregates, including particles of fat and with diffuse intravascular coagulation as a very important component. Indeed, as might be expected, DIC has been indicted as an important part of the patho-physiology of the fat embolus syndrome (Saldeen, 1970).

Pathophysiology

There is no general agreement as to the source of the fat. The earlier mechanical theories, fat being displaced from the long bones and entering the circulation (Gaus, 1916), has been challenged by more recent observations suggesting that fat globules are formed in the blood stream, either by coalescence of serum triglycerides (Gurd, 1970) or as a result of lipolysis of depot fat, induced by catecholamines (O'Driscoll and Powell, 1967). The role of diffuse intravascular coagulation is mentioned above; it has been shown that experimentally, thrombo-plastin intravenously produces a histological picture in the lungs similar to that of fat embolisation. It seems clear that there are many factors both mechanical and biochemical, but that DIC will emerge as the most important component.

Treatment

The diversity of treatments suggested for this syndrome implies that there is no single satisfactory regime. Drugs used include intravenous alcohol, low molecular weight dextran, clofibrate, heparin, steroids and even aprotinin. However the single most important factor is to increase the arterial oxygen saturation. Correction of hypoxaemia may prevent structural brain damage by cerebral fat emboli (Benatar *et al.*. 1972).

Serial blood gas estimations are mandatory, and if hypoxaemia cannot be corrected by adding oxygen to the inspired air, IPPV should not be delayed, with PEEP if necessary.

Drug therapy

We always use heparin intravenously, believing that DIC is an essential part of the syndrome. Steroids are generally advised, but, as is so often the case with this form of therapy, their use is based on animal experiments which are often unwisely extended to man. In cases with extensive cerebral changes a reduction in cerebral pressure might occur with dexamethasone.

In general, however, the treatment of fat emboli should be predominantly pulmonary, i.e. the correction of hypoxaemia, along with the general management of the shocked patient.

BURNS

Patients with severe burns are usually treated in Regional Centres, but first aid measures have to be applied at the time of the incident and patients are usually transferred initially to the nearest district hospital.

Injured tissues which must be considered are the *skin* and the *respiratory tract*.

Skin

Three degrees of damage are recognized:
(1) Erythema. This is reversible.
(2) Partial thickness skin loss. Healing will occur.
(3) Full thickness skin loss. Grafting will be required.

As soon as the injury has occurred it may be advantageous to cool the skin. This affords symptomatic relief, but is unlikely to affect the extent of a burn. Chemical burns may benefit from specific treatment, e.g. 1% copper sulphate to identify phosphorus particles or 10% calcium gluconate subcutaneously for hydrofluoric acid.

In hospital, patients are best isolated in single rooms if they have major areas of trunk burns since these can then be managed without dressings. Blisters are usually removed. Circumferential full thickness burns can cause problems of venous obstruction and may require incision to prevent scar contraction. Hands should be kept moving to prevent scar contractures and may be enclosed in a polythene bag.

Shock

When the area of skin loss is extensive, fluid is lost from the circulation. Capillary permeability is increased with loss of plasma. It is possible for the healthy adult to compensate for loss of up to 15% of body surface area (10% in children).

The *rule of nine* is used to estimate the percentage of surface area. Each arm accounts for 9%, the head 9%, each leg 18% and the front and back of the trunk 18% each. 1% is allowed for the genitalia bringing the total to 100%. In the infant this is modified to allow for the larger relative head size. 10% is allowed for each limb, 20% for the head and 20% each for the front and back of the trunk.

Systemic effects

The stress response to a severe burn includes an increase in circulating catechol-amines, blood cortisol, antidiuretic hormone, renin, insulin and glucagon (Sevitt, 1974). The result may be vasoconstriction of skin and visceral vessels, rise in blood pressure, bradycardia, pupil dilatation and bowel atony. Bowel ischaemia with mucosal breakdown has been reported. Liver function may be impaired. In the kidneys a reduction in glomerular filtration rate results in oliguria while sodium retention occurs as a result of hormone effects.

Fluid requirements

There is very great loss of fluid from the circulation in the first 12 hours follow-ing injury. This gradually lessens and some is eventually reabsorbed into the circulation. There is need for massive intravenous infusion to match this in the initial period. Muir and Barclay (1962) have recommended that a volume can be calculated by multiplying the body weight in grams by the area of burn as a percentage, and then dividing by 2. This calculated volume is given every 4 hours for the first 12 hours, then every 6 hours for 12 hours, and finally over a third 12 hour period. Clinical considerations may of course modify the regime.

The logical replacement fluid is plasma. Human plasma protein fraction contains little globulin or fibrinogen so this preparation should not be used exclusively and a ratio of one unit of fresh frozen plasma to two of human plasma protein fraction has been recommended (Diamond *et al.*, 1975). In addition to plasma expander, a fluid intake of 50 ml/kg per 24 hours will also be required. Oral fluids should be allowed in small amounts frequently so that problems do not arise as a result of reduced gut function as a result of stress.

Intravenous fluid therapy can be monitored by:

(1) Central venous pressure measurement.
(2) Haematocrit estimation.
(3) Measurement of urine volume and specific gravity.

Calorie requirements

The basal metabolic rate is increased by up to 100% in patients with extensive burns as a result of hypercatabolism and preparations such as Vivonex can be given, via a nasogastric tube if necessary. Where oral ingestion is not possible, intravenous nutrition is required.

Warmth is also necessary when large areas of body surface are uncovered. The body loses ability to retain heat when there are large areas of skin loss. The room atmosphere should be warm (32°C) and dry.

The respiratory injury

This may be caused by heat itself, or by inhalation of smoke or chemical fumes. The increasing use of plastic materials in home furnishings increases the chances of inhalation of toxic fumes in domestic fires.

Thermal injury affects mainly the upper air passages, causing oedema which may lead to respiratory injury of such intensity as to make tracheal intubation difficult or impossible so that tracheostomy has to be considered. Inhalation of toxic chemicals causes damage to the tracheobronchial tree down to alveolar level. There may be damage to mucosal surfaces with sloughing (Harrison, 1968), bronchospasm, loss of surfactant, atelectasis and oedema (Zikria *et al.*, 1968). Myocardial damage may occur from release of toxins and smoke inhalation may result in increase of blood carboxyhaemoglobin levels (Mellins and Park, 1975).

Diagnostic procedures include the use of X-rays, blood gas analysis and fibre-optic bronchoscopy to assess the extent of damage (Hunt *et al.*, 1975; Moylan *et al.*, 1975).

Ventilation must be supported by tracheal intubation and early IPPV when respiratory distress is seen (Vivori and Cudmore, 1977). Arterial hypoxaemia is likely to occur as a result of a reduction in functional residual capacity and increased intrapulmonary shunting. The alveolar-arterial oxygen tension difference is a measure of the success or otherwise of IPPV (Armstrong *et al.*, 1977). When general anaesthesia is required the elevation of serum potassium following suxamethonium may result in ventricular fibrillation, especially between the 20th and 60th day following major burns (Bush *et al.*, 1962).

The use of large doses of steroids is controversial. A single large dose has been recommended (Stone *et al.*, 1967), while others recommend administration over a 48 hour period (Moylan *et al.*, 1975; Armstrong *et al.*, 1977).

Infection

All major burns will become the seat of bacterial colonization. This raises problems in the ITU because of the problems of cross-infection. It is likely that tracheostomy wounds will become infected and pulmonary infection may arise in patients on IPPV. The nursing load is heavy and when patients have to be nursed on general wards it will probably be necessary to close part of that ward to other admissions (Diamond *et al.*, 1975).

REFERENCES

Armstrong, R. F., Mackersie, A. M., McGregor, A. P. and Woods, S. D. (1977), The respiratory injury in burns. An account of the management. *Anaesthesia*, 32, 313.

Benatar, S. R., Ferguson, A. D., Goldschmidt, R. B. (1972), Fat Embolism— Some Clinical Observations and a review of Controversial Aspects. *Q. J. Med.*, 161, 85.

Burford, T. H. and Burbanks, B. (1945), Traumatic Wet Lung. *J. Thor. Surg.*, 14, 415.

Bush, G. H., Graham, H. A. P., Littlewood, A. H. M. and Scott, L. B. (1962), Danger of suxamethonium and endotracheal intubation in anaesthesia for burns. *Brit. med. J.*, ii, 1081.

Campbell, D. (1977), Immediate hospital care of the injured. *Brit. J. Anaesth.*, 49, 673.

Campbell, D. (1979) in *Recent Advances in Anaesthesia and Analgesia*–13 ed. Hewer, C. L. and Atkinson, R. S., Churchill Livingstone, Edinburgh.

Diamond, A. W., Pigott, R. W. and Townsend, P. L. G. (1975), Immediate care of burns. *Anaesthesia*, 30, 791.

Diagnosis of Brain Death. Statement issued by the Honorary Secretary of the Conference of Medical Royal Colleges and their Faculties in the United Kingdom (1976), *Brit. med. J.*, 2, 1187.

Daniel, R. H. and Cate, W. R. (1948), Wet Lung. An experimental study. *Ann. Surg.*, 121, 836.

Dittman, M., Keller, R. and Wolff, G. (1978), A rationale for epidural analgesia in the treatment of multiple rib fractures. *Int. Care Medicine*, 4, 181.

Eason, M. J. and Wyatt, R. (1979), Paravertebral block–a reappraisal. *Anaesthesia*, 34, 638.

Editorial (1976), Brain Death. *Brit. med. J.*, 2, 1157.

French, L. A. and Galichich, J. H. (1964), The use of steroids for control of cerebral oedema. *Clin. Neurosurg.*, 10, 212.

Gaus, H. (1916), Studies in cerebral fat embolism with reference to the pathology of delirium and coma. *Arch. Int. Med.*, 18, 76.

Gordon, E. (1971), Controlled respiration in the management of patients with traumatic brain injuries. *Acta. Anaesth. Scand.*, 15, 193.

Greenbaumm, R. (1976), General Anaesthesia for Neurosurgery. *Brit. J. Anaesth.*, 48, 773.

Gurd, A. R. (1970), Fat embolism: an aid to diagnosis. *J. Bone Jt. Surg.*, 52B, 732.

Harrison, H. N. (1968), Respiratory tract injury, pathophysiology and response to therapy among burned patients. *Ann. N.Y. Acad. Sci.*, 150, 627.

Hoffman, E. (1976), Mortality and morbidity following road accidents. *Ann. R. Coll. Surg. Engl.*, 58, 233.

Horton, J. M. (1975), The immediate care of head injuries. *Anaesthesia*, 30, 21.

Horton, J. M. (1976), The Anaesthetist's Contribution to the Care of Head Injuries. *Brit. J. Anaesth.*, 48, 767.

Hunt, J. L., Agee, R. N. and Pruitt, B. A. (1975), Fibre-optic bronchoscopy in acute inhalation injury. *J. Trauma*, 15, 641.

Hunter, A. R. (1975), *Neurosurgical Anaesthesia*, 2nd Edn. Blackwell, Oxford, London, Edinburgh, Melbourne.

Illingworth, G. and Jennett, W. B. (1965), The shocked head injury. *Lancet*, ii, 511.

Jamieson, K. G. and Yelland, J. D. N. (1968), Extradural haematoma: report of 167 cases. *J. Neurosurg.*, 29, 13.

Keen, G. (1974), Chest injuries. *Ann. R. Coll. Surg.*, 54, 124.

Keen, G. (1975), *Chest Injuries*. Wright, Bristol.

Klinger, M., Kazner, E., Grumme, T. H., Amtenbrink, V., Graef, G., Hartmann, K. H., Hopman, H., Meese, W. and Vogel, B. (1975), Clinical experience with automatic mid-line echo-encephalography: cooperative study of three neuro-surgical units. *J. Neurol. Neurosurg., Psychiat.*, **38**, 272.

Lassen, N. A. (1966), The luxury-perfusion syndrome and its possible relation to acute metabolic acidosis localised within the brain. *Lancet*, ii, 1113.

Lundberg, N., Kjallquist, A. and Bien, C. (1959), Reduction of increased intra-cranial pressure by hyperventilation. *Acta.psychiat. neurol. scand.*, **34**, 139.

McDowall, D. G. (1976), in *Recent Advances in Anaesthesia and Analgesia*–12 (Hewer, C. L. and Atkinson, R. S. eds), Churchill Livingstone, Edinburgh, London, New York.

Mellins, R. B. and Park, S. (1975), Respiratory complications of smoke in-halation in victims of fires. *J. Paediat.*, **87**, 1.

Moylan, J. A., Adib, K. and Birnbaum, M. (1975), Fiberoptic bronchoscopy following thermal injury. *Surg. Gyn. Obst.*, **140**, 541.

Muir, I. F. K. and Barclay, J. L. (1962), *Burns and their treatment*. Lloyd-Luke, London.

Norman, J. and Moles, M. (1977), Editorial: Trauma and immediate care. *British J. Anaesth.*, **49**, 641.

O'Driscoll, M. and Powell, F. J. (1967), Injury, serum lipids, fat embolism and clofibrate. *Brit. med. J.*, **4**, 149.

Potter, J. M. (1967), Head injuries today. *Postgrad. Med. J.*, **43**, 574.

Registrar General's Statistical Review of England and Wales for the Year 1973 (1975), Part I (A) Tables, Medical, London, H.M.S.O.

Rossanda, M., Selenati, A., Villa, C. and Beduschi, A. (1973), Role of auto-matic ventilation in treatment of severe head injuries. *J. Neurosurg. Sci.*, **17**, 265.

Saldeen, T. (1970), Fat embolism and signs of intravascular coagulation in a post-traumatic autopsy material. *J. Trauma*, **10**, 273.

Scully, R. E. (1956), Fat embolism in Korean Casualties. Its incidence clinical significance and pathological aspects. *Am. J. Pathol.*, **32**, 374.

Sevitt, S. (1974), *Reactions to Injury in Burns*. Heinemann, London.

Snook, R. (1977), Transport of the injured patient. Past, present and future. *Brit. J. Anaesth.*, **49**, 651.

Stone, H. H., Rhame, D. W., Corbitt, J. D., Given, K. S. and Martin, J. D. (1967), Respiratory burns: A correlation of clinical and laboratory results. *Ann. Surg.*, **165**, 157.

Sugg, W. C., Rea, W. J., Ecker, R. R., Webb, W. R., Race, E. F. and Shaw, R. R. (1968), Penetrating wounds of the heart. *J. Thoracic Cardiovasc. Surg.*, **56**, 531.

Teasdale, G. and Jennett, B. (1974), Assessment of coma and impaired conscious-ness: a practical scale. *Lancet*, ii, 81.

Turner, J. M. and McDowall, D. G. (1976), The measurement of intracranial pressure. *Brit. J. Anaesth.*, **43**, 735.

Vivori, E. and Cudmore, R. E. (1977), Management of airway complications in burned children. *British med. J.*, **2**, 1462.

Zikria, B. A., Sturner, W. Q., Astarhan, N. K., Fox, C. L. and Ferrer, J. M. (1968), Respiratory tract damage in burns: pathophysiology and therapy. *Ann. N.Y. Acad. Sci.*, **150**, 618.

THIRTEEN

Renal disease

INTRODUCTION

This chapter will deal with those problems relating to the kidneys, likely to be encountered in very many of the patients admitted to any intensive care unit.

It will be necessary to have a clear understanding of some of the basic pathophysiological concepts involved, but no attempt will be made to give a comprehensive description of the physiology of the kidney, merely to describe those facts necessary for the understanding of the abnormalities which may occur in the intensive care situation, in order for the physician to be able to treat them more logically and correctly.

Furthermore, there is no intention to produce a detailed list of the whole of renal disease but it is hoped to explain the essentials of the management of a patient presenting acutely with renal problems and then to further expound on some of the more rare, but important, syndromes which may be seen occasionally in such a clinical setting.

MANAGEMENT OF ACUTE URAEMIA

A common problem presenting to an intensive care unit is a patient gravely ill with a high blood urea of unknown origin. Many of these patients will have a form of acute reversible renal failure (acute intrinsic reversible renal failure, commonly known as acute tubular necrosis) or glomerulonephritis. Others may have had asymptomatic renal disease for years which has suddenly become worse because of intercurrent illness or surgical operation (acute, on chronic renal failure).

A third group of patients will be seen who are severely ill with multi-system disease who, whilst in the intensive care unit, may develop a rising urea the cause for which might initially not be clear.

Differential diagnosis

The first problem to be discussed therefore, is the differential diagnosis of acute uraemia. Classically, this is categorized as pre-renal, renal or post-renal; accepting that in the real situation 'pre-renal' problems such as haemorrhage, shock etc. always show some evidence of functional renal impairment and often actual structural damage may be seen on biopsy. Equally the term 'post-renal' is always associated with changes in the kidney produced by the obstruction.

However, the categorization of acute uraemia into these three aetiologies is of use when considering management of the patient in the acute situation.

History and examination

Relevant points in the history might include previous information (e.g. from old notes or routine medicals) or pre-existent hypertension or proteinuria. A past history of urinary tract disease, e.g. recurrent infection, calculi, is obviously important as would be a history of recent sore throat or exposure to toxic drugs or chemicals. Enquiries should always be made into the possibility of analgesic abuse. Family history also could be relevant, particularly with regard to hypertension, polycystic disease, etc.

Specific points to look out for on physical examination include, in addition to the routine clinical examination, body weight if at all possible. This is extremely valuable, as body weight is a far better guide than supposedly complete urine collections which are almost always incorrect. Another important sign to look for is band keratopathy which might suggest long standing calcium problems. Observation of the skin for rashes, scratch marks, micro-infarcts etc. is obviously important as is examination of the fundus to look for evidence of long standing retinopathy. Careful observation of the fluid state of the body, particularly looking for the possibility of salt and water overload, i.e. the presence of raised neck veins and oedema; or salt and water deficiency, where careful measurement of blood pressure is *vital* not only lying, but also standing or at least sitting propped up if necessary. Postural hypotension is one of the earliest signs, and in the severely ill patient perhaps the only reliable sign of volume depletion. Classically described signs are often valueless in severely ill patients—thus a dry tongue is more often due to mouth breathing, e.g. acidosis. Reduced skin turgor, though possibly of some value in the previously fit young individual, is more often the result of age alone or malnutrition. To expand on the importance of *postural* hypotension, there is virtually no patient in whom it is impossible (even if inconvenient to the intensive care unit nurses!) to check the blood pressure in a lying and upright position (standing or sitting) and any postural fall will strongly suggest the possibility (if drugs are excluded) of hypovolaemia. This is, perhaps, the most important physical sign of all to look for in this situation.

Whilst the presence of oedema may well suggest salt and water overload, one should not forget that in severely ill patients it is quite common, particularly if the illness is long standing, that the plasma albumin might fall and the oedema be partly at least hypo-oncotic in nature and, although the extra-cellular fluid space may be abnormally large, the patient may still be uraemic because of lack of *circulating* blood volume.

It is obviously important to look particularly for signs of septicaemia or endocarditis, and also pericarditis which may cause a rise in neck veins and give a false impression of fluid overload when the patient may in fact still be hypovolaemic. Finally, it is essential not to forget a full pelvic examination as carcinoma of the cervix is a not uncommon cause of the apparently unexplained acute renal failure.

PRACTICAL DIFFERENTIATION BETWEEN PRE-RENAL AND INTRINSIC RENAL FAILURE

Many doctors will still think plasma sodium concentration is an important indicator of the sodium state. By itself it is of no value in assessing total body sodium and really indicates the ratio of solute to water in the body, and changes of plasma sodium are therefore more closely related to change in body water than in sodium content. Hyponatraemia may occasionally be a sign of sodium deficiency but this has to be considerable before it shows in this way and a low sodium is more often seen in oedematous patients suffering from sodium overload in whom water excess is even greater than that of sodium. Hypernatraemia usually indicates a water deficiency because of obligatory losses and may often be seen in the intensive care situation when the patient is unable to complain of thirst and has not been given enough water intravenously in the form of 5% Dextrose. Hypernatraemia itself does not exclude the possibility of an additional sodium deficiency. It is unfortunately still quite common to see uraemic patients in whom saline problems have been incorrectly interpreted, mainly on the basis of the plasma sodium.

The demonstration that renal underperfusion not only reduces urine volume and increases its concentration but also reduces urinary sodium concentrations (Mueller *et al.*, 1951) stimulated interest in urinary sodium concentration as a measurement of pre-renal failure. However, variations in urine sodium concentration from 10 to 110 mmol/l occur in patients with established tubular necrosis and it is now accepted that the measurement of urinary sodium concentration is of limited value in the differential diagnosis of acute renal failure (Platts, 1966).

A considerable number of diagnostic suggestions have been made to aid in the differentiation of oliguria due to pre-renal circulatory inadequacy and established acute reversible intrinsic renal failure, and there is little doubt that no single laboratory test is absolutely invariably diagnostic but the most useful is probably a comparison of the urine and plasma osmolality of the urine.

Maximum urine osmolality during dehydration in normal subjects lies between 800 and 1400 mmol/kg water (Miles *et al.*, 1954). Concentrating ability is depressed up to 24 hours after surgery and, in the experimental animal, during and soon after trauma to something like 400 to 700 mmol/kg (Gullick and Raisz, 1960).

In the normal individual when sodium and water depleted, if one takes the plasma osmolality as 300 mmol, the urine/plasma osmolality ratio will be therefore between 2.7 and 4. It is now well established that in the later stages of the acute reversible intrinsic renal failure the urine/plasma osmolality ratio approximates to 1 (Bull *et al.*, 1950).

Thus in theory at least, and also to some extent in fact, the patients with pre-renal circulatory insufficiency, i.e. pre-renal failure, have a urine/plasma osmolality ratio usually greater than 2, and the diagnosis of incipient renal failure may be based on the finding of a urine/plasma osmolality ratio less than this and approaching 1. In patients with established organic intrinsic renal failure the urine/plasma osmolality ratio is usually 1 to 1.15. Although this is found to be very useful investigation in practice, many exceptions do arise particularly in patients undergoing prolonged cardiac by-pass operations, in patients who have pre-existing renal disease, or in patients who have already been given some form of diuretic therapy; furthermore the duration of the oliguria may also be important (Luke *et al.*, 1970).

Other measurements often performed, and based on the same theoretical principal is the urine/plasma urea ratio, when a U/P urea ratio of greater than 20 : 1 almost always implies that the oliguria is still a physiological renal response to hypovolaemia, whereas if the ratio falls to around 5 or lower it is strongly suggestive that acute intrinsic reversible renal failure has become established. (Table 13.1)

Table 13.1 U/P ratios as an aid to differentiating pre-renal from intrinsic renal failure

	U/P ratio urea	U/P ratio osmolality
Pre-renal uraemia	>20:1	>1.8-2
Established A.T.N.	<10:1	<1.05

N.B. Tests invalidated if mannitol or frusemide have already been administered (or high dose of contrast for IVP.)

It is important that these indices are considered in relation to urine volume as obviously in the face of high urine volume the ratio will fall in the absence of renal impairment. It has been the authors practice to use, in the main, urine/plasma osmolality ratio, partly because this is very easily and quickly measured and also because there is some evidence (Luke *et al.*, 1970) that the U/P osmolality ratio is more reliable than the U/P urea ratio.

Other investigations claimed to be of some help include proteinuria, urine microscopy, blood urea level. Proteinuria is not a helpful finding in differentiation as it may be present in pre-renal circulatory inadequacy as well as in acute tubular necrosis, though usually in pre-renal uraemia the degree of proteinuria is less. Routine urine microscopy has proved less helpful than was originally hoped although it does remain true that the finding of haematuria with red cell casts is highly suggestive, though not diagnostic, of acute glomerulitis, particularly in the early stage.

The level of the blood urea itself is not of any value in differentiating between pre-renal and intrinsic renal failure and levels as high as 100 mmol/l may be seen in patients sodium and water depleted with an extremely high protein in-take.

The presence of oliguria should always alert one to the possibility of acute reversible intrinsic renal failure but urine volumes of apparently normal proportions, particularly where catabolism is severe such as after multiple injuries, should not be taken as excluding renal impairment as acute intrinsic reversible renal failure may occur with high volumes of urine in these circumstances. Similarly care must be exercised when high protein in-take is given to patients as it should be remembered for practical purposes that each 3 g of ingested protein produces 1 g of urea, that a high urea out-put produces an osmotic diuresis and in the absence of appropriate replacement, water and possibly also sodium depletion may further impair renal concentrating ability (Luke and Kennedy, 1967).

In summary, when acute intrinsic reversible renal failure is suspected the most useful laboratory measurement is probably the urine/plasma osmolality ratio, particularly if the ratio is measured early in the course of the renal failure.

RENAL RADIOLOGY IN ACUTE RENAL FAILURE

The single major advance in the differential diagnosis of acute renal failure in the past few years has been the introduction of high dose excretion urography. Until 10 to 15 years ago excretion urography was considered both valueless and dangerous with the blood urea exceeded 16 mmol/l. Subsequently however the availability of non-toxic contrast media and the demonstration of their safe use in patients with renal failure has combined to make excretion urography routine in the investigation of patients presenting with acute renal failure. Several studies have now shown no significant or permanent impairment of renal function after urography using doses of hypaque 45% up to the order of 2 mls/kg (Fry and Cattell, 1971; Doyle *et al.*, 1967). It should be recognized that large doses of these contrast media usually entails giving the patients some 100 mmol of contrast medium and there is a serious risk of fluid overload in the subjects unless care is taken. The methyl glucomine salt of Gyatrizoic or Iothalamic acid may have minor advantages over the sodium salt in patients where sodium retention should be avoided.

There have undoubtedly been reports of high doses of these contrast media leading to further impairment of renal function; careful review of the details of the reported cases usually indicates other contributing factors such as hypotension or dehydration, although a special situation may exist with patients who have myelomatosis, liver disease or diabetes. Again however, even in these latter three situations it seems that dehydration is probably the critical predisposing factor.

So far as interpretation of the results is concerned this is well summarized by Fry and Cattell (1972) who have described four nephrographic patterns in acute renal failure (see Table 13.2).

In conclusion it must be emphasized that experience with high dose excretion

Table 13.2 Nephrographic patterns in acute renal failure

Type 1	Immediate faint persistent nephrogram Chronic Glomerular Disease ↓ Number of functioning nephrons ↓ G.F.R. ↓ Rate of excretion of contrast ↓ Non-reabsorption results from over perfusion of remaining nephrons →Osmotic diuresis

Type 2	Delayed but increasingly dense nephrogram
	A Acute extra-renal obstruction
	B Ischaemia or hypotension
	  ↓ G.F.R. → ↑ Na & H_2O reabsorption
	  Tubular stasis

Type 3	Immediate dense persistent nephrogram
	A Acute Tubular Necrosis
	  ? Back diffusion of tubular fluid
	    containing contrast medium and leadage
	    with continuing glomerular filtration
	B Acute oliguric pyelonephritis

Type 4	No nephrogram Renal infarction

urography in patients which acute renal failure is still very limited and further work is needed to define more clearly the validity of the interpretation of the nephrographic patterns. It would seem however, on the evidence thus far available, that this may give valuable help in the diagnosis of patients presenting with acute renal failure providing suitable care is taken during the procedure, and in interpretation of the results.

ANGIOGRAPHY IN ACUTE RENAL FAILURE

Renal angiography is of very limited value for routine investigation. The only indication for immediate arteriography is in a patient suspected of having renal artery occlusion when although the results of surgery in such cases remain fairly disappointing, treatment with Streptokinase may occasionally yield surprisingly good results.

However, in the routine management of patients presenting with acute uraemia angiography has little part to play.

VALUE OF RENAL BIOPSY IN ACUTE URAEMIA

Renal biopsy is of value in selected patients who present with acute uraemia. It may be indicated to assist prognosis, confirm the clinic diagnosis, or to form the basis for attempting treatment. If the clinical features suggest a lesion other than acute tubular necrosis an early biopsy is indicated to permit a better appreciation of the probable out-look, and treatment of some lesions, e.g. Goodpastures syndrome (where plasmapharesis may be helpful). Thus if none of the usual precipitating factors of acute tubular necrosis are present, or there are features to suggest a different cause, the precise diagnosis is essential for management and although clinical features and laboratory examination of blood and urine may help, ultimately a renal biopsy is the best method of diagnosing the origin of acute renal failure. When the history and clinical features strongly suggest a diagnosis of acute tubular necrosis, renal biopsy should only be considered if the oliguria is prolonged. If there is doubt about the precipitating factors or if there are features to suggest a different cause for the syndrome, biopsy should be performed. It must be remembered however that renal biopsy anyway carries some morbidity, especially unless performed by an experienced physician in the technique and in uraemia renal biopsy carries an even higher morbidity so that its value must be assessed against the risks.

In a recent series from Guy's Hospital (Wilson *et al.*, 1976) the effects of renal biopsy in acute uraemia on specific treatment had a small but significant bearing. Two of their patients had myeloma which had not been diagnosed before, presenting with acute renal failure and in only two out of ten patients whose biopsy had showed afferent arteriolar capillary thrombi had the diagnosis been made from the initial blood smear.

Thus renal biopsy has a part to play in the investigations in the acute uraemic syndrome, but only in selected patients such as prolonged oliguria when acute tubular necrosis is suspected or if the clinical features are not classical of, or suggest a lesion other than, acute tubular necrosis. However, it should only be undertaken after due consideration of the not insignificant risk involved and the possible benefit to the patient and then only by a physician experienced in the technique. Furthermore it is desirable that electron microscopy and immuno-fluorescent techniques should be available, as examination using light microscopy only might be misleading.

PHYSIOLOGICAL CONCEPTS IN THE DEVELOPMENT OF ACUTE INTRINSIC REVERSIBLE RENAL FAILURE

It will already have come to the readers notice that in this chapter the emphasis has been made on volume rather than pressure. The traditional view was that glomerular filtration required a pressure in the glomerular capillaries which exceeded that in Bowman's space by more than 25 mm mercury in order to overcome plasma oncotic pressure, and when systolic pressure fell below 60 mm of mercury during haemorrhage, urine formation ceased and this was attributed to a drop in filtration pressure to below 25 mm of mercury. However, there are many clinical conditions in which urine formation can continue in spite of very low blood pressure. During hypotensive anaesthesia for example, or, during the use of ganglion blockers, renal blood flow may be well preserved and glomerular filtration, though reduced, is far from negligible, and post-operative renal function excellent in spite of reduction of blood pressures often below the level of 60 mm of mercury. It therefore seems likely that the vaso-constriction which accompanies shock, whether oligemic, endotoxic or cardiogenic, plays a more important part in the temporary renal shut down, than does pressure alone, i.e. hypotension. It has been shown in animals that shock starves the renal cortex of blood by reflex vaso-constriction shunting blood from the outer cortex to the juxta medullary region and medulla of the kidney (Alpha adrenergic induced). In humans with acute renal failure, diversion of the blood from the cortex in this way, has been shown by angiographic studies (Shaldon *et al.*, 1964, Hollenberg *et al.*, 1968) and by dye dilution curves. In the early stages of shock, the fall in GFR and urine volume can be reversed by restoration of blood volume and, or, by the administration of Phenoxybenzamine to overcome the Alpha adrenergic phase of constriction. However, Phenoxybenzamine, has many hazards including the precipitation of cardiac failure and, more commonly now, a beta adrenergic stimulator such as Isoprenaline may be used. The differential diagnosis of this 'physiological' oliguria due to circulatory inadequacy (i.e. pre-renal uraemia) from 'pathological oliguria' due to acute reversible intrinsic renal failure has been mentioned already in the paragraph on investigations; in a patient following a prolonged period of renal under perfusion the differential is extremely difficult clinically and really the condition of pre-renal uraemia shades into acute intrinsic renal failure. There is no definite dividing line.

The stimulus to the prolonged vaso-constriction and resultant shunting of blood leading to acute intrinsic renal failure, is unknown. High plasma renin levels are often found during acute tubular necrosis and it has been postulated that hyper-secretion of renin within the kidney has been responsible for the renal vaso-constriction (Brown *et al.*, 1970). There is some experimental evidence to back this up in that acute tubular necrosis has been produced in animals by infusion of Angiotensin. However, the doses used in the experiments were very large compared with the modest elevations of plasma renin found in man with acute tubular necrosis. Alterations in renal haemodynamics as explained above may well explain the persistent oliguria and it is currently felt that the development of true intrinsic renal failure may be perpetuated by transient glomerular thrombosis, i.e. intra-renal intra-vascular coagulation and this concept is supported by the findings of raised levels of fibrin degradation products in plasma during the oliguria phase and also in the urine during the diuretic phase (Wardle and Taylor, 1968; Clarkson *et al.*, 1970; Haanen *et al.*, 1970) and by the demonstration of fibrin and platelets in the glomeruli on electron microscopy (Clarkson *et al.*, 1970). The hypothesis has been put forward that renal vasoconstriction leads to intra-renal thrombosis causing acute tubular necrosis (Vassalli and Ricket, 1960) but it remains uncertain whether intravascular coagulation is the cause of, or an epiphenomenon of, acute tubular necrosis.

THERAPEUTIC MANAGEMENT OF ACUTE URAEMIA

Prevention of acute reversible intrinsic failure

Prevention of acute reversible intrinsic renal failure commences with early and efficient treatment of the primary abnormality causing the reduced renal blood flow, thus it is essential to correct any deficit of circulating blood volume by infusion of the appropriate fluid which has been lost, blood plasma or salt. Monitoring of the central venous pressure with a CVP line may be useful and helpful in the acute situation, particularly in ill patients where the JVP may be difficult to see, or in the elderly where over transfusion may be very hazardous. It should be realized that, particularly if the pump, i.e. the heart, is not working efficiently it is quite easy to push the patient into pulmonary oedema with the CVP still not markedly raised so that use of repeated chest X-rays if infusion of large amounts of fluid is indicated is mandatory, to assess the 'circulation and fluid balance' in the right side of the heart.

If one is still undecided after full clinical examination and measurement of U/P osmolalities etc. about whether the uraemia is prerenal or intrinsic renal failure has become established, it is justified cautiously under careful monitoring to infuse the appropriate fluid, watching carefully for signs of fluid overload such as the appearance of sacral oedema, any evidence of pulmonary oedema, rapid gain in weight and particularly in the young, hypertension. Up to three litres saline retention may exist without apparent oedema, but this may well contribute to hypertension.

DIURETICS IN ACUTE RENAL FAILURE

Considerable controversy still reigns regarding the value of diuretics for the prophylaxis and treatment of acute renal failure. Greatest experience has been obtained with mannitol infusion but frusemide and ethacrymic acid are now being used increasingly.

Mannitol

There is good evidence that the infusion of mannitol to induce an osmotic diuresis can maintain the urine flow in animals with haemorrhagic shock (Murphy, Gagnon and Teschan, 1963; Coleho and Bradley, 1964) and reduce or prevent acute renal failure in experimental models (Dawson, 1964; Wilson *et al.*, 1967). This protective effect has been variously attributed to blood volume expansion, a direct vasodilatory effect, increased renal blood flow, increased tubular perfusion, reduction in endothelial cell swelling resulting from ischaemic injury, and to maintainence of the urine flow in the region of the macula densa preventing the activation of vaso constriction via the renin angiotensive system. Evidence of a similar protective role in clinical practice is less satisfactory partly due to the difficulty in obtaining control studies.

In most of the studies suggesting the beneficial effects of Mannitol probably equal in importance has been the continued awareness of the investigators of a potential for acute renal failure in such high risk patients with immediate replacement of blood volume. However, used correctly, Mannitol is safe, although used without attention it is potentially extremely dangerous. The major hazard is further fluid overload in oedematous patients and the adverse osmotic effects of Mannitol if it is not excreted by patients with established renal failure, when it may result in red cell damage, hyponatraemia, cellular dehydration, cerebral damage and over expansion of the extra cellular fluid compartment resulting in acute pulmonary oedema. Despite its hazards however, used cautiously such complications can be avoided. The usual practice is to give a trial of Mannitol in a dose of 100 mls of 20% mannitol intravenously over 15 to 20 minutes with a maximum of 300 mls over 6 hours. The usual indication is that if less than 50 hours has lapsed since the onset precipitating the oliguria and if the urine/plasma osmolality ratio is greater than 1.15. If there is no definite response there is no point in persevering with mannitol and it is in just such circumstances that it could be extremely dangerous. It should be pointed out that it is highly important that Mannitol should not be given until any volume depletion has been corrected.

The potential hazard of fluid and osmotic overload following mannitol infusion stimulated interest in the use of the powerful diuretics frusemide and ethacrynic acid. It is now generally accepted that frusemide in very large doses may induce a diuresis in the presence of severely reduced glomerular function in chronic renal failure but its role of prophylaxis and treatment of acute renal failure is less well established. Again it is difficult to find well controlled trials to support the claim that high dose frusemide has any prophylactic effect on incipient acute renal failure, but the careful administration of large doses of frusemide appears to be relatively safe and has lead to its widespread use. It would seem reasonable to administer 500 mg frusemide intravenously to total dose of 2 g in a 24 hour period. Frusemide should *not* be given to patients who are simultaneously receiving Cephaloridine because of the recognized nephrotoxic effect of this drug combination (see later section on drugs in renal failure).

The role of ethacrymic acid is even less well documented than that of Frusemide. A significant side effect of ethacrymic acid is persistent deafness and for this reason it seems probable that the use of ethacrymic acid is less acceptable than that of frusemide (although eighth nerve damage has also been associated with frusemide).

TREATMENT OF ESTABLISHED ACUTE REVERSIBLE INTRINSIC RENAL FAILURE

Dietary management of renal failure

Non-catabolic patients with acute renal failure may successfully be managed over short periods of time by conservative regimes employing the restriction of fluid, sodium, potassium and protein. The protein restriction is based on the provision of protein of high biological value and high calorie in-take (Berlyne *et al.*, 1967). It is in just such a situation that high doses of frusemide may facilitate control of fluid and electrolyte balance by maintaining urine output and preventing oliguria. However, because conservative régimes are restrictive and demanding on patients, if it appears at an early stage that dialysis will be necessary, it is now common practice to dialyse early rather than maintain patients on strict diet and fluid balance until the blood urea reaches high levels. This not only discourages the development of the patient feeling subjectively ill, being more at risk from infections, venous thrombosis, pulmonary emboli etc. but also because of the ease (with experience) of peritoneal dialysis one is able to keep the patient fitter, maintaining good morale of the patient, allowing more easily adequate protein and calorie replacement and preventing negative nitrogen balance.

Once renal failure is established and dialysis is likely to become necessary, the policy nowadays is to dialyse early because of the safety both of peritoneal and haemo-dialysis. This allows the provision of adequate protein and calories, particularly in hypercatabolic and post traumatic patients. When oral feeding is not possible, parenteral nutrition must be used (Lee, 1974). As in renal failure where one works out the electrolyte requirements etc. in a balanced fashion, an attempt should be made to calculate the individual patients nitrogen requirements by applying simple clinical nitrogen balance measurements. All that is required is the patient's weight, a 24 hour urine collection and blood samples. The urine urea excretion is multiplied by $2 \times 14/1000$ to convert mmols urea to grams of urea nitrogen. To allow for nitrogen excretion as other compounds, multiply the result by 6/5. To convert this total urine nitrogen excretion to protein equivalent multiply by 6.25. For urea excretion measured in grams the corresponding calculation is $28/60 \times 6.25$, i.e. 3.5. To this figure should be added any unchanged protein in the urine (usually negligible in oliguric renal failure) plus a correction for any change in blood urea (urea being distributed in total body water). The correction for changes in body urea content is calculated as change in plasma urea $\times 60\%$ body weight. Hence estimated nitrogen loss = (urine urea + change in body urea) $\times$ 0.2. A fall in plasma urea implies a negative change. Cutaneous losses will be very small usually, but occasionally considerable protein loss will occur through fistulae, purulent discharges or burns. A rough clinical nitrogen balance can then be obtained, the total protein catabolism, the change in urea and the urinary protein excretion (see Table 13.4).

It should be noted that the increased metabolic expenditure in hypercatabolic patients is probably better met by increasing glucose or carbohydrate intake rather than fat intake if one is feeding the patient by mouth and if using intravenous feeding the recommended limit for fat emulsions intravenously is 2.5 g per kg and in this situation glucose is probably more effective.

In addition to the protein requirement calculated as above, the electrolyte requirements will obviously have to be carefully considered as this will determine which particular amino acid solution would be the most appropriate to use. It should be remembered that the various amino-acid solutions available

Table 13.3 Recommended daily nutrient requirements/kg body weight

	Basal	↑ Metabolic rate
Protein	1 g	1.5–2.0 g
Carbohydrate	2 g	10 g
Fat	2 g	2.5 g
Water	30 ml	60
Calories	30	60

Table 13.4 Rough clinical nitrogen balance

(1) Protein catabolism	= Urea excretion (mmol/24 h)
(2) Blood urea excretion	= Rise in blood urea (mmol) $\times$ 60% body wt (Kg)
(3) Urinary protein excretion	
Total protein catabolism	= $[(1 + 2) \times 0.2] + 3$

Table 13.5 Intravenous calory sources

Preparation	Constituent	Cals/l	Mosmol/l	Cost/l	Cost/1000 kcal
Sorbitol 30%	Sorbitol 30%	1230	2100	2.50	2.03
Glucose 50%	Glucose 50%	2000	3800		
Intralipid 10%	Soyabean oil 10% Glycerol 2.5%	1100	280	13.00	11.82
Intralipid 20%	Soyabean oil 10% Glycerol 2.5%	2000	330	19.00	9.50
Lipiphysen 10%	Cotton seed oil 10% Sorbitol 5%	1240	–	11.00	8.87
Lipiphysen 15%	Cotton seed oil 10% Sorbitol 5%	1780	–	12.00	6.74

commercially vary considerably in the amount of electrolytes they contain and it is very important to take this into account when deciding which solution to use for each individual patient, particularly in the oliguric state. It must not be forgotten to include allowance for gastro-intestinal losses not calculated for in the above equations. If the patient already has a hypo-proteinaemic state at the start of either intravenous nutrition or, even oral feeding, the hypoproteinaemia is best corrected by giving albumen in the form of plasma rather than relying on administration of amino-acids. One important practical point is to ensure that calories in the form of lipid infusions are given during the first 12 hours of any intravenous regime thus lessening the risk of hyperlipemia when blood samples are being withdrawn which will interfere with analysis in the laboratory.

PERITONEAL DIALYSIS

Procedure

Setting up of the peritoneal dialysis initially is a relatively simple procedure. Commercially available peritoneal dialysis sets are now used.

The patient is prepared by lying him supine or slightly sitting up. An area about an inch and a half below the umbilicus and in the mid-line is cleaned in the usual manner and a sterile 'operating field' prepared, with towels, etc. It is absolutely essential that strict sterile technique is used in order to prevent early infection of the peritoneum. After local infiltration a nick with a pointed scalpel is made in the skin to enable the peritoneal catheter to be pushed easily through the skin. The peritoneal catheter with a stilette down the centre is then passed through the skin and muscle into the peritoneal cavity by using a screw-ing pressure action. Once the catheter tip goes through into the peritoneal space the stilette is slightly withdrawn and the catheter then guided into the recto-vesical pouch. This final positioning of the catheter is obviously quite essential to enable dialysis to proceed smoothly because of the syphoning action neces-sary during withdrawal of the fluid from the cavity. Occasionally the patient will complain of pain in the rectal area and one should not worry about this other than slight withdrawal of the catheter as at least it means the catheter is in the correct place!

Once *in situ* the catheter is secured by means of a disc which is passed over the catheter and fixed to the skin to prevent the catheter sliding on further into the abdomen during nursing procedures! A purse-string suture is usually helpful to secure the catheter in place as well and then a simple dressing applied over the catheter.

The giving set is then fixed to the catheter and dialysis may proceed. Usually either one or two litres of fluid is poured into the abdomen (depending on the size of the patient), allowed to remain in the abdomen clamped off for ten to fifteen minutes, and then the fluid allowed to syphon out into the collecting bag; the whole cycle can then be repeated. It has been the author's personal practice to carry out one hourly cycles, even though cycles can be more rapid than this, in order to make it simple for nursing staff.

Choice of fluid used depends on whether it is necessary to withdraw fluid from the patient, i.e. if he is overloaded, and there are commercially available solutions with varying osmolarities to choose from.

Unless the patient is grossly overloaded no more than one hyper-tonic cycle of solution should be used consecutively as a large amount of fluid can be withdrawn rapidly. (Hence its use in intractable pulmonary oedema on occasions.) If in such circumstances it is deemed necessary to use more hyper-tonic fluid to withdraw fluid rapidly it is essential to measure the patient's blood pressure lying down and propped up in order to watch out for postural fall, the earliest sign of volume depletion. Over slightly longer term weighing the patient is much more helpful than collecting the fluid. Only under

187

exceptional circumstances therefore should more than one cycle in every three or four be hyper-tonic fluid. It is also possible to vary the sodium content of the commercially available fluids depending on the sodium status of the patient. In the fluids available there is no potassium and therefore if the patient is not hyperkalaemic potassium chloride should be added to each bag at the required amount, i.e. four to five mmol/l.

Complications

Although in *competent* hands peritoneal dialysis is a relatively simple procedure, there are a number of both minor and major complications which make it essential that it should not be undertaken lightly.

(1) *Failure of drainage* (a) 'overage': In order to comply with legal requirements, manufacturers have to dispense at least a litre when dispensing 'one litre cartons' and this means that they add 'overage' to each bag, hence a one litre bag contained anything from one litre to 1100 ml. It is therefore inaccurate to carry out 'fluid balance' studies by measuring intake and output and relying on that to decide how much weight is being gained or lost. It is essential to weigh the patient regularly and also to measure postural blood pressure, lying and standing, and to do frequent chest X-rays to look at the left side of the heart for overload as mentioned in previous passages in this article. However, it is worth while for the nurses to measure how much drains out in order to get a rough idea that the dialysis is working properly and drainage is occurring and that roughly the right amount is draining, i.e. as much is coming out as is going in otherwise there is the danger of the patient retaining fluid, possibly precipitating heart failure.

(b) Sodium and water depleted: If a peritoneal dialysis is started on a patient who is sodium and water depleted, obviously sodium and water will be retained by the patient by osmotic affect, and by diffusion so that the patient may retain enormous amounts of fluid until they get to the correct fluid state, and this may appear, if the diagnosis of sodium and water depletion has not been made, that the dialysis is not working properly and fluid is being retained in the peritoneal cavity.

(c) Poor position of the catheter: If the catheter is not positioned correctly in the pouch of douglas or equivalent, and if it should for instance slip up and lie under the liver, fluid will be able to be poured into the peritoneal cavity but obviously drainage will not occur as this depends on the syphoning effect. All that is required is for the catheter to be re-positioned and often when fluid has been retained this becomes much easier than when the catheter is originally inserted. It is important not to pour more fluid in, or in the mistaken belief pour in hypertonic fluid in order to 'get more fluid out'. This again could only precipitate heart failure or other catastrophies.

(d) Loculation of fluid: Occasionally due to adhesions etc., it becomes very difficult to peritoneal dialyse the patient because of fluid loculating in various spaces within the peritoneal cavity. In this case it may be necessary to go onto haemodialysis, but occasionally it is possible to dialyse the patient again by re-positioning the catheter. It is in practice very rare that patients cannot be peritoneally dialysed.

(e) Leakage of fluid between the tissue plains: The peritoneal dialysis catheter has numerous holes throughout its length for fluid exit into the peri-toneal cavity. If some of these holes are high up on the catheter and are not actually positioned inside the peritoneal space but lie in tissue plains, fluid will track down into the tissue plains and abdominal and genital oedema will occur, this can be extremely troublesome and lead to cellulitis and infection, and should be avoided if possible at all costs. Again re-position of the catheter should deal with this situation providing it is observed early.

(2) *Infections.* Infections in the peritoneal cavity following peritoneal dialysis in competent hands and good nursing are *extremely rare* in the author's experi-ence. Providing a good technique is used to insert the catheter infections are virtually unknown in the first few days. Provided the nurses are trained well, not to interrupt the circuit more than absolutely necessary and are scrupulous about their technique, infections with even prolonged peritoneal dialysis are a rarity. If they do occur, usually they can be dealt with without stopping dialysis with adding the appropriate antibiotics to the dialysate. Occasionally overt peritonism occurs and withdrawal of the catheter stopping dialysis for a few days usually results in cure and dialysis can then be continued.

It is important to send off daily cultures to the laboratory to spot infections early and also for the nurse to record the visual appearance of the drainage fluid, and on the first suggestion that it has become cloudy, it has been the author's practice to add a broad spectrum antibiotic, in appropriate dosage to the dialysate.

(3) *Withdrawal of the fluid from the patient too rapidly.* This has already been covered to some extent. It is very easy to withdraw fluid very rapidly and this is of use in intractable pulmonary oedema in experienced hands. However, as has already been stated, hyper-tonic fluid should only be given in moderation unless very careful observation is maintained and the patients should always be monitored with postural blood pressures, daily weighing and frequent chest X-rays. It is only very rarely necessary, to use more than one in four hyper-tonic solution.

(4) *Protein depletion.* There is good evidence that prolonged peritoneal dialysis can quite seriously deplete the patients of protein. However, this should be preventable by feeding the patient on a high protein diet and in addition by adding high class amino-acids such as vamin to the dialysate. The dialysate is already high in glucose content and if required a small dose of insulin would help feed the patient with carbohydrates as well, by this method. One should

not be alarmed by high glucose levels in the patient during dialysate and it has not been our practice to measure the glucose level unless the patient happens to be a diabetic or unless there are major problems.

(5) *Chest infections.* These are liable to occur particularly in patients who may be small in stature and who have two litres of dialysate in each cycle added to the peritoneal cavity. The amount added should obviously be decided according to the size of the patient, and one litre cycle for smaller patients are quite adequate, particularly if the patient is on a ventilator. Excessive loading of dialysis fluid into the abdomen can cause quite serious embarrassment of respiration but this should with common sense be preventable. It has been our habit to decide on the quantity of fluid infused depending on the size of the patient and this has continued through to the dialysis of infants when obviously far smaller amounts of fluid are used.

(6) *Perforation of viscera.* In competent hands this is extremely rare. One danger in practise however is, that patients who may have retention of urine with over-flow unknown to the doctors, may be asked to pass urine to empty the bladder prior to a dialysis being set up, and if they have retention and a large bladder it is possible to perforate the bladder with the dialysis catheter. This is not serious in that the catheter can then easily be removed from the abdomen, a urinary catheter put in to empty the bladder, and then dialysis can continue afterwards. But far more sensible obviously is prevention and it is our practice *always* to catheterize the patient prior to dialysis and *always* to remove the catheter im-mediately dialysis is set up. It matters little if the patient is passing a few mils of urine, no urine, or 500 mls of urine once renal failure is established and once the diuretic phase occurs this will become obvious, hence there is no indication to keep the catheter in. Perforation of other viscera is extremely rare.

(7) *Contra-indications.* Finally one is often asked the contra-indications to peritoneal dialysis, and in the author's experience there is virtually none, except extremely severe hyper-catabolic renal failure, in which obviously haemodialysis is indicated. Many surgeons have to be persuaded that their own drainage tubes left in post-operatively can often be used quite successfully for peritoneal dialysis providing one is scrupulous about aseptic technique! This applies of course particularly to arterial surgeons who obviously are very worried about infection reaching grafts. However, we have successfully dialysed many patients following graft surgery and so far have not met major complications. Finally one is often asked the indications for peritoneal dialysis, what level of blood urea, etc. There is no magic level of blood urea at which one should or should not dialyse this is a clinical decision and will depend on numerous factors, the whole state of the patient, the rapidity of rise of blood urea, the original insult, prognosis of the patient, and the condition at the time of assessment. If the

patient looks as if he is going to need dialysis and is catebolic the practice should be to dialyse early rather than late, and to err on the side of dialysing early is better, than to err on the side of dialysing late.

Treatment of hyperkalaemia. Almost the only major medical emergency apart from cardiac arrest is the diagnosis of hyperkalaemia. There are many well known regimes for the management of this. In acute renal failure, when the patient is commonly acidotic, perhaps the most rapid and easy correction is by the infusion of sodium bicarbonate. The major disadvantage of this of course is that this necessitates the administration of large amounts of sodium which may precipitate heart failure, but acute administration may still be indicated to bring the potassium down rapidly and then the sodium removed by the immediate setting up of a peritoneal dialysis. Other regimes which are used include the infusion of glucose and insulin and, in the more long term management, calcium resonium enemas may be administered, the important point being that it should be *calcium* resonium rather than sodium resonium, once again to avoid the risks of sodium overload.

DRUG NEPHROTOXICITY
The whole subject of drug and chemical nephrotoxicity has been extensively reviewed by Shriner and Mayer (1965) and Milne (1967). Since that time, particularly with the introduction of the new and powerful antibiotics, further potential nephrotoxic hazards have been identified.

Cephalosporins
Among this family of drugs cephaloridine appears to have a special nephrotoxic property, the affect is dose-related and reversible. Proteinurea and hyaline casts have been observed in the urine of patients given 6 g of cephaloridine a day though previous renal damage may predispose to further nephrotoxicity, particularly affecting the proximal tubules, and the combination of cephaloridine and frusemide is associated with a significant increase in the incidence of renal damage (Foord, 1969). Simultaneous administration of gentamicin also enhances the nephrotoxicity.

Renal damage may rarely be observed with other members in this group, particularly with the combined use of cephalothin and gentamicin. The use of cephaloridine should therefore be avoided in patients with renal disease and those undergoing diuretic therapy. If antibiotics sensitivities demanded, cephalothin would appear to combine maximum antibiotic affectiveness and minimum toxicity providing it is not used with gentamicin.

Colisitin
In recent years this drug has also been incriminated in causing nephrotoxicity and again there appears to be some synergism when given in conjunction with cephaloridine.

Table 13.6 Amino acid preparations (contents per litre)

Preparation	Constit.	Mosmol	gN	Kcal	mmol/Na+	mmol/K+
Aminosol 1%	Casein hydrolysate 10%	925	12.8	330	160	0.15
Aminosol-fructose ethanol	Casein hydrolysate Fructose 15% Ethanol 2.5%	1043	4.25	880	54	0.15
Vamin	Synthetic L-am ac Fructose 10%	1275	9.4	650	50	20
Aminoplex-5	Synthetic L-am ac Sorbitol 10% Ethanol 5%	–	5	1000	35	15
Aminoplex-14	Synthetic L-am ac	961	13.4	340	35	30
Trophysan 10	Synthetic D&L am ac Sorbitol 10%	–	6.48	564	6	8
Trophysan Cole 10	Synthetic D&L am ac Sorbitol 10%	1416	12.13	724	10	8

Amphotericin B

This drug causes acute tubular damage and may produce a Fanconi-like syndrome with nephrocalcinosis. Renal damage following amphotericin B is not always reversible.

Tetracycline

It has long been known that the administration of tetracycline to patients with renal impairment leads to increasing uraemia, but unfortunately this is commonly still not realized (Phillips *et al.*, 1974). Tetracycline should certainly not be given to any patient with renal insufficiency and if absolutely necessary because of sensitivities, doxycyclin has been reported not to cause a rise in urea.

In summary it is of vital importance when administering *any* drug or combination of drugs to a patient with acute renal failure, to consider the possible nephrotoxic affects as well as deciding on the correct dose schedule both in quantity, and time between dosages, in order to gain maximum benefit from the drug without causing any untoward side effects. This not only applies to antibiotics but all drugs used in such a situation.

USE OF DRUGS IN PATIENTS WITH ESTABLISHED RENAL FAILURE

As a basic principle, it is of vital importance when administering any drug (not only antibiotics) to a patient with impaired renal function to consider the possible toxicity the impairment of excretion of the drug might have. Much work has been done on the modification of the dosage of anti-bacterial agents necessary in patients with renal failure if the development of high and toxic concentrations is to be avoided.

O'Grady reviewed this subject with particular reference to antibiotics and discussed the pharmacokinetics (O'Grady, 1971). In theory, as he demonstrated, it is fairly simple to contrive a regime which will maintain a safe and effective level of the desired antibiotic providing one can measure the concentration of the drug produced by a given dose and the rate at which the drug is eliminated.

This may be simply arranged by giving a primary dose sufficient to produce twice the effective level followed by half that dose at intervals corresponding with the half-life of the drug in the patient.

To put such a scheme into practice it is necessary to know the concentration of drug produced by a given dose, and the rate at which the drug is eliminated.

A useful rough guide may be 'arrived at' by means of some semi-log paper and two blood levels, one shortly after the loading dose and one a few hours later to give a rough idea of the half-life of the drug in that particular patient, but obviously in any drug likely to cause severe toxicity repeated estimations are essential, especially in the usual situation when the renal function may be altering from day to day.

There are now many papers available to give one a rough idea of the likely dosage and half-life of most antibiotics commonly used (Bennett *et al.*, 1970;

193

Kunin, 1967; Kunin, 1972; Bower *et al.*, 1973; Ogg *et al.*, 1968; Drug and
Therapeutic Bulletin, 1969). Any intensive care unit should have a comprehensive
list which are available from the above papers. However, it is still of vital importance in any drug which is likely to cause toxicity of any severity not to rely on
'rule of thumb' but to measure blood levels repeatedly.

One extra word of warning is that the doctor will commonly remember to
adjust the dosage of antibiotics and forget to adjust the dosage of other drugs
probably equally if not more important, e.g. digoxin.

SPECIAL SITUATIONS

Intravascular coagulation

The evidence that intravascular coagulation is an important factor in the
development of acute renal failure has already been discussed. In man the
deposition of fibrin within the kidney vasculature has been described in two
separate situations: those conditions in which the primary abnormality is diffuse
intravascular coagulation with the kidney as the principal end organ affected,
and those conditions in which a lesion of the glomerulo-capillaries may be the
primary abnormality with secondary deposition of fibrin.

(a) Renal disease associated with disseminated intravascular coagulation (See also Chapter 18)

Renal lesions have been demonstrated in a variety of conditions in which intravascular coagulation occurs such as haemolytic uraemia syndrome, thrombotic
thrombocytopaenic purpura, eclampsia, postpartum renal failure and acute
tubular necrosis secondary to haemorrhagic or septicaemic shock. The histological changes observed in these different conditions may vary in degree from
minimal glomerular lesions to diffuse glomerular coagulation and Kincaid-Smith
(1972) postulated that the extent of the glomerular lesions may depend on the
degree and duration of intra-vascular coagulation and the effectiveness of the
local fibrinolytic activity. There is considerable circumstantial evidence supporting a causal relationship between intravascular coagulation and acute renal
failure. Intravascular coagulation is a prominent feature of shock, septicaemia,
septic abortion and postpartum haemorrhage all common antecedents to acute
tubular necrosis.

In haemolytic uraemia syndrome and thrombotic thrombocytopaenia an
abnormal immunological response to a virus or bacterial antigen has been
postulated.

During pregnancy the kidney seems especially susceptible to damage by
mechanisms involving intravascular coagulation and in postpartum renal
failure, an antibody to the products of conception has been suggested.

The classic model associating diffuse intravascular coagulation with renal
disease in animals is the induction of a generalized Shwartzman reaction in
rabbits which is induced by two doses of endotoxin given 24 hours apart, the

second injection precipitating diffuse intravascular coagulation with widespread thrombi in arterioles and capillaries but especially in the kidney. Given the observed association between disseminated intravascular coagulation and acute renal failure and recognizing the possible role of vaso-constriction in tubular necrosis a unifying hypothesis has recently been reviewed by Kincaid-Smith (1972). She suggests that in clinical or experimental shock and in the generalized Shwartzman reaction two important chains of reaction develop. Catecholamines are released into circulation, and disseminated intravascular coagulation develops. It is postulated that the vascular effects of the catecholamines are of the dominant importance and that reduced blood flow with irregular constrictions and dilatations of small vessels occurs. As a result this leads to local thrombus formation in a setting of disseminated intravascular coagulation. Deposition of thrombi distal to areas of segmental constriction is associated with further vaso-constriction and local activation of fibrin deposition. The renin angiotensin system may also play a part in cortical vaso-constriction and this too would predispose to deposition of fibrin in the micro circulation. The subsequent course of the disease; the extent to which thrombi will be formed; the vascular occlusion occur; and proliferative glomerular lesions develop; varies considerably among the different diseases, thus the potential for rapid recovery of kidney function and acute tubular necrosis is usually good. Recovery from pre-eclamptic toxaemia is rapid although histological changes may persist for many months; long term follow up of the haemolytic uraemia syndrome has shown full recovery in less than 50% while some patients have severe progressive uraemia: and patients with postpartum renal failure follow an almost universally fatal course unless the condition can be reversed by heparin.

Thus there seems little doubt that intravascular coagulation occurs to a greater or lesser extent in these various conditions but controversy still exists as to the part it plays in both initiating and maintaining the functional changes of acute renal failure. It would seem extremely unlikely that intravascular coagulation would make the same contribution to the pathogenesis of acute renal failure in each and all of these quite different situations and therefore similarly anticoagulant therapy may or may not affect renal function depending on the importance of intravascular coagulation in the particular situation. Success has been claimed in the haemolytic uraemia syndrome but high recovery rate without anticoagulants has also been reported. Improvement in function has been reported in severe pre-eclampsia and septic abortion and impressive results have been obtained in patients with postpartum renal failure.

However, once again no controlled trial of anticoagulant therapy has been carried out and it is not possible to define the true value of this treatment and it would seem that the case for anticoagulants alone or in combination with anti-thrombotic agents remains to be proved, though on present evidence anticoagulation would seem mandatory in patients with severe postpartum renal failure in whom the prognosis is otherwise universally bad.

Malignant hypertension. Oliguric renal failure is a common feature of malignant hypertension and recognition that this is often associated with intravascular coagulation suggests a rapid development of 'fibrinoid necrosis' in the small vessels of the kidney. This is a consequence of the deposition of fibrin or fibrin degradation products in the vessel wall. On this basis treatment with anti-coagulants has been used and rapid improvement in renal function has been claimed in some cases but not in others. However, the very real hazards of haemorrhage in patients with accelerated hypertension discourage most physicians from using anticoagulants at least until the hypertension is controlled with hypotensive agents. However, the diagnosis is important to make, as recently it has been reported that the local use of anticoagulation via a catheter in the renal artery has lead to some improvement in renal function, and in patients presenting with malignant hypertension there is some argument for urgent renal biopsy and renal angiography when, if the glomeruli appear to be well preserved in the biopsy specimen there may be an indication for intrarenal anticoagulation.

(b) Primary renal diseases with fibrin deposition

Interest in the role of fibrin deposition in the pathogenesis of glomerulonephritis stems from the observation that anticoagulant treatment markedly modifies the renal lesion in experimental nephritis and there is now evidence that patients with rapidly progressive glomerulonephritis, particularly with the presence of epithelial crescents on renal biopsy may well have an element of intravascular coagulation exacerbating the disease. Increased levels of fibrin degradation products in the serum have been reported to correlate well with evidence of active disease. It is postulated that the primary factor in the glomerulonephritis is capillary wall damage due to immunological injury and that this is followed by local deposition of fibrin and platelets (Kincaid-Smith, 1972).

On the basis of these observations, and the uniformly bad prognosis in these patients Kincaid-Smith and her colleagues pioneered the treatment of such cases with anticoagulants (Kincaid-Smith *et al.*, 1968; 1970) and impressive results were observed by Kincaid-Smith though these have not always been confirmed by other observers and there is need for carefully controlled prospective trial of anticoagulant therapy in such cases.

Treatment with anticoagulants and antithrombotic agents have also been given to patients with polyarteritis and systemic sclerosis with evidence of microangiopathic haemolytic anaemia but again further evidence is required to justify the use of potentially dangerous treatment in patients with connective tissue disease and evidence of intravascular coagulation.

Acute uraemia associated with liver disease (See also Chapter 17)

Many patients will be seen particularly in intensive care units who have jaundice and uraemia. These patients are frequently labelled 'hepato-renal syndrome'. Whilst there is undoubtedly a syndrome in which oliguric renal failure often rapidly developing, complicates severe decompensated hepatic cirrhosis, it is vitally important that all patients with jaundice and renal failure do not get labelled with this 'syndrome'. The hepato-renal syndrome usually occurs as already stated when the cirrhosis is severely decompensated and is usually a fatal complication. The pathogenesis of the true hepato-renal syndrome remains obscure. There is no significant histological change in the kidneys at post-mortem and it is felt most likely that the oliguric renal failure observed results from redistribution of blood away from the cortex due to increased cortical vascular resistance (Epstein *et al.*, 1970). The cause of this increased resistance is not known although increased sympathetic tone has been postulated. However, phentolamine infusion into the renal artery failed to alter the blood flow. There is little doubt however that the effect is due to a functional circulatory cause rather than to any intrinsic renal damage. The syndrome is often precipitated by fluid volume shifts following paracentesis or diuretic therapy and the patients usually maintain a concentrated urine with low sodium concentration supporting a functional circulatory basis. Several recent investigations have lent considerable support to this concept and kidneys taken from patients who have died from severe cirrhosis with the 'hepato-renal syndrome' and acute renal failure have been used very successfully on occasion for transplantation. It is therefore important to exclude other causes of a raised urea in patients with a liver disease before labelling the patient as having hepato-renal syndrome.

Classic acute intrinsic renal failure (acute tubular necrosis) may develop in patients with parenchymal liver disease as a result of severe haemorrhage or hypovolaemia and quite often this haemorrhage may be occult unless searched for carefully, particularly in a patient who is jaundiced and ill and therefore it is important to look for signs of hypovolaemia especially if the patient may have oedema due to hypoproteinaemia. Once again it is vitally important to check the blood pressure lying and standing, to get serial measurements of haemoglobin, to watch for blood loss which would give the patient a high protein meal if they bleed into the gastrointestinal tract and thus raise the urea due to pre-renal causes all of which are completely correctable if observed in time. It is worth while noting here that cholecystographic and cholangiographic agents probably damage the kidney, directly causing acute tubular necrosis and high doses in hepatic disease may potentiate the renal damage.

Acute interstitial nephritis

This form of oliguric renal failure is probably often misdiagnosed as acute tubular necrosis as it closely resembles this in clinical course. The disease most commonly results from exposure to drugs classically Phenindione or Penicillin though there is often other, usually cutaneous, evidence of hypersensitivity. Interstitial nephritis is also seen associated with viral infections and in acute exanthemata.

Recovery of renal function is usual after withdrawal of the drug which has precipitated the hypersensitivity reaction. Occasionally corticosteroids have been used to accelerate the recovery.

The mechanism of acute renal failure in interstitial nephritis is uncertain but in the analogous situation of transplant rejection there are haemodynamic changes similar to those in acute tubular necrosis.

Renal biopsy shows the tubules are separated by oedema and a cellular infiltrate often with abundant eosinophilia. The prognosis is good and the main clinical problem is to distinguish it from anuria caused by a sensitivity angiitis (e.g. from sulphonomides) which carried a much graver prognosis.

Weil's disease

The clinical picture seen with Weil's disease is, so far as the renal side is concerned, extremely variable, much more so than the classical accounts suggest. It may vary from slight proteinuria to severe acute renal failure. It is therefore always important to ask the appropriate direct questions about a patient presenting with jaundice and renal failure and to send off the appropriate investigations to exclude this disease. One possible clue to this diagnosis is that the degree of hyperbilirubinaemia is often much more severe than the abnormalities in other liver function tests. However, it is obviously important to exclude this by checking the antibodies as the disease is potentially reversible and although permanent interstitial scarring may occur in survivors, normal renal function is to be expected.

Glomerulonephritis

Acute renal failure severe enough for the patient to become oliguric and possibly require dialysis only affects a very small percentage of patients with acute glomerulonephritis but is obviously responsible for most of the early mortality in this disease. However, as therapeutic benefit has been claimed from corticosteroids (Nakamoto et al., 1965) cyclophosphamide, heparin and dipyridamol (Kincaid-Smith et al., 1968) and because management may well be very different than management from a patient similarly oliguric from acute tubular necrosis, if acute nephritis is suspected early renal biopsy may be indicated. Unfortunately most claims of therapeutic benefit by whatever drugs have been on the basis of uncontrolled trials or case reports, rather than any systematic controlled trial. It should be noted that renal function has returned to normal after periods of oliguria of a considerably prolonged period without specific therapy, well over 28 days, but the chances of recovery diminish with increasing length of oliguria (Persoff, 1965; Connoly et al., 1968).

Episodes of acute renal failure may also complicate nephrotic syndrome with minimal change nephritis and these episodes are not glomerular in origin and may be due to prolonged hypovolaemia (Connoly et al., 1968) or possibly water intoxication (Hamburger et al., 1968).

Other important and treatable causes of glomerulonephritis which must always be excluded are systemic lupus, and sub-acute bacterial endocarditis.

Most cases of subacute bacterial endocarditis producing severe renal failure are due to immune complex disease secondary to the organism causing the SBE and elimination of the antigen, i.e. the causative organism, has resulted in improvement in renal function, similar to that described in children with 'shunt' nephritis when the nephritis is an immunological reaction to a staphlococcal infection on the shunt, and the renal failure has improved on re-operating on the child removing the infected shunt and replacing it with a new one. The measurement of complement is helpful in diagnosis and management of such cases.

Pyelonephritis

Acute renal failure following severe pyelonephritis is rare unless the pyelonephritis is complicated by papillary necrosis. This should always be suspected if there is an abrupt decline in function in a patient with acute pyelonephritis and it can sometimes be confirmed by the demonstration of a ring sign or cavitation of the papilla on intravenous pyelography. Papillary necrosis is of course more commonly seen as a complication of analgesic abuse but in the acute situation may complicate diabetes, obstruction or pyelonephritis. Bilateral papillary necrosis may also complicate gastroenteritis in infancy and in this situation particularly it is compatible with excellent recovery of renal function.

Myelomatosis

Myeloma can result in acute renal failure by at least four different mechanisms: (a) Plasma cell infiltration (b) hyperuricaemia (c) hypercalcaemia (d) hyperviscosity tubular blockage with casts and Bence Jones protein. Much more commonly the renal failure of myelomatosis is slowly progressive and presents with chronic renal failure. However, acute failure precipitated by tubular blockage of Bence Jones protein is probably precipitated by dehydration and it is this dehydration which is more likely to be to blame than the much over emphasized association with intravenous pyelography. With modern contrast media the risk of precipitation of mucoprotein and development of acute renal failure is likely to be very small even in the presence of renal disease provided dehydration is avoided.

Obstruction to urinary out-flow

When presented with any patient with acute renal failure it is obviously of vital importance to exclude any obstructive element which usually is completely reversible, perhaps foremost among those conditions which must be excluded is retroperitoneal fibrosis. Although this classically will present with acute anuria in a patient who has complained of back pain for some months and who on investigation is found to have a raised urea and high ESR and hydronephrotic kidneys with obstruction on IVP; occasionally a patient will present with what appears to be end stage chronic renal failure still passing urine and it is essential to exclude this diagnosis by bulb ureterogram (rather than retrograde pyelogram) in order to make sure that a potentially curable form of renal failure is not overlooked.

The retroperitoneal fibrosis may be idiopathic or associated with drugs such as methysergide or practolol, associated with an aortic aneurysm, or neoplastic disease.

Other causes of obstructive uropathy causing acute renal failure include hypercalcaemic crisis, particularly if this is treated with phosphate infusion when it is thought the probable cause of the acute renal failure is proximal tubular damage and obstruction of the lumina with cellular debris (Duffy *et al.*, 1971).

The usual effects of hypercalcaemia are damage to the loop of Henley causing polyuria, intrarenal hydronephrosis and chronic renal failure.

'Osmotic nephrosis' has been described as the appearance of the proximal tubules whose cells are swollen to several times their normal size and appear to obliterate the lumen. This condition has been described after intravenous administration of large doses of low molecular weight Dextran and occasionally Mannitol. These descriptions have always followed very large doses of these drugs and given usually to patients in whom there may be other possible causes of acute renal failure but in a few patients no other explanation could be found other than the administration of Dextran or Mannitol. There is therefore need for caution with these substances particularly if infused for long periods in large doses.

Distal tubular cast formation may play a part in acute renal failure following shock particularly with crush injuries and myoglobin casts are a prominent feature of renal damage that follows muscular injury even without shock due to a wide variety of insults including generalized fits of a prolonged nature.

Haemoglobin casts are found in the kidney when acute renal failure follows a transfusion reaction, blackwater fever, sickle-cell crisis or haemolysis from various causes. However, it is unlikely that the haemoglobin released plays a major part in the damage and in almost all situations alternative explanations exist; although this may be playing a minor part.

Crystaluria and obstruction of the collecting ducts, pelvis and ureters was a common cause of acute renal failure in the early days of sulphonamide therapy. Drug crystaluria is now however, rare though uric acid crystaluria following a rise in plasma uric acid to very high levels such as in the course of leukaemia, lymphoma or rapidly growing neoplasm, particularly in the few days after treatment of these with cytotoxic drugs, is common. This can of course be completely prevented by giving Allopurinol before the anti-tumour therapy and making sure the urine is kept alkaline. The established condition responds well to dialysis.

The last important cause of obstructive uropathy is ureteric obstruction and the commonest cause of this other than retroperitoneal fibrosis is neoplasm or possibly ureteric calculi.

In any case of suspected obstructive uropathy it is obviously important to exclude this as soon as possible in order to get a good return of function. Recovery of renal function can be expected if the obstruction is removed early and good function has returned after periods of complete ureteric occlusion up to four weeks, with some function returning after occlusion for up to six months (Brunshwig *et al.*, 1964). *Total* anuria raises the suspicion of obstruction.

Good pastures syndrome

This syndrome is the picture of acute nephritis often rapidly progressive associated with haemoptysis. The definitive diagnosis can only be made by renal biopsy and examination of this with immunofluorescence, when the linear pattern of anti-glomerular basement membrane antibody can be seen.

Although this is a rare disease it has become of major importance now to diagnose this condition early as plasma-pharesis has been recently described as causing marked improvement in a number of cases. It is therefore of vital importance to consider this diagnosis early in any atypical cause of oliguria, in order to perform a biopsy to exclude it, as the longer the immunological reaction goes on, the more renal damage will be caused and the less renal function will be available following treatment.

REFERENCES

Bennett, W. M., Singer, I. and Coggins, C. H. (1970), A Practical Guide to Drug Usage in Adult Patients with Impaired renal function. *J. Am. med. Ass.*, **214**, No. 8, 1463–1475.

Berlyne, G. M., Bazzard, F. J., Booth, E. M., Janabi, K. and Shaw, A. B. (1967), The dietary management of acute renal failure. *Q. J. Med.*, **36**, 59–83.

Berlyne, G. M., Jones, J. H., Hewitt, V. and Nilwarangkur, S. (1964), Protein loss in peritoneal dialysis. *Lancet*, i, 738–741.

Berlyne, G. M., Lee, H. A., Giordano, C., de Pascale, C. and Esposito, R. (1967), Amino acid loss in peritoneal dialysis. *Lancet*, i, 1339–1341.

Bowersox, D. W., Winterbaver, R. H., Stewart, G. L., Orme, B. and Barrow, E. (1973), Isoniazid dosage in patients with renal failure. *N. Eng. J. Med.*, iii, 84–87.

Brown, J. J., Gleadle, R. I., Lawson, D. H., Lever, A. F., Linton, A. L., Macadam, R. F., Prentice, E., Robertson, J. I. S. and Tree, M. (1970), Renin and acute renal failure; studies in man. *Brit. med. J.*, 1, 253.

Brunschwig, A., Barber, H. R. K. and Roberts, S. (1964), Return of renal function after varying periods of ureteral occlusion; A clinical study. *J. Am. med. Ass.*, **188**, 5.

Bull, G. M., Joekes, A. M. and Lowe, K. G. (1950), Renal function studies in Acute Tubular Necrosis. *Clin. Sci.*, 9, 379.

Clarkson, A. R., MacDonald, M. K., Fuster, V., Cash, J. D. and Robson, J. S. (1970), Glomerular coagulation in acute ischaemic renal failure. *Q. J. Med.*, 39, 585.

Coleho, J. B. and Bradley, S. E. (1964), Function of the nephron population during haemorrhagic hypotension in the dog with special reference to the effects of osmotic diuretics. *J. clin. Invest.*, **43**, 386–400.

Connolly, M. E., Wrong, O. M. and Jones, N. F. (1968), Reversible renal failure in idiopathic nephrotic syndrome with minimal glomerular changes. *Lancet*, i, 665.

Dawson, J. L. (1964), Jaundice and anoxic renal damage: protective effect of mannitol. *Brit. med. J.*, 1, 810–811.

Doyle, F. H., Sherwood, T., Steiner, R. E., Breckenridge, A. and Dollery, C. T. (1967), Large dose urography. Is there an optimum dose? *Lancet*, ii, 964–966.

Drug and Therapeutics Bulletin (1969), Prescribing for patients with renal failure. 7, No. 14, 53–56.

Duffy, J. L., Suzuki, Y. and Churg, J. (1971), Acute calcium nephropathy. Early proximal tubular changes in the rat kidney. *Arch. Path.*, 91, 340.

Epstein, M., Berk, D. P., Hollenberg, N. D., Adams, D. R., Chalmers, T. C., Abrams, H. L. and Merrill, J. P. (1970), Renal Failure in the patient with cirrhosis. The role of active vasoconstriction. *Am. J. Med.*, 49, 175–185.

Foord, R. D. (1969), Progress in anti-microbial and anti-cancer therapy. Sixth International Congress of Chemotherapy. Tokyo, 1, 597.

Fry, I. K. and Cattell, W. R. (1971), Radiology in the diagnosis of renal failure. *Brit. med. Bull.*, 27, 148–152.

Fry, I. K. and Cattell, W. R. (1972), The nephrographic pattern during excretion urography. *Brit. med. Bull.*, 28, 227–232.

Gjessing, . . (1968), Addition of amino acids to peritoneal dialysis fluid. *Lancet*, i, 1123–1126.

Gullick, H. D. and Raisz, L. G. (1960), Changes in renal concentrating ability associated with major surgical procedure. *N. Eng. J. Med.*, 262, 1309.

Haanen, C., Holdrinet, A. and Wijdeveld, P. (1970), Introvascular clotting and acute renal failure. *Scand. J. Haematol.*, Supplement 13, 337.

Hamburger, J., Richet, G., Crosnier, J., Funck-Brentano, J. L., Antoine, B., Ducrot, H., Mery, J. P. and de Nontera, H. (1968), *Nephrology* (translated by A. Walsh). Saunders, Philadelphia.

Hollenberg, N. K., Epstein, M., Rosen, S. M., Basch, R. I., Oken, D. E. and Merrill, J. P. (1968), Acute oliguric renal failure in man; evidence for preferential cortical ischaemia. *Medicine* (Baltimore), 47, 455.

Kincaid-Smith, P. (1972), Coagulation and Renal Disease. *Kidney Int.*, 2, 183–190.

Kincaid-Smith, P., Laver, M. S. and Fairley, K. F. (1970), Dipyramedole and anticoagulants in renal disease due to glomerular and vascular lesions: a new approach to therapy. *Med. J. Aust.*, 1, 145–151.

Kincaid-Smith, P., Saker, B. M. and Fairley, K. F. (1968), Anticoagulants in 'irreversible' acute renal failure. *Lancet*, ii, 1360–1363.

Kunin, C. M. (1972), Antibiotic usage in patients with renal impairment. *Hospital Practice*, 1, 141–149.

Kunin, C. M. (1967), A guide to use of antibiotics in patients with renal disease. *Ann. Int. Med.*, 67, No. 1, 151–158.

Lee, H. A. (1974), Intravenous Nutrition. *Brit. J. Hosp. Med.*, 1, 719–728.

Luke, R. G., Briggs, J. D., Allison, M. E. M. and Kennedy, A. C. (1970), Factors determining the response to mannitol in acute renal failure. *Am. J. med. Sci.*, 259, 168–174.

Luke, R. G. and Kennedy, A. C. (1967), Prevention and early management of acute renal failure, *Postgrad. med. J.*, **43**, 280–289.

Miles, B. E., Paten, A. and de Wardener, H. E. (1954), Maximum urine concentration. *Brit. med. J.*, ii, 901.

Milne, M. D. (1967), Drugs, poisons and the kidney. In *Renal Disease*, (Black, D. A. K., ed.) p. 546. Blackwell Scientific Publications, Oxford.

Mueller, C. B., Surtshin, A., Carlin, M. R. and White, H. L. (1951), Glomerular and tubular influences on sodium and water excretion. *Am. J. Physiol.*, **165**, 411–418.

Murphy, G. P., Gagnon, J. A. and Teschan, P. E. (1963), Renal haemodynamic effect of mannitol in normotension and hypotension. *Surg. Forum*, **14**, 99.

Nakamoto, S., Dunea, G., Koleff, W. J. and McCormack, L. J. (1965), Treatment of oliguric glomerulonephritis with dialysis and steroid. *Ann. Int. Med.*, **63**, 359.

O'Grady, F. (1971), Antibiotics in renal failure. *Brit. med. Bull.*, **27**, 142–147.

Ogg, C. S., Toseland, P. A., Cameron, J. S. (1968), Pulmonary Tuberculosis in a patient on intermittent Haemodialysis. *Brit. med. J.*, ii, 283–284.

Persoff, D. (1965), Recovery from prolonged oliguria in acute glomerulonephritis. *Lancet*, i, 347.

Phillips, M. E., Eastwood, J. B., Curtis, J. R., Goner, P. E. and de Wardener, H. E. (1974), Tetracycline poisoning in Renal Failure. *Brit. med. J.*, **2**, 149–151.

Platts, M. M. (1966), Electrolyte excretion in Uraemia. *Clin. Sci.*, **30**, 453–471.

Schreiner, G. E. and Maher, J. F. (1965), Drugs and the Kidney. *Ann. N. Y. Acad. Sci.*, **123**, 326–332.

Shaldon, S., Sheville, E. and Rae, A. I. (1964), Angiography in acute renal failure. *Clin. Radiol.*, **15**, 123.

Vassalli, P. and Richet, G. (1960), Nécrose corticale et insufficiance rénale aiguë des états de choc. *Proc. 1st Int. Cong. Nephrol.*, pp. 236–302.

Wardle, E. N. and Taylor, G. (1968), Fibrin breakdown products and fibrinolysis in renal disease. *J. clin. Path.*, **21**, 140.

Wilson, D. M., Turner, D. R., Cameron, J. S., Ogg, C. S., Brown, C. B. and Chantler, C. (1976), Value of renal biopsy in acute intrinsic renal failure. *Brit. med. J.*, **2**, 459–461.

Wilson, D. R., Thiel, G., Arce, M. L. and Oken, D. E. (1967), Glycerol–induced acute renal failure in the rat–III Micropuncture study of the effect of mannitol and isoteric saline on individual nephron function.

FOURTEEN

Metabolic disorders

DIABETIC COMA

Under this heading we will discuss the management of three clinical conditions, though it is very important to appreciate that each may occur in isolation, or more commonly, in co-existence with each other.
(1) Diabetic keto-acidosis
(2) Hyperosmolar non-ketotic diabetic coma
(3) Lactic acidosis

DIABETIC KETO-ACIDOSIS

Diabetic keto-acidosis remains a clinical challenge that requires the ultimate in care and attention—despite modern advances in understanding this metabolic disaster, overall mortality remains between 5–10%. Such patients must be managed in an environment where accurate fluid balance estimation is routine, where biochemistry is rapidly available day and night, and where vital functions can be monitored.

Definition

'Coma', or lack of consciousness, is not an essential pre-requisite of this condition; nor is a high blood sugar; nor a low bicarbonate in isolation. Diabetes becomes a grave threat to life when a number of biochemical abnormalities coalesce.

The following abnormalities have been used to define serious keto-acidosis.
(1) Hyperglycaemia (mean between 27–45 mmol/l)
(2) Bicarbonate less than 9 mmol/l: Hyperventilation
(3) Plasma hyperosmolarity (above 330 mosmol/l)
(4) Disturbance of consciousness
(5) Arterial pH less than 7.3
(6) Positive plasma reaction with Ketostix.

Patho-physiology

The sequence of events in diabetic keto-acidosis is outlined in Figure 14.1. It will be noted that hyperosmolarity is present in all types of diabetic coma.

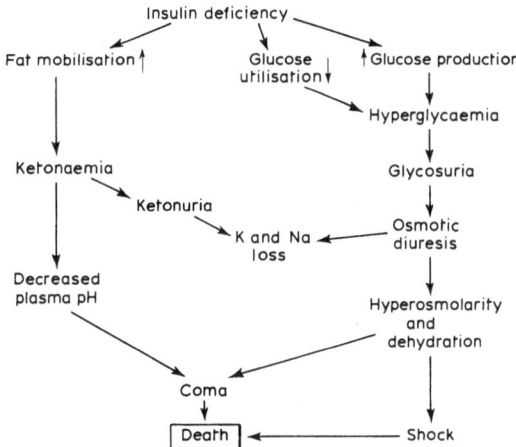

Fig. 14.1 The sequence of events in diabetic keto-acidosis (From Sodeman and Sodeman Pathologic Physiology **V** *Ed Saunders, London, 1974).*

Causes

The causes of diabetic keto-acidosis are often clear, but it should be remembered that coma may be the presenting symptom in the young and also in the elderly. Failure to take insulin is unusual, except where an established diabetic develops an acute gastro-intestinal disturbance with anorexia, nausea and perhaps vomiting; and decides himself, or unfortunately is badly advised to reduce or even omit his insulin because he is not eating. In general sick diabetics require more insulin not less. Infection is a common association, often in the urinary tract, and primary symptoms of this may be absent. In elderly patients progressive arteriosclerosis may lead to gross dietary indiscretions such as the consumption of vast amounts of glucose-containing liquids, e.g. Lucozade.

Clinical picture

Most cases of diabetic ketosis are preceded by a period of increased thirst and polyuria, but, of course, this history may not be available if the patient is first seen with alterations in level of consciousness. The presentation may be very acute, without preceding symptoms, in children. Vomiting and abdominal pain follow, the latter symptom being occasionally severe enough to mimic an acute abdominal surgical emergency. On examination the three cardinal physical signs are:
    (1) dehydration
    (2) hyperventilation
    (3) alteration in level of consciousness
    The blood pressure is low and the pulse volume decreased. It is unwise to rely on smelling acetone on the breath as the ability to recognize this odour is not universal and may be impaired in heavy smokers.

Biochemical findings

Hyperglycaemia

The absolute level of the blood sugar is not of prime importance. Severe metabolic abnormalities can be present even with quite modest increase in blood sugar; and the converse also occurs (i.e. high blood sugar without significant acidosis etc.). Very high levels (over 55 mmol/l) are associated with increased mortality.

Acidosis

Bicarbonate. The serum bicarbonate will be reduced though the level does not correlate well with the severity of the ketosis. In general, levels will be below 15 mmol/l, levels below 9 mmol/l indicate a severe acidosis.

Ketone bodies. Unfortunately estimation of serum ketone bodies is not in the routine repertoire of many biochemistry departments. As a guide to the severity of the condition, and to exclude hyperosmolar non-ketotic diabetic coma, this is a most important investigation. Rapid ketone body estimation can be achieved by the use of Ketostix. In this technique plasma is applied to the test strip and readings (0–+++) taken at 15 seconds.

Where +++ occurs the plasma can be diluted 1 in 2 with tap water and further readings taken.

The results of this method correlate well with the level of aceto-acetate, but other ketone bodies do not react as well.

Table 14.1 Ketostix reaction

Ketone body	Ketostix reaction
Aceto-acetate	good
Acetone	weak
3-hydroxybutyrate	none

The correlation, therefore, with total blood ketone levels may be poor, where large amounts of 3-hydroxybutyrate are present. This investigation should be considered in conjunction with arterial pH—a discrepancy suggesting either the presence of large amounts of 3-hydroxybutyrate, or lactic acid. It is important that the Ketostix are stored properly as inaccurate results occur when they have been allowed to get damp. However, this method still remains useful for the assessment of the severity of the metabolic disorder (Alberti and Hockaday, 1972).

Table 14.2 Values of ketone bodies in diabetic coma

Aceto-acetate	over 1.5 mmol/l (Normal 0.10 mmol/l)
3-hydroxybutyrate	greater than 5 mmol/l
Acetone	greater than 5.0 mmol/l (Normal 0.03 mmol/l)

Arterial pH. This will be lowered. The characteristic acidotic respiration usually appears when the pH falls below 7.25.

Lactic acid. Lactic acidosis is described below. It is appropriate, however, to point out here that lactic acidosis, although liable to occur in many seriously ill patients from other causes, is more common in diabetics, even if not on diguanide therapy (see below).

Significant lactic acidosis is said to be present when the lactic acid is above 7.0 mmol/l and the lactate/pyruvate ratio exceeds 10/1. It should be suspected when severe acidosis is present without sufficiently high levels of ketone bodies. However, in the majority of cases the lactic acid level does not contribute greatly to the acidosis, being around 3.0 mmol/l. It should be noted that lactate levels *rise* after administration of insulin in diabetic keto-acidosis and this is one of the reasons for avoiding electrolyte solutions containing lactate in treatment (Watkins *et al.*, 1969).

Hyperosmolality

This occurs in all cases of diabetic coma, but is greatly raised in non-ketotic hyperosmolar coma, where not only is the blood sugar grossly raised but also there is a high blood urea and hypernatraemia.

The osmolality can be measured direct or derived from the following formula:

Plasma osmolality = 2(Na + K) (mmol/l) + blood glucose (mmol/l)
(mosmol/kg) + blood urea (mmol/l)

Normal osmolality is 280–295 mosmol/l.

Electrolytes

Blood urea is raised in proportion to the dehydration, markedly so in hyperosmolar cases. It should also be noted that impaired renal function may be present *before* the onset of the acute metabolic disturbance.

Sodium will be either normal or low, but high in non-ketotic hyperosmolar coma.

Potassium may be normal, raised or low (see below).

Haematology

The haemoglobin and PCV will reflect dehydration. The white cell count is almost invariably raised, with a polymorph leucocytosis. This may be due to infection, but also occurs when no infection can be demonstrated.

Urine

This will contain sugar and ketones. The presence of albumin may indicate pre-existing renal disease or infection. A centrifuged deposit should always be examined for pus cells. Urine volume will be reduced in most cases of keto-acidosis.

Management of diabetic keto-acidosis (Hockaday and Alberti, 1972; Malins, 1971; Page *et al.*, 1974; Kidson *et al.*, 1974; Semple *et al.*, 1974; Moseley, 1975)

The management of diabetic keto-acidosis is outlined in Table 14.4. Further details are appended after the table. It will be noted that two alternative regimes are outlined, although the principles of management remain similar.

Table 14.3 Principles of management of diabetic keto-acidosis

(1)	Control of blood sugar – Insulin*
(2)	Correction of dehydration
(3)	Electrolyte management

* N.B. Must always be soluble insulin

Further notes on Table 14.4

(1) *Gastric aspiration* Diabetic keto-acidosis is accompanied by acute atony of the stomach. A common cause of death is aspiration of gastric contents. A naso-gastric tube must be left *in situ* with continuous aspiration until the crisis is over.

(2) *Catheterization* Although catheters, especially in-dwelling catheters, are known to produce a great risk of urinary tract infection, and in general is to be avoided—accurate assessment of urinary output, together with urinanalysis is essential in the management of diabetic ketosis. In the unlikely event of a fully conscious and co-operative patient, catheterization may be avoided. Under other circumstances it is mandatory.

(3) *ECG monitoring* Dysrhythmias are common in diabetic coma and are often related to potassium deficiency. Although monitoring cannot replace frequent estimations of the serum potassium it is a useful adjunct and the early changes of hypokalaemia (see Chapter 7) may be recognized in time to avert a fatal dys-rhythmia.

(4) *Oxygen* If the arterial pO_2 is less than 10 KPa.

(5) *Antibiotics* As infection is such a frequent cause of diabetic ketosis it would appear reasonable to recommend antibiotics as routine. However, many cases are precipitated by viral infections. Antibiotics should be reserved for cases where bacterial infection is present, e.g. in the urinary tract, lungs or skin. Indiscriminate use of antibiotics in the Intensive Therapy Unit will only lead to long-term problems (see Chapter 25).

Table 14.4 Management of diabetic keto-acidosis

Preliminary investigation management	Insulin therapy	Low dose	0	2	4	6	8 hrs	
(1) Blood analysis U+E, Hb, PCV, Bl. sugar, ketones, pH, osmolarity	2 hourly blood sugar U+E estimations	Intravenous	6 units/hour by continuous infusion change to s/c insulin after 8 hours or when BS < 200 mg %					8–36 hours sliding scale s.c. insulin
(2) Urinalysis sugar, ketones, protein, microscopy		Intramuscular	20 units stat – then 10 units hourly as above					2–3 days insulin tds–bd

Fluid and electrolytes			
N/saline 1l in 30 min 500ml in 30 min 1l 2–3 hourly } Total 6–7 l in 24 hours			
N/2 saline if hypernatraemia after 4 hours or osmolality > 330 mosol/kg			
Potassium 1G ≡ 13 mmol first hour 2G ≡ 26 mmol hourly afterwards			
Dextrose 5% when blood sugar < 11 mmol/l			

[Average deficit water 6 l
Na^+ 500 mmol/l
Cl^- 400 mmol/l
K^+ 350 mmol/l]

(3) Aspirate stomach leave tube in situ.

(4) Catheterise (unless urine is voided normally)

(5) ECG monitor

(6) 100% oxygen

(7) Antibiotics if evidence of bacterial infection

Indications for bicarbonate

Severe acidosis pH<7
Severe acidotic symptoms
100 mmol bicarbone max. (Danger of hypokalaemia)

Frequent check on
(1) Urine output   (2) K   (3) U+E

209

(6) *Insulin therapy.* It would not be appropriate here to discuss the pharmaco-kinetics or biochemistry of insulin in detail. There is no agreement as to the optimum dose of insulin, or by what route it should be given, or at what intervals. Low dose insulin therapy is a recent introduction for the treatment of diabetic keto-acidosis and in a relatively short period of time has acquired a general acceptance which suggests that it is simple and highly effective (Editorial, B.M.J., 1977).

(a) *Conventional.* Soluble insulin is the only type of insulin that is suitable for use in this condition (very occasionally in patients known to be sensitive to standard soluble insulin, neutral soluble insulin can be used—it has exactly the same actions as standard soluble insulin). The intravenous routine is conventional although it is known that the half-life of insulin in the plasma is only a few minutes. Certainly no reliance must be placed on *large* doses of insulin intra-venously alone. In the shocked, hypovolaemic and dehydrated patient the subcutaneous route gives unreliable absorption. For these reasons in the initial 8 hours of therapy it is suggested that at least 50% of the dose is given intra-muscularly.

Hypoglycaemia is likely to occur unless frequent blood sugar estimations are being performed. The high dose insulin treatment of diabetic keto-acidosis has now been replaced by the low-dose technique described below and is mentioned because of historical interest.

(b) *Low dose insulin.* It has long been known that insulin requirements drop if frequent doses are given. This has been extended to the treatment of diabetic keto-acidosis. In every sense it is a more physiological approach to a very difficult problem. In normal subjects maximum hypoglycaemic activity is achieved by blood insulin levels of between 20–200 μU/ml and the same levels have been found to be effective in uncontrolled diabetics. By giving 6 units/hour intra-venously a plasma steady-state level of 100 μU/ml is achieved. However, there are difficulties associated with low dose intravenous insulin infusion. The dose must be monitored accurately and this can be difficult if a syringe pump, or infusion pump is not available. A paediatric giving set can be used. Another problem with intravenous insulin infusions is that the insulin can be adsorbed onto the plastic of the giving set. This can be prevented by the addition of human albumin 0.5 g/100 ml of the infusion. This should not, however, be a serious problem if excessively dilute insulin solutions are avoided. Concentra-tions of 1 unit of insulin in 1-10 ml saline produce a negligible loss.

Low dose intramuscular insulin. 10 units hourly—has been shown to be equally effective and the difficulties of insulin infusion are avoided.

Using this technique, the same dose is given to all patients and the risks of hypoglycaemia and hypokalaemia are considerably reduced. The method has the great advantage of simplicity.

However, frequent monitoring of blood sugar, serum potassium and urine output are mandatory and the technique's basic simplicity does not mean that diabetic keto-acidosis should be relegated to the position of a less demanding emergency.

(7) *Fluid and electrolytes.* The average deficits are stated in Table 14.4. There are innumerable electrolyte cocktails recommended for treatment of diabetic ketosis. In our view there is no place for the use of these solutions in a hospital where junior staff change frequently and it is suggested that routine i.v. fluids available in all hospitals should be used, with additions where appropriate. N/Saline is the i.v. fluid of choice.

Although it is known that there is proportionally more water than electrolyte deficit there are risks of producing cerebral oedema if hypotonic solutions are used. Half-strength saline should be reserved for cases where hypernatraenia or osmolality > 330 mosmol/l occurs. Over-rapid correction of hyperosmolality is undesirable. However, correction of dehydration is of paramount importance, and an i.v. line must be started even before biochemistry is available.

Potassium. Many cases of diabetic keto-acidosis succumb in the small hours of the morning of cardiac dysrhythmias produced by hypokalaemia. There is *no* alternative to regular 2 hourly checks of serum K during the first critical 8–10 hours of treatment, and the biochemistry department must be informed of this as soon as the case is admitted.

The serum potassium falls suddenly when treatment is instituted, and a high serum potassium (in the absence of renal failure) at the onset may not accurately reflect a total body deficit of potassium. It is therefore suggested that in all save the most seriously ill patients, potassium replacement is commenced at the onset of treatment, and thereafter monitored 2-hourly.

Bicarbonate. The indications for bicarbonate are stated in the table. Lactate solutions are no longer used because the lactate level is already raised in many cases of diabetic keto-acidosis, and the previous objection to bicarbonate was a technical one, due to the difficulty in preparation and sterilization of stable solutions. Over-enthusiastic use of bicarbonate is contra-indicated for three reasons

(1) a potentially lethal fall in potassium can occur

(2) a metabolic alkalosis occurs if the usual formula for calculation of bicarbonate requirements is used

(3) due to its effect on the CSF pH a disequilibrium situation leading to cerebral dysfunction may occur.

(8) *Glucose.* In the form of dextrose 5% should be given when the blood sugar has fallen below 11 mmol/l. It is illogical to use it before. If it is considered that water is the principle deficit half strength saline can be used (subject to consideration of inducing cerebral oedema by over-rapid correction of hyper-osmolality as mentioned above).

(9) *Sliding scale insulin.* When the acute metabolic maelstrom has subsided,

insulin can be given on a sliding scale. This will normally be after about 8-36 hours, at which time the patient will still be having i.v. fluids and nil by mouth.

A sliding scale at this stage must take account of ketonuria. The figures for insulin dosage should be based on blood sugars and not pure guess work. Only too often a sliding scale constitutes an abdication of clinical responsibility and tends to preclude any further constructive thought on the problem. It should be remembered that the period on a sliding scale is a brief interlude between the crisis period and stabilization on soluble insulin tds and then twice daily (and ultimately the definitive future regime).

Table 14.5

Urine test	Soluble insulin in units	
		Ketonuria ++ to +++
2% (Orange)	24	30
1% (Yellow)	16	20
½% (Green)	12	16
0% (Blue)	8	10

Complications of diabetic keto-acidosis

Cerebral oedema

Mention has already been made of this complication, which may be due to over-rapid correction of hyperosmolarity, the use of excessive amounts of alkali and too rapid lowering of the blood sugar. The exact mechanism is however obscure. It usually occurs as the biochemical parameters are returning to normal and is recognized as a relatively sudden loss of consciousness, or failure to regain consciousness. Intravenous mannitol or dexamethasone may help (though the latter may aggravate the diabetes), but the mortality rate is very high.

Renal failure

If the period of shock and hypovolaemia is long, diagnosis is delayed, or admission to hospital delayed acute tubular necrosis may develop (see Chapter 13). Early recognition is paramount because of the risk of gross fluid-overloading in a patient with renal failure. The oliguria of dehydration, however, must not be confused with the oliguria of acute tubular necrosis. If adequate rehydration has been achieved; and the urine output falls with a rise in blood urea it must be assumed that acute renal damage has occurred.

It should also be noted that diabetics are prone to renal disease and that if there is evidence of pre-existing renal disease the fluid and electrolyte regime outlined in Table 14.4 will need modification, especially in respect of potassium supplements.

Cardiac failure

Many patients in diabetic 'coma' will be elderly and large quantities of intravenous fluids may provoke cardiac failure. This risk is increased if potassium levels are allowed to fall. If it is considered that there is risk of inducing cardiac failure during treatment a CVP line should be inserted and fluid therapy monitored in this way.

Disseminated intravascular coagulopathy

This has been rarely reported and may respond to heparin therapy as in other causes of the condition (see Chapter 18) (Nicholson and Tomkin, 1974).

Diabetic keto-acidosis in children

The principles of management are exactly the same as in adults. However, fluid requirements must be modified for the age and weight of the child.

500 ml can be infused at the following rates

in 2-3 hours < 2 years of age
1 hour   2-5 years
15-30 minutes 6 + years

subsequently these rates are cut to one-third.

Potassium supplements are in the order of 10 mmol per 500 ml N/saline.

A modification of the insulin infusion method described above using *intramuscular* small doses of insulin has been shown to produce excellent results (Moselely, 1975). Using this technique the dose of insulin is as follows:

Initial dose 0.25 unit/kg body wt
followed by 0.1 unit/kg body wt hourly until keto-acidosis was relieved and plasma glucose had fallen below 11.1 mmol/l (200 mg/100 ml).

HYPEROSMOLAR NON-KETOTIC DIABETIC COMA (Gerich *et al.*, 1971; Arieff and Carroll, 1972)

This condition is differentiated from keto-acidosis, as described above, by little or no ketonaemia or ketonuria. It occurs mainly in elderly patients, where it may be the presenting symptom of diabetes. The characteristic presentation is with stupor or coma. Convulsions are common. The striking physical sign is intense dehydration. Acidotic respiration is absent.

Biochemical findings

(1) extreme hyperglycaemia, often in excess of 55 mmol/l and levels of 150-220 mmol/l have been reported
(2) hypernatraemia
(3) hyperosmolality (> 300 mosmol/l)
(4) bicarbonate normal or only slightly reduced.

Treatment

(1) These patients tend to be insulin-sensitive and large initial doses should be

avoided. *Low dose* insulin will be the therapy of choice in this group of patients (see page 210).

(2) Intravenous therapy should be with N/2 saline, very large volumes may be required—up to 20 l in the first 24 hours. Under these circumstances, in elderly patients, monitoring of the CVP is desirable.

(3) Potassium supplements may be necessary in larger doses than advised above.

(4) Because of the intense dehydration, and possibly other factors, these patients are liable to thrombotic episodes and anticoagulant therapy is indicated.

Prognosis

The mortality rate is between 40–50%. Those patients who survive differ greatly from the keto-acidotic group in that many do not require insulin treatment, but are maintained on oral hypoglycaemic agents or even dietary restriction only. (Diabetic keto-acidosis is an absolute contra-indication to attempts at control with oral agents after recovery.)

DIFFERENTIAL DIAGNOSIS OF DIABETIC COMA

Diabetics can present in coma due to other causes. Cerebro-vascular disease, uraemia, poisoning, etc., are unlikely to be confused, but it must be remembered that these other conditions may provoke an episode of keto-acidosis. *Hypoglycaemia* is unlikely to be confused—if for any reason there is some doubt as to the nature of coma in a diabetic, no harm can be done by the i.v. administration of 20 g of glucose. It is, however, important that blood is taken for glucose estimation *before* i.v. glucose is given.

Occasionally cerebro-vascular catastrophes are accompanied by glycosuria but blood sugars will not be grossly elevated and no acidosis will be present.

Table 14.6 Differential diagnosis of diabetic coma (Hockaday and Alberti)

Diagnosis	Dehydration	Hyper-ventilation	Ketosis	Acidaemia	Insulin requirements
Ketotic coma	+++	+++	+++	+++	+++
Hyperosmolar coma	+++	+	0–+	0	++
Lactic acidosis	+	+++	0–+++	+++	?+
Hypoglycaemia	0	0	0	0	0

LACTIC ACIDOSIS (Watkins *et al.*, 1969; Woods, 1971)

This severe metabolic abnormality is discussed here because it is often associated with diabetic keto-acidosis, but there are many other associations.

In addition to the above disease states, lactic acidosis may occur in association with drug therapy, though usually not in 'fit' patients.

Table 14.7 Associations with lactic acidosis

Diabetes mellitus
Uraemia
Hepatic disease
Acute pancreatitis
Bacterial infections and septicaemia
Leukaemia and lymphoma

Table 14.8 Drugs associated with lactic acidosis

Phenformin
Ethanol
Salicylate

Definition and diagnosis of lactic acidosis

Unfortunately, there is no clearly defined condition of 'lactic acidosis'. Different criteria have been used. The two most commonly used biochemical parameters are the blood lactate level, and the lactate/pyruvate ratio. If the lactate level is raised above 7 mmol/l without corresponding increase in pyruvate so that the normal lactate/pyruvate ratio of 10:1 is exceeded, clinical lactic acidosis may be said to be present. Under these circumstances a clinical metabolic acidosis will develop. The clinical picture consists of an increase in the rate and depth of respiration with a deterioration in the level of consciousness progressing to coma.

The diagnosis of lactic acidosis should be suspected when clinical acidosis is present without any obvious cause such as diabetic keto-acidosis, salicylate poisoning or uraemia. It is generally associated with tissue hypoxia and circulatory failure.

The blood lactate can be measured direct but suspicion should be alerted to the presence of lactic acidosis when there is increased *anion gap*, without any other known cause.

$$(Na^+ + K^+) - (Cl^- + HCO_3^-)$$

Normally this is less than 20 but will be increased in metabolic acidosis.

Management

Treatment must be directed at relief of tissue hypoxia in a shocked patient (see Chapter 2) and the correction of the acidosis. The amount of bicarbonate that needs to be administered may be very large—as much as 1000 mmol. The amount required may be calculated from the following formula

$$\text{Dosage (mmol/l)} = 0.3 \times \text{Body wt (kg)} \times \text{Base deficit (mmol/l)}$$

The prognosis of lactic acidosis, occurring in patients critically ill from other causes, is very high.

215

SURGERY IN THE DIABETIC PATIENT

Emergency surgery may be necessary in the diabetic patients, without time for adequate preparation; and many diabetic patients will be admitted to an Intensive Therapy Unit for reasons other than their diabetes. It is therefore, briefly, necessary at this stage to discuss something of the management of such cases.

(1) Hypoglycaemia is more of a risk than hyperglycaemia, assuming that no ketosis is present.

(2) Ideally all such patients should be on a soluble insulin b.d. or t.d.s. regime before surgery, and in the convalescent period, after oral feeding has commenced.

(3) Carbohydrate can be given in the form of intravenous fluids (5% Dextrose ≡ 25 G CHO in 500 ml, 4% Dextrose ≡ 20 G CHO in 500 ml in 1/5 N. Saline).

(4) If ketosis is present and the patient requires emergency surgery (possibly to treat the cause of ketosis, e.g. perforation or intestinal obstruction), the operation should be delayed for 2–3 h, if possible, to allow rehydration, control of blood sugar and electrolyte control at least to be commenced.

Elective surgery

Preferably the patient should be first on the list so that a reasonably accurate assessment of starting time can be made. This will allow the insulin to be given so that the period of starvation before a general anaesthetic will not produce hypoglycaemia, or allow the blood sugar to rise if delayed. In general about 1/3 the usual morning dose of insulin can be given and at the same time an intravenous infusion set up to allow administration of 25–30 g of carbohydrate. Through surgery most anaesthetists prefer to use the type of insulin infusions described on page 210. Modern techniques of general anaesthetics do not cause a significant rise in blood sugar.

The post-operative period

If the blood sugar rises there should be no panic as long as no ketosis develops. Blood sugar estimations can now be made rapidly and with reasonable accuracy in the post-operative ward, the Intensive Therapy Unit and the ward by use of a reflectance meter (Schersten *et al.*, 1974). Ketonaemia can be detected by applying plasma to Ketostix.

At this stage, until parenteral fluids are discontinued it is reasonable to use a sliding scale of insulin, an example is on page 212. However, this form of insulin therapy does not preclude regular blood sugar estimations as it should be remembered that renal thresholds for sugar vary, and may be modified by dehydration etc., furthermore 2% glycosuria may indicate a blood sugar of anything over 14 mmol/l. As the patient recovers the carbohydrate intake should be adjusted to approach what seems appropriate for the metabolic situation or his normal needs and the sliding scale modified to 8 hourly with the doses of insulin before breakfast, lunch and evening meal arranged in a ratio of 3/6:1/6: 2/6 of total 24 h requirement. In this way a rapid transition to s.c. soluble insulin tds and then bd can be made; with an ultimate return to his normal regime. Patients lying around in hospital will need to have their insulin dosage reduced when they leave the ward and assume normal daily life.

The patient on oral agents

Many 'mild' diabetics can be submitted to surgery without recourse to insulin. It is wise to omit oral agents on the day of surgery and maintain i.v. fluids with insulin if necessary until normal oral feeding is recommenced. Insulin may need to be continued if sepsis is present. It should be remembered that chlorpropamide can cause severe relapsing hypoglycaemia for up to 24 hours after administration.

THYROID DISEASE

Thyrotoxic crisis

Thyroid storm is an exacerbation in intensity of the features of thyrotoxicosis, it is usually precipitated by surgery and is most likely to occur in patients who have not been adequately treated pre-operatively. This life-threatening metabolic crisis may become even more uncommon with the growing use of beta-receptor adrenergic blocking agents in the pre-operative treatment of thyrotoxic patients (Levey, 1975). It is more likely to occur when thyroidectomy has been difficult and there has been prolonged handling of the gland.

The clinical features are as follows:
(1) fever, sweating–leading to dehydration
(2) tachycardia, with low output, heart failure (thyrotoxic cardiomyopathy)
(3) confusion, agitation
(4) tachypnoea

Pathophysiology. The manifestations of thyrotoxic crisis are probably due to exhaustion of the body to circulating thyroxines rather than a sudden increase in their concentration (Jacobs *et al.*, 1973) (raising the possibility of plasmophoresis as an adjunct of therapy of thyroid crisis). Relative adrenal insufficiency contributes to the clinical picture (Waldstein *et al.*, 1960).

Treatment (Havard, 1974)

(1) Correction of sympathetic over-activity
　　(a) Propranolol 40 mg 6-hourly by mouth or 2 mg i.v. 6-hourly*
　　(b) Reserpine 2.5 mg 6-hourly i.m.
(2) Correction of relative adrenal insufficiency, hydrocortisone 200 mg i.v.
(3) Blocking further thyroid hormone synthesis and release:
　　Sodium iodide 1–2 g by slow intravenous infusion
　　(?plasmaphoresis)

---

* *Beta-adrenergic receptor blockers must be used cautiously if heart failure is present.*

oral antithyroid drugs
(Neo-mercazole 100 mg as a stat dose maintenance dose 15 mg tds for 72 hours)
(4) General measures
  (a) antipyretic measure—tepid sponging
     cooling fans
     ice-packs (if hyperpyrexia)
     aspirin
  (b) oxygen
  (c) i.v. glucose infusion (quite severe dehydration may be present)
(5) Heart failure may require digitalization and diuretics

MYXOEDEMIC COMA AND HYPOTHERMIA

These two conditions have many points of management in common, and of course myxoedema is a potent cause of hypothermia.

MYXOEDEMIC COMA

This condition is virtually confined to the elderly—arising when a patient with established, but untreated or neglected, hypothyroidism is exposed to cold or sedative drugs. Co-existent degenerative cerebro-vascular disease is a contributory factor in many cases.

Clinical features

Relatives may give a history of weight gain, general slowness, voice changes, dementia, deafness and cold intolerance. However, many cases will occur in elderly patients living alone in poorly heated accommodation, who are found unconscious by chance. In these cases suspicion should be alerted to the existence of myxoedema by the general appearance of the patient, bradycardia, low voltage ECG and myotonic tendon reflexes. Body temperature (which must be taken rectally) will usually show a reduction. Levels below 30°C (86°F) carry a high mortality, with a great risk of ventricular dysrhythmias.

Pathological findings

There is little time to organize the full galaxy of thyroid function tests but a T_3-T_4 (Thyopac) result can usually be obtained rapidly from a single blood specimen. It must, however, be emphasized that there is no time to waste in the treatment of this condition and appropriate therapy should be commenced as soon as blood is taken for biochemical investigation. A respiratory acidosis due to alveolar hypoventilation is usually present and blood gas estimations should be made. The reasons for this are not clear and may be due to the following factors:

(1) Alteration of metabolic needs, i.e. reducing O_2 consumption and CO_2 excretion.

(2) Alteration of the mechanism for control of respiration.

(3) Alteration of gas solubility and transport.

(4) Alteration of mechanical properties of the lung, muscular weakness.

Hypoventilation therefore results in hypoxaemia and respiratory acidosis (Zwillick *et al.*, 1975; Buchanan *et al.*, 1967; McNicol, 1967). Pancreatitis, with a rise in serum amylase, and occasionally leading to diabetic keto-acidosis occurs; but some patients show hypoglycaemia, which may be profound (Maclean *et al.*, 1973).

Treatment

(1) Thyroid replacement therapy. This must be by the use of rapid acting Tri-iodothyronine. Thyroxine is too slow in action. There is, however, a grave risk of inducing cardiac problems. Severe atherosclerosis occurs with long-standing untreated myxoedema and myocardial infarction, dysrhythmias and heart failure may be induced by over-rapid acceleration of the metabolic rate. Patients should be on continuous ECG monitoring and special attention paid to serum potassium levels (especially as many elderly patients are on digoxin therapy).

The dose of tri-iodothyronine should be between 20–40 μg daily initially, increasing to perhaps 60 μg after 2–3 days. Rapid intravenous injection may be very dangerous and if oral administration (via naso-gastric tube) is not possible the drug should be given by slow intravenous infusion (Buchanan *et al.*, 1967; de Groot and Stanbury, 1975).

(2) Treatment of hypothermia (see below).

(3) Oxygen and assisted respiration if PaO_2 is low.

(4) Intravenous steroids. Even in primary myxoedema relative adrenal insufficiency exists as the metabolic rate is increased, and i.v. hydrocortisone 200–300 mg daily should be given.

(5) Glucose if hypoglycaemia is present, but beware of cases who may develop severe keto-acidosis related to acute pancreatitis (see above).

(6) Antibiotics—if infection is present, or when respiratory infection develops.

(7) Diuretics, ? digoxin if cardiac problems occur.

Hypothermia (Hockaday, 1972)

Hypothermia is most common in the very young and the very old. In the old it is particularly associated with socio-economic problems and myxoedema. Also it occurs in patients in diabetic coma, after high spinal cord injuries, cerebro-vascular accidents, in association with drugs, especially chlorpromazine and alcohol drug overdose, and secondary to excess environmental stress, such as exposure or near-drowning. It must be emphasized that hypothermia will be missed if low reading rectal thermometers are not used.

Re-warming

The rate and method of re-warming will depend on the age of the patient and the reason for the hypothermia. In general rapid re-warming is safe in previously fit young patients whose hypothermia is secondary to an obvious external factor, e.g. immersion.

Rapid re-warming

Before admission to hospital the patient should be given hot drinks and warm clothing. During transfer to hospital he should be carried supine because of the risks of severe postural hypotension. As soon as possible the patient should be immersed in hot water at a temperature of 40–44°C. In order to avoid problems with a severe drop in central core temperature during rapid re-warming, this should be stopped once body temperature has reached 35°. At this stage gentle external warmth in an ambient temperature of about 38–40°C should be continued. Ledingham and Mone (1980) suggest that active re-warming using radiant heat cradle over the torso can be used even in the elderly.

Slow re-warming

In the young, and very old, where temperature-regulating mechanism may be impaired; or in patients whose hypothermia is secondary to other diseases, gradual re-warming is indicated. A rate of about 0.6°C an hour is suggested. This may be achieved by warming the body with hot water bottles or a thermostatically controlled electric blanket. The patient should be well insulated and in ambient temperature of about 25–29°C. Active internal warming by use of a heart-lung machine or artificial kidney has been suggested—but this facility is rarely available.

Other measures

The risk of dysrhythmias is very great and ECG monitoring is essential. It should be noted that many drugs routinely used in treatment of cardiac dysrhythmias are dangerous or ineffective at low body temperatures. Calcium i.v. can be used, but at lower dosage. If DC defibrillation has to be performed the voltage used should be lower than usual.

There is no place for the routine use of tri-iodothyronine unless the patient has myxoedema, or if there are reasonable clinical grounds for thinking so.

Oxygen, assisted respiration, steroids, glucose and fluids may be administered as described under the treatment of myxoedemic coma (above).

DISORDERS OF CALCIUM METABOLISM

Hypercalcaemia

Hypercalcaemia may require urgent treatment in the Intensive Therapy Unit, untreated serum calcium levels in excess of 4 mmol/l are likely to provoke a hypercalcaemic crisis, which carries a high mortality rate.

Table 14.9 Symptoms of hypercalcaemia

CNS	headache, lethargy, confusion, coma, muscle weakness
Renal	polyuria, thirst, deterioration in renal function, renal calculus
Gastro-intestinal	acute pancreatitis, peptic ulcer, vomiting
Cardiovascular	ECG changes
Symptoms of *primary disease*, e.g. bone pain	

The most common causes of hypercalcaemia are

(1) primary hyperparathyroidism
(2) malignant bone disease, e.g. myelomatosis, bone secondaries, reticulosis
(3) vitamin D intoxication
(4) sarcoidosis
(5) milk-alkalis syndrome
(6) immobilization (unlikely to cause severe problems)

Diagnosis

With the routine use of multi-channel auto-analyzers unsuspected hypercalcaemia is an increasingly common unexpected finding, but this type of case is unlikely to cause acute problems. It is worth pointing out, at this stage, that the interpretation of a serum calcium estimation must be made with some caution. This point is particularly relevant to hypocalcaemia (below). The serum calcium level must be corrected to take into account the serum albumin level.

Treatment

The treatment of hypercalcaemia will depend on the underlying cause and the degree of renal impairment. In primary hyperparathyroidism the definitive treatment is parathyroidectomy. In malignant bone disease emergency treatment may save the patient to allow time for treatment with either radio-therapy or cytotoxic agents.

(1) *Calcitonin.* This is available commercially as porcine ('Calcitare') or synthetic salmon type ('Calsynar').

It is the treatment of choice where renal function is impaired. Calcitonin lowers the serum calcium in two ways: by inhibition of bone calcium resorption, and this is its principal action. Its other effect, of inhibiting renal tubular reabsorption, is of much less significance.

Table 14.10 Dosage of calcitonin preparations

Porcine calcitonin (calcitare)	4 international units/kg/day
Salmon calcitonin (calsynar)	400 international units 6–8 hourly

This drug is given by intramuscular injection. It has a rapid hypocalcaemic action in hypercalcaemia due to disseminated malignant disease, vitamin D intoxication, idiopathic hypercalcaemia of infancy (and other conditions in which the hypercalcaemia is unlikely to cause a crisis situation). Dosage should be monitored by at least daily serum calcium estimations (Buckle *et al.*, 1972; Woodhouse, 1974).

(2) *Sodium phosphate* is effective, but metastatic calcification can occur and this is potentially hazardous where renal impairment is present.

(a) Oral phosphate therapy can most conveniently be achieved by the use of Phosphate-Sandoz tablets. Up to six tablets daily are dissolved in water, and the dose monitored by frequent serum calcium estimations. Renal function must always be monitored carefully when phosphate therapy is used.*

(b) Intravenous therapy

500 ml 0.1 M phosphate buffer

= disodium phosphate (0.081 M)

  monosodium phosphate (0.019 M)

given over 12 hours (Goldsmith and Ingbar, 1966; Thalassinos and Joplin 1968).

(3) *Steroids* reduce the calcium in hypercalcaemic states but their action is slow and in emergency use calcitonin can now be considered the treatment of choice.

(4) *Mithramycin.* This cytotoxic agent has been used for the emergency treatment of hypercalcaemia. Although it has marked bone marrow toxic effects when used in high dosage, in low dose these do not occur (Stamp *et al.*, 1975).

Hypocalcaemia

The comments above on correction of serum calcium estimations in relation to the plasma proteins are particularly important in this context. Hypocalcaemia is unlikely to cause florid symptoms until the level approaches 1.5–1.8 mmol/l.

Symptoms

Muscle cramps and paraesthesiae in the extremities, and around the mouth occur in the early stages and this progresses to severe spasms which are unpleasant if confined to the arm (carpo-pedal spasm) but dangerous when cramps in the jaws and respiratory muscles lead to acute respiratory insufficiency. More severe spasms can involve the laryngeal musculature. If hypocalcaemia is prolonged, dementia, toxic delirium and coma have been described. Papilloedema can occur. It is important to note that the neurological symptoms may occur without tetany.

* *If the proprietary preparation Phosphate-Sandoz is not available the formula for oral Phosphate mixture is as follows*
Na_2HPO_4 (anhydrous) 3.66 g
$NaH_2PO_4 \cdot 2H_2O$ 1 g
Orange syrup 16 ml
Water to 60 ml   (60 ml 8 hourly)

Causes

Hypocalcaemia is most likely to be seen after thyroidectomy when transient or permanent damage to the parathyroid glands has been inflicted. It also occurs after removal of a parathyroid tumour when the bones take up large amounts of calcium. Idiopathic hypoparathyroidism and pseudo-hypoparathyroidism may present with tetany and neurological signs.

Treatment

Acute. Where frequent tetanic spasms occur and respiratory insufficiency or laryngeal stridor is present the emergency treatment must be parenteral in order to raise the serum calcium to normal levels. *i.v. calcium gluconate* is given—100 ml 10% calcium gluconate in 900 ml 5% dextrose daily by slow infusion.

Long term. Most cases of post-operative tetany are transient. However, the serum calcium may remain low for days or months (particularly after removal of parathyroid adenoma) and these cases will require oral vitamin D therapy.
The preparation of choice is dihydrotachysterol (ATIO). The initial dose is 1-2 mg daily and the maintenance dose 0.5 mg daily. Frequent monitoring of the serum calcium is essential when vitamin D or its analogues are being given.

ADRENAL DISORDERS

Phaeochromocytoma

We have seen two patients admitted in deep coma, considered to have hypertensive encephalopathy, unresponsive to conventional therapy, who, at postmortem have been shown to have phaeochromocytomas. It is therefore necessary briefly to review this subject.

Pathology

Tumours of chromaffin tissue, which cause hypertension by secreting catechol amines. They usually occur in the adrenal medulla but can occur at many other sites; and may be multiple. There is an association with neurofibromatosis (which also may be associated with meningiomata).

Clinical features

The symptoms are directly due to the excess secretion of catechol amines. The prime symptom is hypertension which is classically paroxysmal but is often sustained. The blood pressure however does not show the normal variations that occur in other causes of hypertension; this is particularly marked at night, where there is little or no drop (Littler and Honour, 1974). In the classic attack the blood pressure rises sharply, there is tachycardia, pallor and sweating, apprehension and headache. Shortness of breath and anginal pain may be prominent symptoms. The patient may present in coma with fixed hypertension. The attacks may be precipitated by a variety of insults, including citrus fruits and, importantly, diamorphine (Chaturvedi *et al.*, 1974) (which produces histamine release). Ganglionic and post-ganglionic blocking drugs sensitize peripheral receptors to circulating catecholamines and are therefore contra-indicated.

Diagnosis

The diagnosis of phaeochromocytoma is made by finding an excess of catecholamines or their metabolites in the urine. It should be noted that a careful drug history should be taken before relying on these results: not only may the patient be taking ephedrine in patent cold-cures, but be established on hypotensive agents such as methyl-dopa or clonidine both of which interfere with the estimation.

The usual metabolite that is estimated is vanilmandelic acid (VMA), which is normally less than 6.5 mg in an accurate 24 hour urine collection.

If a comatose patient with severe hypertension is admitted a history should be obtained from a relative if possible and careful consideration given before any drugs are given (e.g. bethanidine, guanethidine, diamorphine—see above) if there is a possibility of phaeochromocytoma.

Treatment

The treatment of the hypertension due to phaeochromocytoma is by combined alpha and beta adrenergic receptor blocking agents. The alpha receptor blocker *phenoxybenzamine* up to 100 mg daily is given with the beta receptor blocker *propranolol* 40–160 mg daily. This regime must be continued through surgery to the tumours. The manipulation and removal of these tumours can cause very wide swings in the blood pressure and hypotension may be acute in the post-operative phase.

Hypoadrenalism

Acute adrenal insufficiency may occur as a complication of septicaemia, as a secondary phenomenon in patients who are on steroids or should have had steroid cover in the course of an intercurrent severe illness or traumatic episode, and most rarely as a presenting symptom in a case of primary adrenal insufficiency.

Clinical picture

The characteristic features are abdominal pain, which may be severe enough to mimic an acute surgical emergency, with vomiting, severe weakness and hypotension. If the patient has Addison's disease abnormal pigmentation may be observed, particularly on the skin creases, pressure areas and on the buccal mucous membranes. In these cases a preceding history of overwhelming apathy, anorexia and weight loss is usually present.

In those cases who are suffering from secondary adrenal insufficiency it may be important to identify a steroid card in their possession. If no history is available the stigmata of steroid therapy—a Cushingoid appearance, hypertension, fluid retention, plethora, acne and purple striae—may be present. But adrenal insufficiency can occur in patients whose steroid therapy has been discontinued up to a year previously (see below), and a careful drug history should be obtained, from relatives if necessary. Adrenal insufficiency in this highly susceptible group is generally provoked by a serious intercurrent illness or major surgical (or traumatic) procedure.

A condition often treated with steroids should always be searched for. These would include rheumatoid arthritis, asthma and ulcerative colitis or regional ileitis. It should also be remembered that carcinoma of the breast or bronchus frequently metastasise to the adrenals.

Biochemical findings

Characteristically the sodium is low, but, as has been noted in Chapter 2, this is not an uncommon finding in severe illness. The potassium and urea are elevated, the glucose low and calcium high.

Serum cortisol levels are not readily available as an emergency measure, and levels need to be interpreted with caution as a 'normal' level in a severely stressful situation may in fact represent a serious deficiency. If a diagnosis of acute adrenal insufficiency is made, blood should always be taken for cortisol estimation, before steroid therapy is started (but steroids should not be delayed until the result is available).

Treatment

Steroid therapy

(1) Hydrocortisone 100 mg 6-hourly until the patient's condition has improved enough to commence oral therapy (cortisone 25–37.5 mg daily).

(2) Aldosterone. The salt-retaining steroid can be given parenterally (i.v. or i.m.) 1 mg and followed by oral therapy (Fludrocortisone 100–200 μg daily).

Electrolyte replacement. Normal saline must always be given, preferably with CVP control. When these patients present severe dehydration is usually a feature and 0.5–1 l N/saline can be given rapidly.

Further electrolyte therapy will depend on frequent blood estimations, remembering that sodium will be retained if a mineralocorticoid has been given.

Management of patients on steroids

Steroid therapy represents a serious potential hazard to patients suffering from serious illness, surgery or trauma. A particularly careful history must be obtained from this group, particularly with reference to the dosage and duration of steroid treatment.

(1) *Normal pituitary-adrenal axis function* may not return for up to a year after steroid therapy. This depends largely upon the dosage and duration of therapy,

225

but it is probably wise to assume that steroid cover will be necessary (Graber *et al.*, 1965).

(2) *Steroid cover.* It is safer to give steroids than to assume that adrenal function has returned to normal. This applies in all cases, except those who have had an isolated short course. Certainly all patients who have had steroids for a year should have steroid cover in any subsequent operation. In patients actually on steroids, systemic hydrocortisone should always be substituted for the oral therapy. The dosage depends on the oral dose previously being taken. If the oral dose is prednisone 10 mg (or equivalent of other steroid preparations), the usual dose of hydrocortisone (i.m. or i.v.) is 100 mg followed by 50 mg 6 hourly until oral therapy is resumed (in all except the most minor procedures the normal oral maintenance dose should be doubled for several days and then gradually reduced to the usual dose). If the usual dose of steroids is over 10 mg prednisone (or equivalent) daily the dose of hydrocortisone should be increased in proportion. It should be remembered that if inadequate steroid cover is given not only is a relative hypoadrenal state possible, but an exacerbation of the original disease for which the steroids were given might occur.

(3) *Steroid withdrawal.* This is not usually a problem in the ITU. Very short courses of high dose steroids (such as in some shocked patients) can be tailed rapidly or even stopped abruptly without serious consequences (see Chapter 3).

In general the pace of steroid withdrawal depends upon the dosage and length of time during which steroids have been administered. Intercurrent illness during this phase will necessitate a temporary increase in dosage.

If steroids have been given for a long period (e.g. over 2 years) dose reduction should not exceed 2.5 mg prednisone (or equivalent) per month and pituitary-adrenal axis integrity checked at intervals. This can be done by estimating the clinical variation of plasma cortisol, and measuring the adrenal response to ACTH. However these considerations should not be necessary in an ITU where it can be assumed that severe illness would be a contra-indication to a long-term of programme of steroid withdrawal.

THE PORPHYRIAS

This important, but rare, group of metabolic disorders may present in the ITU in a variety of ways, and brief discussion is necessary because of the difficulties of drug prescription in the disease.

A detailed classification and description of the biochemistry would be inappropriate here. The porphyria most likely to be encountered is *acute intermittent porphyria* (Goldberg, 1959).

This condition, which affects women more than men, is inherited as an autosomal dominant, but in up to 30% of cases there appears to be no family history. The presentation may be as follows below.

Neurological

Peripheral neuropathy

Causing severe muscular weakness. This is proximal more than distal and the respiratory muscles are often affected.

Epilepsy

Serious psychiatric disturbances

Gastro-intestinal

Severe abdominal pain radiating to the back and associated with vomiting. Hyponatraemia may be associated with inappropriate secretion of ADH.

Cardiovascular

Hypertension and tachycardia.

Acute attacks of porphyria are often precipitated by drugs and obviously these drugs must be avoided in therapy. Intercurrent infection and pregnancy are other provocative factors.

Drugs that are known to aggravate porphyria are given in Table 14.11.

Table 14.11 Drugs that must not be given in porphyria

Barbiturates, including intravenous anaesthetic agents
Sulphonamides
Chlordiazepoxide (Librium)
Glutethamide (Doriden)
Meprobamate (Equanil)
Sex hormones, including oral contraceptives
Methyldopa (Aldomet)
Alcohol

Management

If respiratory insufficiency develops the patient should be maintained on mechanical ventilation as described in the management of other neurological causes (Chapter 22). Recovery may be delayed for months, and under these circumstances tracheostomy will be indicated. Treatment is essentially symptomatic, avoiding the drugs listed above. Morphine is a safe analgesic and diazepam (valium) can be used as a sedative and to control epileptic fits (phenytoin should not be used). Propranolol (inderal) can safely be used for the cardiovascular manifestations.

Nutrition is an important consideration because an acute attack may be precipitated by low carbohydrate and protein intake. In an acute attack parenteral nutrition will generally be indicated to achieve a high carbohydrate and protein intake (see Chapter 18).

Diagnosis

The condition may be suspected if there is a history of recurrent bouts of neuro-psychiatric symptoms with abdominal pain. The family history may be helpful. A biochemical diagnosis is made by finding a raised urinary prophobilinogen, raised urinary uroporphyrin and a very high urinary excretion of delta-aminolaevutic acid.

REFERENCES

Alberti, K. G. M. and Hockaday, T. D. (1972), Rapid ketone body estimation in the diagnosis of diabetic keto-acidosis. *Brit. med. J.*, 2, 565.

Arieff, A. I. and Carroll, H. J. (1972), Non-ketotic hyperosmolar coma with hyperglycaemia: Clinical features, pathophysiology, renal function, acid-base balance plasma, cerebrospinal fluid equilibria and the effects of therapy in 37 cases. *Medicine*, 51, 73.

Buchanan, J., McKiddie, M. T. and Reid, J. M. (1967), Respiratory acidosis in hypothermia and myxoedemic coma. *Postgrad. med. J.*, 43, 114.

Buckle, R. M., Gamlen, T. R. and Pullen, I. M. (1972), Vitamin D Intoxication treated with Procine Calcitonin. *Brit. med. J.*, 3, 205.

Chaturvedi, N. C., Walsh, M. J., Boyle, D. McC. and Barber, J. M. (1974), Dia-morphine induced attack of paroxysmal hypertension in phaeochromo-cytoma. *Brit. med. J.*, 2, 538.

(Ed) (1977), Insulin regimens for diabetic keto-acidosis. *Brit. med. J.*, 1, 405.

Gerich, J. E., Martin, M. M. and Becant, L. (1971), Clinical and metabolic characteristics of hyperosmolar non-ketotic coma. *Diabetes*, 20, 228.

Goldberg, A. (1959), Acute intermittent porphyria—a study of 50 cases. *Q. J. Med.*, 28, 183.

Goldsmith, R. S. and Ingbar, S. H. (1966), Inorganic phosphate treatment of hypercalcaemia of diverse etiologies. *N. Eng. J. Med.*, 274, 1.

Graber, A. L., Ney, R. L., Nicholson, W. E., Island, D. P. and Liddle, G. W. (1965), Natural history of pituitary-adrenal recovery following long-term suppression with corticosteroids. *J. Clin. Endocr.*, 25, 11.

de Groot, C. J. and Stanbury, J. B. (1975), *The Thyroid and its Diseases*. John Wiley, London, p. 456.

Havard, C. W. (1974), The management of thyrotoxicosis. *Brit. J. Hosp. Med.*, 11, 893.

Hockaday, T. D. (1972), Hypothermia. *Brit. J. Hosp. Med.*, 8, 279.

Hockaday, T. D. and Alberti, K. G. M. (1972), Diabetic coma. *Brit. J. Hosp. Med.*, 7, 183.

Jacobs, H. S., Eastman, C. J., Ekins, R. P., Mackie, D. B., Ellis, S. M. and McHardy-Young, S. (1973), Total and free Tri-iodothyronine and Thyroxine levels in thyroid storm and recurrent hyperthyroidism. *Lancet*, ii, 236.

Kidson, W., Carey, J., Kraegen, E. and Lazarus, L. (1974), Treatment of severe diabetes mellitus by Insulin Infusion. *Brit. med. J.*, 2, 691.

Ledingham, I. McA., and Mone, J. G. (1980), Treatment of accidental hypo-thermia: a prospective clinical study. *Brit. med. J.*, 280, 1102.

Levey, G. S. (1975), The heart and hyperthyroidism. Use of beta-adrenergic blocking drugs. *Med. Clin. N. Am.*, 59, 1193.

Littler, W. A. and Honour, A. J. (1974), Direct arterial pressure, heart rate and ECG in unrestricted patients before and after removal of Phaeochromocytoma. *Q. J. Med.*, 171, 141.

Maclean, D., Murison, J. and Griffiths, P. D. (1973), Acute pancreatitis and diabetic keto-acidosis in accidental hypothermia and hypothermic myxoedema. *Brit. med. J.*, 4, 757.

Malins, J. M. (1971), The management of diabetic coma. *J. Roy. Coll. Physns. (Lond.)*, 6, 75.

McNicol, M. W. (1967), Respiratory failure and acid-base balance in hypothermia. *Postgrad. med. J.*, 43, 674.

Moseley, J. (1975), Diabetic Crisis in children treated with small doses of intramuscular Insulin. *Brit. med. J.*, i, 59.

Nicholson, G. and Tomkin, G. (1974), Successful treatment of D.I.C. complicating diabetic coma. *Brit. med. J.*, 4, 450.

Page, M. Mc. B., Alberti, K. G. M., Greenwood, R., Gumma, K. A., Hockaday, T. D., Korvy, C., Nabarro, J. D., Pyke, D. A., Sonshen, P. M., Watkins, P. J. and West, T. E. (1974), Treatment of Diabetic Coma with continuous low-dose infusion of Insulin. *Brit. med. J.*, 2, 687.

Schersten, B., Kuhl, C., Hollender, A. and Ekman, R. (1974), Blood glucose measurement with Dextrostix and new reflectance meter. *Brit. med. J.*, 3, 384.

Semple, P. F., White, C. and Manderson, W. G. (1974), Continuous Intravenous Infusion of small doses of Insulin in Treatment of Diabetic Keto-acidosis. *Brit. med. J.*, 2, 694.

Stamp, T. C. B., Child, J. A. and Walker, P. G. (1975), Treatment of osteolytic myelomatosis with mithramycin. *Lancet*, I, 719.

Thalassinos, N. and Joplin, G. F. (1968), Phosphate treatment of hypercalcaemia due to carcinoma. *Brit. med. J.*, 4, 14.

Treatment with Calcitonin (Editorial) (1973), *Brit. med. J.*, I, 371.

Waldstein, S. S., Slodki, S. J., Kaganiec, G. J. and Bronsky, D. (1960), A Clinical Study of Thyroid Storm. *Ann. Int. Med.*, 52, 626.

Watkins, P. J., Smith, J. S., Fitzgerald, M. G. and Malins, J. M. (1969), Lactic acidosis in diabetes. *Brit. med. J.*, I, 744.

Woodhouse, N. J. (1974), Clinical applications of Calcitonin. *Brit. J. Hosp. Med.*, 11, 677.

Woods, H. F. (1971), Some aspects of lactic acidosis. *Brit. J. Hosp. Med.*, 6, 668.

Zwillick, C. W., Pierson, D. J., Kofeldt, F. D., Lufkin, E. G. and Weil, J. V. (1975), Ventilatory Control in myxoedema and hypothyroidism. *N. Eng. J. Med.*, 292, 662.

FIFTEEN

Nutritional care: intensive nutrition

Maintenance of nutrition is another way in which many intensive care patients are unable to fend for themselves. Since intensive care can be defined as the support of vital functions until some life-threatening disease process is treated then nutritional support is certainly important.

Not only is it important in maintaining metabolic balance in those merely unable to feed themselves but since the healing process requires metabolic units, materials and considerable energy, then in the injured, post surgical or infected patient it is even more important.

The science of nutrition applied to starving and ill patients is reaping rich rewards in the area of intensive therapy. The particular requirements of the patient differ at various stages of the disease process. Most trauma and infections produce similar metabolic responses. These responses are different from those of simple starvation and this distinction will be made repeatedly throughout this chapter. Except in special circumstances, starvation should not be allowed to co-exist with disease. The reaction of the patient to his disease affects his metabolism, and not least in the way in which he is able to handle energy substrates at various stages of illness. This reaction can be divided into ebb and flow phases (Cuthbertson, 1942).

THE EBB PHASE

The fear, fight and flight response is designed to preserve life, maintaining circulation in the face of haemorrhage and other physical and chemical factors such as cold, fever and toxaemia. Maintenance of circulation to vital organs such as brain, heart, kidneys and liver may be at the expense of blood flow to other organs, resulting in lactacidaemia, and acidosis, from anaerobic glycolysis (MacLean et al., 1967).

The ebb phase is of limited duration and depends on catecholamine release which results from sympathetic nerve stimulation. The catecholamines mobilize glucose from the liver and initiate gluconeogenesis as well as antagonising insulin release (Porte and Bagdade, 1970; Lerner and Porte, 1971).

As the body compensates for the particular injury, metabolism enters the Flow Phase.

FLOW PHASE

This phase itself is characterized by two separate stages, known as the 'acute phase' and the 'adaptive phase'. The key hormones of the acute phase are catecholamines which have the following metabolic actions:

(1) Inhibit release of insulin (Porte and Bagdade, 1970).

(2) Elevation of blood glucose level resulting from glucose mobilization from the liver.

(3) Mobilization of triglycerides from adipose tissues.

These calorie rich energy substrates are well utilized in the presence of the relatively limited glucose flow from the liver and are quite adequate to meet energy requirements in the first day or two after injury (Flatt and Blackburn, 1974), or early simple starvation)Cahill, 1970).

Effective nutritional support in this phase is limited to administration of glucose to maintain glucose flow. 100 grams of glucose per 24 hours is the maximum requirement (Gamble, 1946). Others dispute the value of even this (Giddings, 1974). It must be stressed that this does not prevent mobilization of the body's protein during the acute phase (Cahill, 1970). Amino acid administration at this stage, for gluconeogenesis, is not only wasteful but because the specific dynamic action is greater than 1, actually increases energy demand (Bistrian *et al.*, 1975).

These metabolic effects of catecholamines are mediated by both alpha and beta receptors and can be blocked by the concurrent use of both alpha and beta blockers (Tanaka *et al.*, 1976).

The acute phase gives way to the adaptive phase in which glucocorticoids become the dominant hormones. The adaptive phase is the one where therapeutic nutrition has the greatest importance to the recovery of the patient. In a straightforward case of major surgery, the transition may occur at about 1-3 days after the operation (Blackburn and Flatt, 1975). The transition may be detected by a sudden or gradual (Moore and Brennan, 1975) fall from the hyperglycaemia of the acute phase to normal or low blood sugar levels. At the same time the low blood insulin level of the acute phase gives way to a high insulin level (Johnston, 1973; Den Besten *et al.*, 1973; Shambaugh and Beisel, 1967).

Administration of dextrose solutions during the transition stage will mask the changes in the blood glucose level.

During the adaptive phase, the net protein utilization is up to 70% (Rutten *et al.*, 1975), assuming that concurrent calorie intake is adequate. The adaptive phase after trauma is characterized by increased blood glucocorticoid levels, (which is nothing other than the well recognized steroid response to stress) and high blood insulin levels. The circulating glucocorticoid hormones moderate the response of the tissues of the body to insulin. This produces a balance between catabolism, due partly to glucocorticoids (Munck, 1970) and anabolism due partly or wholly to insulin (Fulks and Goldberg, 1975). These two processes should not be considered as antagonistic but rather they should be seen as complimentary. Catabolism produces the metabolic building blocks for healing and repair, whilst anabolism is the building process involved in healing and repair. An analogy may be made between this process and a building site, where old houses are dismantled to produce bricks to build new homes.

Inevitably, in such a process, there will be a waste of materials and extra energy and effort required to prepare the bricks for building. It would be far easier to have a large pile of new bricks of various types, and in the right proportions, delivered ready for building.

Catabolism sacrifices some less vital structures in order to provide a ready supply of circulating metabolic substrates for healing tissues (Ryan, 1976), production of serum albumin, fibrinogen, immune globulins (Bistrian *et al.*, 1975; Blackburn *et al.*, 1975), and lymphocytes.

The relatively crude methods used for many years to measure the overall balance between anabolism and catabolism, for example, nitrogen balance (Blackburn and Flatt, 1975), have nearly always shown resultant excess catabolism (Moore, 1971) with negative nitrogen balance. This has been deplored (Moore and Brennan, 1975), and rightly so, for it represents a somewhat wasteful physiological process aimed at repair of injured tissues. It is wasteful because skeletal muscle protein is mobilized to provide both amino acids and energy. Fat stores, surprisingly, are used very little to provide energy at this adaptive phase of the body's attempt to heal its injuries. This may be due to the high circulating insulin level. Because of the hormones involved in the adaptive phase following injury, hyperalimentation tends to produce lipogenesis (frequently best seen in the liver) rather than skeletal muscle replacement (Ryan *et al.*, 1974b).

During simple starvation there is a similar acute phase and adaptive phase. The differences are that the acute phase lasts a day or so longer and the protein mobilization during the early adaptive phase is primarily from the liver and visceral organs and only after some days does skeletal protein depletion develop (Waterlow and Stephen, 1967).

More important, in simple starvation, ketones, derived from triglyceride metabolism are widely mobilized and used for energy throughout the body, including brain (Cahill, 1970). Skeletal protein is spared in this process thus: 100 grams of glucose per 24 hours is all that is required in early simple starvation (Gamble, 1946). In a previously well nourished individual, energy requirements during simple starvation may be met from body reserves. Moreover, in a malnourished individual, administration of fat emulsion could be expected to supply the major energy requirement. After trauma, however, the role of fat emulsions in energy supply is not so obvious.

In practice, of course, surgical and infective trauma are usually followed by starvation of greater or lesser degree. In such circumstances, each compounds the problems of the other, resulting in excess catabolism, delayed healing, reduced immunocompetence and susceptibility to infection (Fisher, 1975). Nutritional therapy is employed to combat these. Whether such therapy is given orally or intravenously, or both, the principles are the same in each case. The energy requirement of the 'ideal adult' during the flow phase is up to 3000 kcal (12.6 MJ) (Cairnie *et al.*, 1957) and the protein nitrogen requirement up to 15 G (100 G protein) (Kinney and Roe, 1962).

THE AGENTS USED

Carbohydrates: Glucose is the most physiological, the most widely available and the cheapest energy substrate. It is also one of the least toxic when delivered in large quantities.

It is metabolized via the Embden-Mayrhof pathway through trioses to pyruvate with the production of a few high energy bonds. This process is anaerobic. Insulin is required for the entry of glucose into cells and entry into this pathway. Pyruvate is then aerobically oxidized via the Krebs cycle, with the production of very many high energy bonds, and waste products carbon dioxide and water. Each gram of glucose when fully oxidized in the body will produce about 4 kcal (17 kJ) of energy (McCance and Widdowson, 1960).

Glucose is easy to dissolve in water (even above 50% solution), is stable, and can be stored for long periods in glass or PVC containers. It is easy to sterilize by autoclaving, due to formation of minute amounts of caramel. This has been called the Maillard reaction. It is important because it is responsible for the compounding of amino acids when mixtures are autoclaved and for chelation of zinc and copper (Freeman *et al.*, 1975). In modular nutrition therapy glucose has distinct advantages.

It does, however, possess some drawbacks:

(1) The intravenous solutions required for delivery of 2000–3000 kcal (8.4–12.6 MJ per 24 hours) are considerably hypertonic and thus highly irritant to veins. Moreover, the rapid intravenous injection of hypertonic glucose depresses blood pressure and peripheral perfusion in the circulation. The same osmotic effect may produce diarrhoea when strong glucose solutions are administered enterally.

(2) Insulin is required for assimilation of glucose into cells and metabolic processes. Diabetic and injured patients in the acute phase may be unable to produce this.

(3) When administered parenterally, large infusions of glucose may cause enough hyperglycaemia, especially in shocked states, to exceed the renal threshold, resulting in glycosuria. This may be corrected by the concurrent administration of soluble insulin, either subcutaneously or, better, from a continuous infusion pump to maintain a blood glucose of 8-12 mmol/l. The insulin requirement varies enormously, but 1 unit per hour is a reasonable starting point.

A simple regime providing 2000 kcal (8.4 MJ) would be 1 l of 50% glucose given (via a drip controller) over 15 hours. Alternatively, 3 l of 20% glucose provide 2400 kcal (10 MJ).

Fructose is a normal metabolite of sucrose but is not directly utilized by muscle, heart or brain (only after conversion to glucose in the liver). Fructose uptake and phosphorylation by the liver is an extremely rapid process with a large load capacity. This may, however, be exceeded in starved infants with resultant dangerous lactacidosis. It stores well and can be autoclaved.

The results of fructose administration are thus similar to those of glucose. When given by mouth it will be noted to be exactly twice as sweet as glucose (Moskowitz, 1974). Hereditary fructose intolerance is a contraindication to its use.

It has the same calorific value as glucose, i.e. 4 kcal/g (or 17 kJ per gram) and the same disadvantages except that insulin is not necessary for its uptake into the liver. However, after conversion to glucose 6-phosphate, it is fully dependant on insulin. It has no advantages over glucose, is more toxic and more expensive and is mainly of historical interest.

Sorbitol (D-glucitol) is the hexahydric polyalchol prepared by hydrogenation of D-glucose.

It is converted via fructose to glucose in the liver and is normally found in brain, nerve, kidney, red blood corpuscles and aorta. It is fully and efficiently metabolized in the body, having a calorific value of 4 kcal/g (17 kJ/g). It is, however, just as liable as fructose to produce dangerous lactacidosis. This effect is potentiated by ethyl alcohol.

The maximum recommended rate of infusion before renal overspill into the urine occurs for glucose, fructose and sorbitol is 0.33 g/kg/h. Sorbitol is expensive and is mainly of historical interest.

Overload of the circulation with hypertonic carbohydrate solutions may produce the *hyperosmolar syndrome*, in which the blood pressure, cardiac output and peripheral perfusion fall dramatically, the patient becomes disorientated and the serum sodium level rises.

Ethanol (Atwater and Benedict, 1897) is a well-proven (Robles *et al.*, 1974) energy source with a high energy value of 7 kcal/g (30 kJ/g).

It is easily stored in glass or plastic containers, easily autoclaved, and has a long shelf life. If administered as a 5% solution it is not irritant to veins and has been given up to a maximum of 150 g/day in the adult. Teenagers and children tolerate smaller doses on a weight for weight basis before pharmacological effects appear. These are drowsiness, and disorientation, and flushed face (especially in teenagers and children) with diuresis. Ethanol is liable to produce metabolic acidosis, particularly when given with fructose or sorbitol, and this effect has led to a discontinuation of its use for intravenous feeding.

Disaccharides and oligosaccharides have been developed to overcome the osmotic diarrhoea effects of strong sugar solutions in enteral feeding programmes. They are easily digested, even by a mildly failing gastrointestinal tract and provide a high calorie source without a heavy osmotic load. The disaccharides have also been used for intravenous feeding.

Dextrins (very low molecular weight oligosaccharides) are also being evaluated, and if successful, would overcome one problem of the monosaccharides

*Table 15.1 A simple regime for a 70 kg adult with uncomplicated gastro-
intestinal failure in an intensive care unit. A and B given intravenously
simultaneously using a Y-connection.*

(A)	50% dextrose	1000 ml plus 120 mmol KCl via central line	18 h
(B)	Aminoplex 14 or Vamin or any equivalent preparation	500 ml	6 h
	Hartmann's solution	500 ml plus sodium phosphate 20 mmol	6 h
	Aminoplex 14 or Vamin or any other equivalent preparation	500 ml via a Y connector	6 h
Also	multivitamin preparation 1 ampoule daily as a bolus intravenous injection. (Must contain vitamins A, B_{1-6} and B_{12}, C, D, K and folic acid)		
Also	Trace elements 1 ampoule daily as a bolus intravenous injection		
Also	Soluble insulin, 1 unit, hourly by subcutaneous injection		

(e.g. glucose) which is the high osmotic concentration required to carry ample
calories in a reasonably small quantity of solution.

Butanediol and propanediol are as good a calorie supply as glucose, but
hepatotoxic in large amounts. They must be well diluted with glucose.

Proteins The protein food which has the most complete utilization in normal
man is egg albumin. For this reason, many of the available products attempt to
follow the amino acid pattern found in this protein, or in another highly utilized
protein from milk, i.e. Casein. For intravenous administration, amino acids must
be used and preparations should contain all the essential amino acids as well as a
balanced quantity of the non-essential ones (see Table 15.2).

Oral preparations

These are based on Casein, casein hydrolysates, egg albumin, hydrolyzed beef
protein or crystalline amino acids. (See Table 15.3) The choice between amino
acids and proteins depends on the degree of gastrointestinal failure. Low
molecular weight peptides are more efficiently absorbed from the gastro-
intestinal tract than amino acid preparations. The use of an enteric coated
pancreatic enzyme capsule may render the use of oral protein preparations more
effective (Blackburn *et al.*, 1976). Many of the available preparations contain
carbohydrates and fats and salts in addition. In maintenance diets 8% of the
calories are supplied as protein, while in the adaptive phase after injury, 16% of
the calories are supplied as proteins (Hallowell *et al.*, 1976). Where amino acids
are used, concentrations greater than 8% are not very palatable (Blackburn *et al.*,

235

Table 15.2 Composition of some intravenous preparations

Preparation	Constituents	Contents per litre						Remarks
		Kcal	N(g)	Na⁺ mmol	K⁺ mmol	PO₄ mmol	pH	
Aminoplex 14	synthetic l-amino acids	340	13.4	35	30	0	7.0	Reliable basic preparation.
Vamin 7%	l-amino acids	650	9.4	50	20	0	5.2	Reliable basic preparation.
Amigen 800	casein hydrolysate fructose/ethanol	800	6.0	35	18	0.4	5.6	Fructose is the chief caloric source.
Aminosol 10%	casein hydrolysate	330	12.8	160	0.15	0.5	5.0	Reliable basic preparation. High ammonia content.
Trophysan conc 10	synthetic d, and l- amino acids	724	12.1	10	8	0	6.3	d-Amino acids poorly utilized. Glycine excess.
Aminofusin L 1000	synthetic l-amino acids sorbitol/ethanol	1000	7.6	40	30	0	6.8	Basic combined preparation. The sorbitol and ethanol content has drawbacks.
Aminoplex 5	synthetic l-amino acids, sorbitol/ethanol	1000	5.0	35	15	0	7.0	Basic combined preparation. The sorbitol and ethanol content has drawbacks.

Note: In the table above, the Na⁺, K⁺, and PO₄ columns are expressed in mmol.

Table 15.3 Composition of some enteral preparations

| Product | (kcal/l) | % calories from: | | | Protein source | CBH source | Fat source |
		Protein	Carbo-hydrate	Fat	Essential fatty			
Vivonex	1000	8	90	1.3	1.0	l-amino acids	maltose, dextrins	safflower oil
Vivonex-hn.	1000	16	84	0.8	0.6	l-amino acids	glucose, maltose	safflower oil
Jejunal	900	9	90	0.8	0.6	l-amino acids	glucose	safflower oil
Hy-cal	2300	5	87	8	–	–	glucose	–
Clinifeed 400	1066	16	61	33	–	milk, egg	maize, soya, wheat, sugar, honey	maize oil, soya oil
Clinifeed 500	1330	24	55	21	–	milk	corn, sugar	soya oil
Triosorbon MCT.	484	15	48	37	–	milk	monooligo, and polysaccharides	medium chain triglycerides

1976), and parenteral supplements will be required. When gastrointestinal failure is complete, or enteral feeding is contraindicated, parenteral nutrition is indicated.

Intravenous preparations

These contain amino acids. The choice includes casein hydrolysates and crystalline amino acids (Table 15.2). It is important that the preparation used contains the essential amino acids (Buse and Reid, 1975; Border *et al.*, 1976) and that these contribute 40% of the total amino acids (Munro, 1970).

It is also important that the non-essential amino acids are in reasonably balanced proportions. A gross excess of one, e.g. glycine, may prove toxic. Many of the available preparations contain calorie sources, e.g. sorbitol, glucose, fructose and ethanol, often in the ratio of 200 kcal (850 kJ)/g of amino acid nitrogen. This ratio is in the middle of the range of nitrogen/calorie ratios which extend from 150 kcal/g N (anabolic diets) through 300 kcal/g N (maintenance diets) to 700 kcal/g N (severe renal and hepatic failure diets). Because of the simplicity of the balanced solutions, they may conveniently be used as the mainstay of parenteral nutrition therapy with modification by modules of amino acids, carbohydrate, fat, vitamins and salts.

Fat emulsions are excellent as a rich energy source (9 kcal (38 kJ)/g) without a heavy osmotic load. As shown above, in the simple starved state they are the preferred energy source, and carry the strong advantage of providing additional phosphates, and the essential fatty acids, linolinic and linoleic acid.

In the post-traumatic state, e.g. adaptive phase, they are less easily utilized, and smaller quantities should be given (e.g. up to 500 ml 20% soyabean emulsion in 24 h). Fat administration may prevent hypophosphatemia with its unpleasant symptoms (Travis *et al.*, 1971), confusion and disorientation, with an erythrocyte P 50 below 25, resulting in poor oxygen transport in blood (Lichtman *et al.*, 1971), hypoxia, pulmonary oedema and lactic acidosis and poor lymphocyte function (Craddock *et al.*, 1974). If hypophosphatemia occurs, it may be treated by direct administration of phosphate.

Where there is some degree of gastrointestinal failure, fat digestion is frequently the most affected of the various activities of the gut. Enteral fat administration may in these circumstances lead to profuse offensive diarrhoea because of malabsorption. This situation may be helped by use of medium chain triglycerides for enteral nutrition therapy, which are very easily absorbed, apparently without need for further digestion and are oxidized directly in the liver (Senior, 1968). They are available in modular and compound products. Mono and diglycerides are also available. As with all enteral therapy, fats should be started at half strength and increased to full strength (Moore and Brennan, 1975; Bury *et al.*, 1971; Stephens and Randell, 1969) after 24–48 h.

Vitamins and trace elements

Many of the apparent complications of prolonged parenteral nutrition in the past, e.g. hypochromic anaemia (Sanders *et al.*, 1977), macrocytic anaemia, hypoprothrombin-anaemia and capillary fragility, have now been shown to be due to deficiency of vitamins and trace elements. These may now be administered with comparative ease since preparations have become available which may be given by mouth or intravenously. One of the advantages of using liquidized ordinary hospital food for enteral feeds is that these elements will almost certainly be present, together with dietary fibre. Table 15.4 gives the daily requirements.

Table 15.4 Daily electrolyte & vitamin requirements

			Adult	Children
Sodium	80 mmol	Vitamin A	3000 IU	2000 IU
Potassium	100 mmol	B		
Magnesium	15 mmol	Thiamine B_1	3 mg	1.5 mg
Calcium	15 mmol	Riboflavin B_2	3 mg	1.5 mg
Phosphorus	40 mmol	Niacin	40 mg	20 mg
Iron	100 mmol	B_6	4 mg	1 mg
Zinc	30 mg	Pantothenic acid	15 mg	5 mg
Manganese	5 mg	Folic acid	1 mg	1 mg
Copper	2 mg	B_{12}	0.03 mg 1 kg	0.2 mg 1 kg
Chromium	0.2mg	Biotin	5 mg 1 kg	30 mg 1 kg
Cobalt	0.05 mg	C	100 mg	80 mg
Iodine	0.5 mg	D	200 IU	400 IU
		E *a* tacopherol	10 IU	5 IU
		K *phytylmenaquinone	2 mg 1 kg	50 mg 1 kg

Note: There is wide variation in the recommended allowances by different authorities. The above are average figures.
* Menadione may cause haemolysis and enzyme inhibition and should not be used in intravenous therapy.

ASSESSMENT OF CALORIFIC REQUIREMENTS

Ideally, daily measurement of actual energy expenditure would provide the information for matching intake of calories to requirements. Daily nitrogen balances should indicate the recommended protein nitrogen intake. In the absence of Kjeldahl estimations, a simple clinical formula for the nitrogen loss is:

$$\text{Nitrogen loss} = \frac{(35 \times \text{daily urine output} \times \text{urinary urea})}{100} + 1.2 \text{ g}$$

The Harris–Benedict equations are simpler and for practical purposes are accurate enough for calculations of the Basal Energy Expenditure (BEE).

To relate the calorie intake of the patient to the energy expenditure, the basis provided by Rutten *et al.* (1975) is useful. It may be seen that for uncomplicated post surgical cases, i.e. 1st and 2nd degree catabolism, the Resting Metabolic Expenditure is similar to the Basal Energy Expenditure calculated

239

from the Harris-Benedict equations (Harris and Benedict, 1919; Rutten *et al.*, 1975).

Males: BEE = 66.473 + 13.7516(W) + 5.0033(H) − 6.7550(A)
Females: BEE = 655 + 9.6534(W) + 1.8496(H) − 4.6756(A)

where H = Height in cm, W = Weight in kg and A = Age in years.

For oral (enteral) nutrition the calorie requirement is 1.54 × Basal Energy Expenditure per day.

For intravenous (parenteral) nutrition, the calorie requirement is 1.76 × Basal Energy Expenditure per day. (See Table 15.5.)

Table 15.5 Daily calorie and nitrogen requirement for an average 70 kg adult.

	Daily calorie requirement	Daily amino acid nitrogen requirement
Normal	1500–2000	5 g
After major surgery, (uncomplicated)	2000–3000	5–10 g
Moderate burns, or major infective focus.	2500–3000	10–15 g
Major burns, septicaemia.	3000–3500	15 g

The higher caloric requirement during parenteral nutrition is due to the mild degree of hyperinsulinism which follows constant infusion of strong glucose solutions, resulting in diversion of some of the infused glucose into lipogenesis. These calorie intakes have been shown to produce a high net protein utilization of 72%.

Moderate catabolism, for example, in surgery complicated by infection may require a calorie intake of 2 × Basal Energy Expenditure and 4th degree (severe catabolism) such as that found in major burns, may require 2.5 × Basal Energy Expenditure per day (Wilson *et al.*, 1974). The nitrogen/calorie ratios are those indicated in the section on protein sources.

CYCLICAL (INTERMITTENT) ADMINISTRATION OF PARENTERAL NUTRITION THERAPY

It is long established that better net protein utilization occurs when amino acids, fats and carbohydrates are given concurrently. This has led to the use of 24 h continuous drip regimes. However, to allow a conscious patient periods of the day when his drip line is *not* in use carries two important advantages.

First, it may improve patient morale and diurnal rhythm. These areas are only recently receiving attention in intensive care units, and cyclical nutritional therapy is one way in which they may be forwarded.

To give parenteral solutions only at night, or only during the day, or in two separate periods, gives the patient a welcome break from the dreary round of intensive intravenous therapy. The giving set is disconnected, the catheter filled with heparinised saline and closed off with a sterile tap or rubber cover.

Secondly, constant infusions of carbohydrates, especially glucose, usually produce considerable reflex secretion of insulin, the anabolic hormone, one of the actions of which is lipogenesis, especially hepatic (O'Connell *et al.*, 1973) and the prevention of lipolysis of existing body fat stores (Flatt and Blackburn, 1974). Lipogenesis may consume about 70% of the administered metabolic energy (Blackburn and Bistrian, 1976).

Cyclical therapy thus allows periods of lipolysis to occur, providing phosphate and essential fatty acids to be liberated into the circulation. (This does not apply in the marasmic patient who would require exogenous fat administration (Jeejeebhoy *et al.*, 1974).) It would appear to increase the efficiency of utilization of administered calories (Maini *et al.*, 1976).

Cyclical therapy calls for care in not exceeding the maximum rates of carbohydrate administration, and may require the use of a drip set with a Y-piece which delivers solutions from two different bottles concurrently into the same intravenous cannula or catheter. (See also Bennotti *et al.*, 1976.)

PREVENTION OF COMPLICATIONS

In parenteral nutrition, thrombophlebitis of veins into which the nutrient solutions are delivered remains the commonest problem of this therapy. Scrupulous care in setting up the infusion is required, drip sets should be changed daily and the dripsite inspected daily (just like any wound), and sprayed with a suitable antimicrobial spray. Antibiotic sprays should not be used as they merely encourage the development of antibiotic resistant bacteria which may then gain access to the bloodstream. The drip site should be kept dry (Dillon *et al.*, 1973; Winters *et al.*, 1972).

Leg veins should not be used because of the greater risk of phlebothrombosis and thromboembolism.

The drip site may be changed every day before signs of thrombophlebitis appear, although the speed of onset of this condition is largely determined by the individual response of the patient's veins, some being irritated in a few hours and others showing no problems for weeks or even months (Ryan *et al.*, 1974a; Wilmore and Dudrick, 1969).

Central venous catheters are most useful, being inserted from median cubital, internal jugular and subclavian veins, using full aseptic technique.

A drip entering the patient through an infected drip site must be removed to prevent bacteraemia and septicaemia. Serial blood cultures are helpful in the early diagnosis of septicaemia due to *Candida*.

SPECIAL CIRCUMSTANCES

In enteral nutrition, *diarrhoea* often heralds the overload of a failing gastrointestinal tract. It may be due to carbohydrate or amino acid induced osmotic load, or to inadequate protein digestion and absorption in the proximal small

241

bowel. Poor digestion of fats without absorption throughout the small bowel is common and may be associated with bacterial overgrowth, causing further gastrointestinal failure. Reduction of the offending elements or bowel rest is indicated.

The problems in *renal failure* are discussed in Chapter 13.

In *severe hepatic failure*, there is reduced ability to deaminate branched (Munro *et al.*, 1975) amino acids, especially tryptophan. Other, aromatic, amino acids are inadequately synthesized (Fischer *et al.*, 1975). The aim of therapy is to correct this situation while avoiding anything which may hamper hepatic function further. Thus, ethanol is contraindicated, fats are given in minimal amounts and amino acid preparations are specially formulated (Aguirre *et al.*, 1974). Carbohydrate calories are given to meet the calculated energy requirement exactly, as excess calories give the added work of lipogenesis. Ammonia-containing solutions should be avoided (Stein *et al.*, 1976).

In *diabetes*, insulin requirements may be increased after trauma and insulin resistance may be encountered especially in severe or prolonged infective states. Very frequent, even hourly, monitoring of blood sugar levels may be required (Porte and Bagdade, 1970; Ryan *et al.*, 1974). Ketoacidosis is always a potential problem in diabetes.

In neonates, the calorie intake may be over 100 kcal/kg/day, falling to half this figure when body weight exceeds 10 kg.

The infant protein intake is 3 g/kg per day, giving a nitrogen/calorie ratio of 1/200, similar to the adult ratio.

Neonates and infants accept fats well by both enteral and parenteral routes and their veins, though small, tolerate amino acid, fat emulsion and glucose solutions (Winters and Hasselmey, 1975). Fats may with advantage be used to contribute over 50% of the calorie intake. Fructose carries the risk of lact-acidaemia.

Hyperaminoacidaemia, hyperosmolar syndrome and infected dripsites are complications to be avoided by frequent monitoring and scrupulous care.

Anaemia may call for blood transfusion and *hypo-albuminaemia* may require plasma or albumin infusion.

Circulatory overload, particularly in the elderly, is avoided by reduction of the water and salt load, perhaps with CVP and frequent electrolyte monitoring, and careful maintenance of the serum protein level. *Lactic Acidosis* resulting from overinfusion of fructose, ethanol and sorbitol is detected by daily acid/base estimations, and treated with bicarbonate if necessary. Urine testing for glucose is of limited value since *glycosuria* is a common accompaniment of serious disease. However, glycosuria does indicate increased insulin requirement.

ENTERAL NUTRITION

Indications

(1) To feed a patient who has normal gastro-intestinal function but is

unable to swallow due to unconsciousness, paralysis, psychiatric disease, senility or upper gut abnormality.

(2) In combination with parenteral feeding in patients whose gastrointestinal function is recovering from failure.

(3) In continuing partial gastrointestinal failure from various causes.

Partially predigested or completely digested (elemental) diets may be given by mouth, by nasogastric tube, by gastrostomy or by jejunostomy, depending on the patient's condition. By mouth, palatability is important. The presence of more than 8% aminoacids or ketoacids in a mixture will probably render it unpalatable. A nasogastric tube may with advantage be a fine-bore radio-opaque 60 cm length with internal diameter 1 mm. A lubricated Seldinger wire stiffens it for insertion via the nose, pharynx and oesophagus to the stomach, leaving 2–3 cm projecting from the nose. The guide wire is withdrawn with moderate traction. The correct position of the tube is verified by air injection and auscultation over the stomach or by X-ray. The feed is then dripped or pumped continuously down the tube during daytime hours.

The diet

The normal 200 kcal/g of nitrogen ratio is satisfactory for most patients, and this is easy to achieve with combinations of the available products.

Liquidized hospital food, either from the hospital daily menu, or specially prepared is easy, cheap and effective, but is not sterile and may be the route by which pseudomonas and other bacteria gain access to ill patients. Its strong advantage is that it contains dietary fibre.

Commercially available conventional diets, e.g. *Clinifeed* (particularly suited for fine-bore oral feeding) and *Complan*, if made up or diluted with sterile water are effective, safe and of relatively low osmolarity. Other calorie sources are saccharides, e.g. *Hycal* and polysaccharides, e.g. *Caloreen*.

Elemental diets are prepared from protein hydrolysates or amino acids combined with glucose (or its polymers), lactose or dextrins. They are of low residue, and have been recommended for inflammatory bowel disease, gastro-intestinal fistulae, exocrine pancreatic failure, short-gut syndrome, preparation for surgery and radiology, and space travel! They have high osmolarity however and may cause diarrhoea, nausea, vomiting, dumping syndrome, osmotic diuresis and hyperosmolar coma. Some contain medium chain (8 carbon atom) tri-glycerides, e.g. *Triosorbon*, added vitamins and electrolytes. They are expensive, e.g. *Vivonex, Aminutrin, Calonutrin, Flexical, Albumaid*.

Pancreatic enzymes may be given by mouth for the specific treatment of exocrine pancreatic deficiencies, e.g. *Nutrizym*.

Problems with enteral (oral) diets

(1) Osmotic overload with diarrhoea. Prevented by gradual introduction of diluted feed over 3 days. Otherwise it may be treated by codein phosphate, 30 mg twice daily.

243

(2) Introduction of infection. Reasonable care should be exercised in preparation and storage. It should be remembered that tap water contains bacteria.

(3) Inadvertent intravenous administration. Containers of these feeds should be clearly labelled 'not for intravenous use'.

(4) In chronic renal failure, protein intake is restricted to 40 g/day or less. Below 20 g/day, essential amino acids are indicated, e.g. *Kidnamin, Nefranutrin, EAS Perlen*. Ketoacid analogues of essential amino acids have theoretical advantages here. Sodium intake is severely reduced and diuretics may help. Iron supplements are usually required. Hyperphosphataemia may be controlled by oral aluminium hydroxide.

(5) In diabetes, the usual careful monitoring and insulin therapy is required.

SUMMARY

The rewards of adequate nutritional therapy are greater resistance to infection, accelerated wound healing (Moss *et al.*, 1976), maintenance of body mass with positive nitrogen balance, increased immunocompetence (Bistrian *et al.*, 1975) and even increased host resistance to carcinomas (Ota *et al.*, 1977). These are rich rewards for the expenditure of a little therapeutic care.

REFERENCES

Abel, R. M., Abbott, W. M. and Fischer, J. E. (1971), Acute renal failure. Treatment without dialysis by total parenteral nutrition. Archives of Surgery, 1971; 103: 513.

Aguirre, A., Yoshimura, and N. Westman, T. (1974), Plasma Amino Acids in dogs with two experimental forms of liver damage. *J. Surg. Res.*, 16, 339.

Atwater, W. O. and Benedict, F. G. (1897), An experimental enquiry regarding the nutritive value of alcohol. *Memoranda Nat. Acad. Sci.*, 8, 235.

Bennotti, P. *et al.* (1976), Cyclic Hyperalimentation Comprehensive Therapy.

Blackburn, G. L. and Flatt, J. P. (1975), Metabolic response to illness. Role of protein-sparing therapy. *Comprehensive Therapy*, 1, 23.

Blackburn, G. L., Bistrian, B. R. and Flatt, J. P. (1975), Restoration of the visceral component of protein malnutrition during hypocaloric feedings. *Clin. Res.*, 23, 315A.

Blackburn, G. L. and Bistrian, B. R. (1976), Nutritional care of the injured and/or septic patient. *Surg. Clin. N. Am.*, 56, 1195.

Blackburn, G. L., Williams, L. F. and Bistrian, B. R. (1976), New approaches to the management of severe acute pancreatitis. *Am. J. Surg.*, 131, 114.

Blackburn, G. L. and Bistrian, B. R. (1976), In Nutritional Support of Medical Practice (ed Schneider, H.). Harper and Row, New York.

Bistrian, B. R., Blackburn, G. L., Scrimshaw, N. S. and Flatt, J. P. (1975), Cellular immunity in semi-starved states in hospitalised adults. *Am. J. Clin. Nutr.*, 28, 1147.

Border, J. R., Chenier, R. and McMenamy, R. H. (1976), Multiple Systems Organ Failure. Muscle fuel deficit with visceral protein malnutrition. *Surg. Clin. N. Am.*, 56, 1147.

Bury, K. D., Stephens, R. V. and Randall, H. T. (1971), Use of a chemically defined liquid elemental diet for nutritional management of fistulas of the alimentary tract. *Am. J. Surg.*, **121**, 174.

Buse, M. G. and Reid, S. S. (1975), Leucine: A possible regulator of protein turnover in muscle. *J. clin. Invest.*, **56**, 1250.

Cahill, A. F. (1970), Starvation in man. *N. Eng. J. Med.*, **282**, 668.

Cairnie, A. B., Campbell, R. M., Pullar, J. D. and Cuthbertson, D. P. (1957), The heat production consequent to injury. *Brit. J. exp. Path.*, **38**, 504.

Craddock, P. R., Yawata, Y., Van Santen, L., Gilberstadt, S., Silvis, S. and Jacob, H. S. (1974), Acquired phagocyte dysfunction resulting from parenteral hyperalimentation. *N. Eng. J. Med.*, **290**, 1403.

Cuthbertson, D. P. (1942), Post shock metabolic response. *Lancet*, i, 433.

Den Besten, L., Reyna, R. H. and Connor. W. E. (1973), The different effects on serum lipids and faecal steroids of high carbohydrate diets given orally or i.v. *J. clin. Invest.*, **52**, 1384.

Dillon, J. D., Schaffner, W. and Van Way, C. W. (1973), Septicaemia and total parenteral nutrition. *J. Am. Med. Ass.*, **223**, 1341.

Fischer, J. E. (1975), *Total Parenteral Nutrition*. Little Brown and Co., Boston.

Fischer, J. E., Funovics, J. M. and Aguirre, A. (1975), The role of plasma amino acids in hepatic encephalopathy. *Surgery*, **78**, 276.

Flatt, J. P. and Blackburn, G. L. (1974), The metabolic fuel regulatory system: Implications for protein sparing therapies during caloric deprivation and disease. *Am. J. clin. Nut.*, **27**, 175.

Freeman, J. B., Stegink, L. D. and Meyer, P. D. (1975), Excessive Urinary Zinc losses during parenteral Alimentation. *J. Surg. Res.*, **18**, 463.

Fulks, R. M., Li, J. B. and Goldberg, A. L. (1975), Effects of insulin, glucose and amino acids on protein turnover in the rat diaphragm. *J. Biol. Chem.*, **250**, 290.

Gamble, J. L. (1946), Physiological information gained from studies on the life raft ration. *Harvey Lectures*, **42**, 247.

Giddings, A. E. (1974), The control of plasma glucose in the surgical patient. *Brit. J. Surg.*, **61**, 787.

Go, V. L., Hofman, A. F. and Summerskill, W. H. (1970), Pancreozymin bio-assay in man based on pancreatic enzyme secretion. Potency of specific amino acids and other digestion products. *J. clin. Invest.*, **49**, 1558.

Hallowell, E., Sasvary, D. and Bistrian, B. R. (1976), Factors determining optimal use of defined (elemental) formula diets. *Clin. Res.*, **24**, 500A.

Harris, J. A. and Benedict, F. G. (1919), A Biometric Study of basal metabolism in man. *Publication 279, Carnegie Institution*, Washington.

Hiebert, J. M., Celik, Z., Soeldner, J. S. and Egdahl, R. H. (1973), Insulin response to haemorrhagic shock in the intact and adrenalectomised primate. *Am. J. Surg.*, **125**, 501.

Jeejeebhoy, K. N., Anderson, G. H., Sanderson, I. and Bryan, M. H. (1974), Total Parenteral Nutrition. Nutrient needs and technical tips. *Mod. Med.*, Canada, **29**, 1.

Johnston, I. D. A. (1973), The metabolic and endocrine response to injury—a review. *Brit. J. Anaesth.*, **45**, 252.

Kinney, J. M. and Roe, C. F. (1962), *Annals of Surgery*, **156**, 610.

Lerner, R. L. and Porte, D. (1971), Epinephrine: Selective inhibition of the acute insulin response to glucose. *J. clin. Invest.*, **50**, 2453.

Lichtman, M. A., Miller, D. R. and Cohen, J. (1971), Reduced red cell glycolysis, 23DPG and ATP concentration and increased haemoglobin oxygen affinity caused by hypophosphataemia. *Ann. Int. Med.*, **74**, 562.

MacLean, L. D., Mulligan, W. A., MacLean, A. P. H. and Duff, J. H. (1967), Patterns of septic shock in man—a detailed study of 56 patients. *Ann. Surg.*, **166**, 543.

Maini, B., Blackburn, G. L. and Bistrian, B. R. (1976), Cyclic hyperalimentation, an optimal technique for preservation of visceral protein. *J. Surg. Res.*, **20**, 515.

McCance, R. A. and Widdowson, E. M., The Composition of Human Foods, M.R.C. Special Report Series No. 297, London HMSO, 1960.

Moore, F. D. (1971), in *Manual of preoperative and postoperative care*. ed Kinney, J. M., Egdahl, R. H. and Zuidema, G. D. W. B. Saunders Co., Philadelphia.

Moore, F. D. and Brennan, M. F. (1975), *Manual of Surgical Nutrition*. eds Ballinger, W. F. *et al.* W. B. Saunders Co., Philadelphia, p. 169.

Moskowitz, H. R. (1974), in *The Psychology of Sweetness of Sugars in Nutrition*. eds Stipple, H. D. and McNutt, K. W. Academic Press, New York.

Moss, G., Bierenbaum, A. and Bova, F. (1976), Postoperative metabolic patterns following immediate total nutritional support: hormone levels, D.N.A. synthesis, nitrogen balance, and accelerated wound healing. *J. Surg. Res.*, **21**, 383.

Munck, A. (1971), Glucocorticoid inhibition of glucose uptake by peripheral tissues. Old and new evidence. Molecular mechanisms and physiological significance. *Perspect. Biol. Med.*, **14**, 265.

Munro, H. N. (1972), in *Intravenous Hyperalimentation*. eds Cowan, B. and Sheetz, H. L. Lea and Febiger, Philadelphia, p. 34.

Munro, H. N. (1970), in *Mammalian Protein Metabolism* Vol. 4, p. 299. Academic Press, New York.

Munro, H. N., Fernstrom, J. D. and Wurtman, R. J. (1975), Insulin, plasma amino acid imbalance and hepatic coma. *Lancet*, i, 722.

O'Connell, R. C., Morgan, A. P. and Aoki, T. T. (1973), Nitrogen conservation in starvation; Graded responses to intravenous glucose. *J. clin. Endocrin. Metabol.*, **89**, 555.

Ota, D. M., Copeland, E. M. and Strobel, H. W. (1977), The effect of protein nutrition on host and tumour metabolism. *J. Surg. Res.*, **22**, 181.

Porte, D. and Bagdade, J. D. (1970), Human insulin secretion: An integrated approach. *A. Rev. Med.*, **21**, 219.

Robles, E. A., Mezey, E., Halsted, C. H. *et al.* (1974), Effect of ethanol on motility of the small intestine. *Johns Hopkins Med. J.*, **135**, 17.

Rose, W. C. (1949), Amino acid requirements of men. *Fedn Am. Socs exp. Biol.*, **8**, 546.

Rutten, P., Blackburn, G. L. and Flatt, J. P. (1975), Determination of optional hyperalimentation infusion rate. *J. Surg. Res.*, **18**, 477.

Ryan, J. A., Abel, R. M., Abbott, W. M., Hopkins, C. C., Chisney, T., Colley, R.,

Phillips, K. and Fisher, J. E. (1974), Catheter complications in total parenteral nutrition. A prospective study of 200 consecutive patients. *N. Eng. J. Med.*, **290**, 757.

Ryan, N. T., Blackburn, G. L. and Clowes, G. H. A. (1974), Differential tissue sensitivity of elevated endogenous insulin levels during experimental peritonitis in rats. *Metabolism*, **23**, 1081.

Ryan, N. T. (1976), Metabolic Adaptations for Energy Production during Trauma and Sepsis. *Surg. Clin. N. Am.*, **56**, 1073.

Sanders, R., Sheldon, G. F., Garcia, J. *et al.* (1977), Erythropoietin synthesis in rats during total parenteral nutrition. *J. Surg. Res.*, **22**, 649.

Senior, J. R. (1968), *Medium Chain Triglycerides*. University of Pennsylvania Press, Philadelphia.

Shambaugh, G. E. and Beisel, W. R. (1967), Insulin response during tularaemia in man. *Diabetes*, **16**, 369.

Stein, T. P., Leskin, M. J. and Wallace, H. W. (1976), Metabolism of parenterally administered ammonia. *J. Surg. Res.*, **21**, 17.

Stephens, R. D. and Randall, H. T. (1969), Use of concentrated, balanced liquid elemental diet for nutritional management of catabolic states. *Ann. Surg.*, **170**, 642.

Tanaka, N., Sakaguchi, S., Oshige, K. *et al.* (1976), Effect of chronic administration of Propranolol on lipoprotein composition. *Metabolism*, **25**, 1071.

Travis, S. F., Sugerman, H. J., Ruberg, R. L. (1971), Alteration of red cell glycolytic intermediates and oxygen transport as a consequence of hypophosphataemia in patients receiving intravenous hyperalimentation. *New Eng. J. Med.*, **285**, 763.

Walser, M. (1974), Urea Metabolism in chronic renal failure. *Journal of Clinical Investigation*, **53**, 1385.

Waterlow, J. C. and Stephen, J. M. (1967), The measurement of total lysine turnover in the rat by intravenous infusion of L ($U^{14}C$) lysine. *Clin. Sci.*, **33**, 489.

Wilmore, D. W. and Dudrick, S. J. (1969), Treatment of Acute Renal failure with intravenous essential L-amino acids. *Arch. Surg.*, **99**, 669.

Wilmore, D. W., Long, J. M. and Mason, A. D. (1974), Catecholamines: mediator of the hypermetabolic responses to thermal injury. *Ann. Surg.*, **180**, 653.

Winters, R. W., Santulli, T. V., Heird, W. C., Schillinger, J. N. and Driscoll, J. H. (1972), Hyperalimentation without sepsis. *N. Eng. J. Med.*, **286**, 321.

Winters, R. W. and Hasselmey, E. G. (1975), *Intravenous Nutrition in the High Risk Infant*. John Wiley and Sons, New York.

SIXTEEN

Poisoning

Self poisoning is increasing in incidence and in many units is among the commonest reasons for admission.

Only in a few cases is a specific antidote available or necessary, so emphasis must be placed on the general principles of maintaining vital functions and only after this can attention move to specific or pharmacological antidotes, and techniques to enhance elimination of the drug.

Table 16.1 Principles of management of drug overdose

Maintenance of vital functions	Airway
	Circulation
	Fluid and electrolytes
	Hypothermia
Elimination of drug	induced vomiting/gastric lavage*
	other techniques
Antidotes	Specific
	Pharmacological

(1) Never when corrosive agents have been taken
  (2) Never in unconscious patients, unless cuffed endotracheal tube in position.

DIAGNOSIS OF SELF-POISONING

Frequently the diagnosis will be apparent if a note has been found with the patient or if she has announced her intention of taking an overdose; if conscious, a history (often very unreliable) may be obtainable. However, unconscious patients may be a problem and it must be remembered that a history of psychiatric illness does not provide immunity to meningitis, subarachnoid haemorrhage or other causes of unconsciousness, including, of course, head injury.

Examination is unlikely to be productive of diagnostic physical signs, however assessment of ventilating function is essential and should be done immediately. Superficial *blistering* occurs in barbiturate poisoning and rarely in other overdoses. *Venepuncture* marks, often with evidence of recurrent thrombophlebitis, may lead to suspicion of serious narcotic overdose. *Pupil size* may be misleading, in particular fixed dilated pupils are a common finding in Mandrax (methaqualone with diphenhydramine) poisoning. In this condition other abnormal neurological signs may be present (see below) leading to a mistaken diagnosis of organic neurological disease. Similar neurological signs may be present and equally misleading in glutethamide (Doriden) poisoning. *Papilloedema* also occurs in children who have taken Nalidixic acid (Negram). An unconscious patient with no lateralising signs in the CNS, and no evidence of head injury, can be regarded as suffering from drug poisoning while investigations into the circumstances of the coma are proceeding. In this respect information from the police or ambulance personnel may be valuable.

IDENTIFICATION OF DRUG

The current trend is towards the deliberate ingestion of a cocktail of anti-depressant and sedative drugs, often with the help of alcohol. These mixtures may produce a confusing picture. Any tablets or bottles found with the patient should be identified (however, it is unwise to assume that an empty bottle has contained the drug that its label states). Early identification of the drug can be of great importance, particularly if paracetamol has been taken, and it should be noted that many analgesics, e.g. Distalgesic, contain paracetamol.

The constituents of proprietary drugs can always be checked in a reference book such as Martindale's Extra Pharmacopea. Unlabelled tablets should be identified in the Pharmacy.

However it is a mistake to waste a great deal of time in identification of drugs and, generally, full scale blood and urine forensic biochemistry is not indicated as the results will not influence the management of the case when they arrive many hours or days later. Blood should however be taken if there is any suspicion of salicylate poisoning, as the level is important, and the estimation quick and relatively easy. There is no reason for routine blood barbiturate estimation in unconscious patients as barbiturates are less popular as overdose agents; may frequently be taken in conjunction with other drugs; and the result may be misleading, e.g. in patients with epilepsy who tolerate high levels of barbiturate without loss of consciousness. Prognosis and management in paracetamol poisoning depends to some extent on the blood level, and blood should always be taken, with a note of the approximate number of hours after ingestion.

TREATMENT

Immediate measures

(1) *Respiration.* Respiratory function must always be checked immediately. This is best checked by use of an anenometer which can be attached to a face mask or endotracheal tube—a tidal volume of less than 300 ml will be an indication for assisted ventilation.

An endotracheal tube, passed through the mouth or nose will be necessary in most patients unconscious through hypnotic or narcotic overdose. If gastric lavage (see below) is to be used in an unconscious patient the cuff must be inflated to prevent aspiration of gastric contents.

It is unwise to wait for blood gas estimations before diagnosing respiratory insufficiency. The diagnosis is clinical—if there is any doubt it is better to institute IPPV. Many patients left to 'sleep off' their 'trivial' overdose in the corner of a ward have inadequate ventilation.

If respiratory function is adequate the patient should be put on his side and an oro-pharyngeal airway inserted.

(2) *Circulation*. Maintenance of adequate tissue perfusion is of great importance and hypotension occurs in many cases of coma due to drug overdose. The first line of treatment when this happens is to elevate the legs to prevent pooling.

If hypotension (systolic less than 80 mmHg) is not improved by elevation of the foot of the bed a central venous line should be introduced and cautious plasma expansion with plasma or plasma substitute started under CVP control. (See Chapter 3).

It should be remembered that inadequate oxygenation is an important cause of shock and attention is again drawn to the importance of maintaining respiratory function.

Rarely, vasopressor drugs are justified if these measures do not control hypotension. Metaraminol (Aramine) can be given intravenously. The dose is 5 mg and it should not be repeated more than twice at 20 minute intervals.

Cardiac dysrhythmias may complicate some drug overdoses (see below) and appropriate treatment started.

(3) *Fluid and electrolytes*. An intravenous line should always be set up in unconscious patients. Sufficient i.v. fluid is given to produce a urine output of around 1.5 l/day. If the patient has been unconscious for some time before admission some dehydration may be present initially, but if no complication, such as renal failure, develops, electrolyte and fluid control is not difficult. Hyperpyrexia will require infusion rates to be increased.

If urine output drops and the CVP indicates adequate hydration, the amount of fluid may need reduction to avoid overload, while renal function is assessed. Acute tubular necrosis can follow prolonged hypotension.

(4) *Body temperature*. The importance of this is frequently overlooked. Hypothermia is common and may only be identified if rectal temperatures with a low reading thermometer are taken. Gradual rewarming should be started using unheated blankets, or in more severe cases, with a foil 'space blanket'.

Hyperpyrexia most frequently occurs following barbiturate poisoning, and the temperature may rise in many other overdoses during recovery. It is important to recognize this and not prescribe antibiotics unless infection is present.

Elimination of the drug

Physical measures

(1) *Induced vomiting.* This, and gastric lavage (below), must never be attempted if (a) the patient has ingested a corrosive poison, (b) he is unconscious, unless intubated.

Many patients can be induced to vomit by irritating the pharynx with the fingers or blunt spoon. If this fails 15 ml of syrup of ipecacuanha can be given. Saline solutions should not be used.

(2) *Gastric lavage.* The same contraindications apply. If performed in an un-conscious patient a cuffed endotracheal tube must be *in situ*. The indications for gastric lavage are unclear. If the drug has been ingested recently (within 4 hours) it is indicated. However, if salicylates, paracetamol or tricyclic antidepressants have been taken lavage should always be done. Under other circumstances its therapeutic value is in doubt. However the aspirated material (which should always be retained for analysis) might give useful information and the benefits outweigh the risks.

The impression that a punitive gastric lavage will prevent further suicide attempts is fallacious.

A wide bore tube (30 English gauge Jacques) should be used and the lavage performed using warm water. The stomach should be emptied at the end of the procedure.

Other techniques

Before a decision is taken to try and eliminate the drug by forced diuresis, dialysis or other means, the question should always be asked if the technique is appropriate to the drug ingested. It must never be forgotten that the general measures outlined above are mandatory and the improved survival figures for drug overdose depend far more upon maintenance of vital functions than ingenious techniques which may be, in themselves, often dangerous and even more frequently totally inappropriate.

(1) *Forced diuresis.* The theory is that by increasing urine flow a drug that is normally excreted by the kidney will be more rapidly eliminated. In addition, by modifying the pH of urine, certain drugs (notably aspirin in alkaline urine) will be excreted in larger quantities.

The dangers of a forced diuresis are that a large volume of fluid is infused rapidly and pulmonary oedema can readily be provoked in elderly patients with heart disease, or where renal function is reduced. Electrolyte disturbances can result, notably hypernatraemia.

Indications

(a) Aspirin poisoning

(b) Phenobarbitone overdose

(c) Meprobamate overdose

(d) Amphetamine overdose (forced acid diuresis)

(2) *Dialysis.* Haemodialysis (not peritoneal) may be indicated in severe barbiturate poisoning, but the principal indication is renal failure consequent upon the nature of the poison, or secondary to shock.

Antidotes

Specific antidotes, where available—and there are very few—are discussed under the individual drugs below, as are drugs to counteract the effects of the agent ingested.

General care

Coma might be protracted and intensive nursing care is essential to prevent bedsores and the other complications of prolonged unconsciousness.

Prophylactic antibiotics are not indicated. Antibiotics should only be used where there is clinical evidence of infection.

Tracheotomy may be necessary if IPPV through a cuffed tube has to be maintained for 72 hours or more, although modern endotracheal tubes are relatively less irritant to the tracheal mucosa and some anaesthetists would not consider tracheostomy for 5-6 days.

The *psychiatric* element of drug overdose must not be overlooked. Often the ITU is not the appropriate environment for a psychiatric consultation, but it must be remembered that even the most 'trivial' overdose is an indication for help from the psychiatrists. Generally this will be after the patient has been transferred back to the general ward.

POISONING BY SPECIFIC SUBSTANCES

The remaining part of this chapter is devoted to specific poisons. It is not intended to be a complete list. It should be noted that Poison Information Centres have been set up in different parts of the British Isles and full and up to date advice on the management of poisoning can always be obtained from them. These centres will be able to provide details of the composition and toxic hazards of any substance or chemical to which the patient has been exposed. If there is any doubt about the management of a case the Poison Centre should always be contacted.

Poison Information Centres

Belfast	0232 30503
Cardiff	0222 33101
Dublin	Dublin 45588
Edinburgh	031-229 2477
London	01-407 7600
Leeds	0532 32799
Manchester	061-740 2254
Newcastle	0632 25131

INDEX TO SPECIFIC POISONS

	Page		*Page*
Aconite	272	Hydrogen sulphide	270
Alcohols	262	Imipramine	259
Amitriptyline	259	Insecticides	267
Antimony	265	Iron	264
Arsenic	268	Lead	265
Arsine	268	Librium	261
Aspirin	255	Limbritol	259
Ativan	261	Lithium	260
Barbiturates	253	Lorazepam	261
Benzodiazepines	261	Mandrax	262
Bleaches	269	Meprobamate	261
Carbon monoxide	269	Mercury	265
Carbon tetrachloride	269	Miltown	261
Chlorate	269	Mogadon	261
Chlordiazepoxide	261	Monoamine oxidase inhibitors	259
Cresol	269	Morphine	260
Cyanide	265	'Mushrooms'	271
DDT	268	Nitrazepam	261
Deadly nightshade	272	Opiates	260
Dextropropoxyphene	258	Oxazepam	261
Diazepam	261	Paracetamol	257
Digoxin	264	Paraquat	266
Dihydrocodeine	260	Pentazocine	260
Disinfectants	269	Pethidine	260
Distalgesic	257, 258	Phenol	269
Doriden	262	Phenothiazines	261
Ethylene glycol	263	Plant poisons	271
Equanil	261	Serenid	261
Fortral	261	Snake bite	270
Glutethamide	262	Solvents	269
Gold	265	Tofranil	259
Halogenated hydrocarbons	269	Tranzene	261
Haloperidol	262	Tricyclic antidepressants	259
Heavy metals	265	Tryptyzole	259
Heroin	260	Valium	261

BARBITURATE POISONING

There appears to be a decrease in the incidence of self-poisoning by the barbiturate groups of drugs. This probably reflects changes in prescribing habits, possibly due to the campaign to limit the prescription of barbiturates in favour of the benzodiazepines, which although more expensive, are much less dangerous if taken in overdose. Howevere there is a large reservoir of patients, particularly epileptics, on chronic barbiturate therapy; and many elderly patients still prefer them for night sedation.

Clinical picture

Barbiturates are depressants. Examination shows coma with flaccid limbs, arreflexia, shallow depressed respiration, bradycardia and hypotension. The effects of barbiturates overdose are aggravated by alcohol and patients who have taken both are particularly at risk.

Management

In the past a great deal of emphasis has been placed on blood levels, but the relationship between blood levels and severity of the overdose is not certain. Furthermore, addicts and epileptics are tolerant of blood levels that produce coma in other patients, and the levels may, therefore, be a misleading guide to the severity of the problem. However, if blood levels fail to fall, especially if renal impairment occurs, it could be an important factor in deciding on haemodialysis. As a general guide a level of 3.5 mg/100 ml with a long-acting agent, or 8 mg/100 ml with the others, indicates severe intoxication.

Type of barbiturate

Barbiturates are conventionally divided into three groups: long, medium and short-acting. This is of some practical importance in the management of overdose as the excretion of the long-acting agent, phenobarbitone, may be enhanced by the use of forced diuresis (see below). Most patients are prescribed medium or short-acting barbiturates either alone or in combination, e.g. Tuinal.

(1) *General management* is as described above. Particular attention to ventilation function is essential. Coma might be protracted and acute tubular necrosis occur if profound hypotension persists. There is no indication for the use of analeptic agents such as Bemegride.

(2) *Forced diuresis.* This technique is indicated *only* in barbitone (Veronal), which is 100% renally excreted (but very rarely prescribed), or phenobarbitone overdose. Phenobarbitone is 25% renally excreted.

The other barbiturates are mainly detoxicated in liver and rapidly protein-bound. Forced diuresis should therefore not be used as a routine for all cases for barbiturate overdose. It is a potentially dangerous technique and moreover it is pharmacologically useless unless a long-acting barbiturate has been taken.

(3) *Dialysis.* The indication for dialysis in barbiturate poisoning is renal failure. Only with long acting agents will much barbiturate be removed from the blood by the use of haemodialysis. Peritoneal dialysis is not an efficient technique for the removal of barbiturates. Therefore dialysis will only be indicated when a

Table 16.2 Forced diuresis for long-acting barbiturate poisoning

(1)	Catheterise – Empty bladder Test urine pH and specific gravity Check for adequate renal output hourly
(2)	2 Intravenous infusions using a Y connection 1st i.v. Mannitol 20% 4 hourly 2nd i.v. Dextrose 5% Sodium bicarbonate 2.74% Normal saline

(2) 2 Intravenous infusions using a Y connection
     1st i.v.   Mannitol 20% 4 hourly
     2nd i.v.   Dextrose 5%   ⎫ 500 ml of each to run in
                Sodium bicarbonate 2.74% ⎬ 20 minutes.
                Normal saline   ⎭ Complete cycle hourly

(3) Potassium supplements 6 g KCl given IVI in divided doses
     during each 4 hour period.
                4 g KCl in 500 ml Mannitol
                0.5 KCl to alternate bottles of 2nd infusion
                until 4 doses (2 g) have been given in 4 hours

(4) Monitor urine output, watch JVP
     Continue until level of consciousness improves.

long acting barbiturate has been taken and forced diuresis cannot be undertaken due to renal failure secondary to hypotension, or if renal failure occurs in any barbiturate poisoning, when the object of the treatment is to treat the renal failure rather than remove barbiturates.

SALICYLATE POISONING

Salicylate poisoning is an important condition, with a significant mortality, and particularly dangerous because the patient is usually conscious, which may lead to a false impression of the severity of the condition.

Aspirin is freely available without prescription and is an ingredient of many analgesics and 'cold cures'. It is probably the most widely taken drug, and most households will have some in one form or another. Particularly dangerous are the 'junior aspirins' which have been pleasantly flavoured to make the bitter taste acceptable to children. Aspirin poisoning is therefore common, and dangerous, in children.

Clinical features

The patient with salicylate poisoning is restless, sweating and usually hyperventilating. Vomiting occurs frequently. Tinnitus and deafness soon develop. Adults are often conscious but children may be comatose, due to metabolic acidosis, which tends to occur more rapidly and at lower salicylate levels in the young.

Hyperpyrexia and sweating can readily lead to dehydration. It should also be remembered that aspirin is irritant to the gastric mucosa and haematemesis can occur.

The *diagnosis* is made from salicylate levels which should be done in all suspected cases. The clinical picture may mimic other causes of acidosis such as

255

uraemia or diabetic ketoacidosis (the latter may be suspected if the ferric chloride test is used to detect ketones in the urine as salicylates give a false positive).

Biochemical findings

Salicylate levels

These must be performed in all cases as there is a close association between the level and mortality. The levels, should, however, be interpreted with caution as the drug can still be absorbed up to 12 hours after ingestion, and an early low level may therefore not truly indicate the severity of the poisoning.

In adults a level of over 3.6 mmol/l, and in children over 2.1 mmol/l is an indication for active therapy. Levels over 8.6 mmol/l carry a high mortality.

Effects on acid-base balance

The initial effect of salicylate is to stimulate the respiratory centre which leads to hyperventilation and a respiratory alkalosis, often with associated hypo-kalaemia. The salicylic acid in the blood leads to a metabolic acidosis. The over-all picture, therefore, is a mixture of respiratory alkalosis and metabolic acidosis. Under these circumstances the serum bicarbonate level will fall due to both the respiratory and metabolic components of the disturbance (see Chapter 2). Full blood gas and pH estimations will be necessary to assess the true state of affairs and in this respect it is important to emphasise again that in children severe metabolic acidosis occurs earlier than in adults.

Prothrombin levels

These may drop considerably, increasing the risk of gastro-intestinal haemor-rhage.

Management

(1) Gastric lavage should always be carried out regardless of the time stated to have elapsed between ingestion and treatment.

(2) *Forced diuresis* should always be instituted if the drug has been taken within 12 hours and levels of over 3.6 mmol/l (2.1 mmol/l in children) are present.

N/Saline—500 ml
5% Dextrose—1 l
1.26% Sodium Bicarbonate—500 ml
(Potassium Chloride 1 g
   in every alternate 500 ml)

} Given in sequence
2 l/h for 3 hours*
1 l/h until salicylate
level 2.5 mmol/l (1.5 mmol/l in children)

*In children 30 ml/kg/h.

During forced diuresis the serum potassium and electrolytes should be monitored frequently, blood gas and pH estimations performed and urine pH checked. More bicarbonate will be necessary if the urine pH falls below 7. If an adequate urine flow does not develop i.v. frusemide 40 mg can be given, but if positive fluid balance persists or indications of fluid overload (CVP, JVP, pulmonary oedema) develop the forced diuresis should be discontinued and haemo or peritoneal dialysis commenced. If intense acidaemia is present initially this should be corrected with 8.4% bicarbonate, the dose calculated as on page 000.

(3) *Vitamin* K_1 (Konakion) 25 mg i.m. should be given if the prothrombin time is abnormal.

PARACETAMOL POISONING

Paracetamol poisoning is of increasing importance because, in overdose, it can cause acute centrilobular hepatic necrosis. It is one of the commonest causes of acute hepatic failure in the UK. The drug is available without prescription and is often part of the analgesic cocktail in proprietary preparations for headache, dysmenorrhoea and cold 'cures'. It should also be noted that popular analgesics such as Distalgesic contain paracetamol.

Individual susceptibility varies considerably but the lethal dose can be as little as 6.2 g.

Clinical picture

Vomiting can occur but there is no alteration of consciousness and physical examination is initially negative. If liver damage occurs abdominal pain, vomiting and jaundice develop within 4-5 days. Some patients will rapidly progress to hepatic failure. If liver damage occurs the liver is enlarged and tender. Renal failure frequently occurs at this stage and a rise in blood urea is common in all but the mildest cases.

Biochemical findings

(1) *Paracetamol levels.* There is a good correlation between plasma levels and hepatotoxicity. Plasma concentrations above 1.6-2.0 mmol/l at 4 hrs after ingestion, or above 0.3 mmol/l at 12 hours carry a high risk of liver damage. Blood should always be taken for paracetamol level and the result considered in relation to the time of ingestion.

(2) *Liver function tests.* Blood should be taken for liver function tests and prothrombin time on admission to act as a baseline. The abnormalities of liver function develop between 3-5 days after ingestion. Bad prognostic signs include a prothrombin ratio of greater than 2.2 and a bilirubin of over 70 μmol/l at this stage. The rise in the hepatic enzymes (SGOT, SGPT) may be very large, exceeding 10 000 units, although the alkaline phosphatase shows no, or only a slight rise. Generally liver function returns to normal within 2-3 weeks.

Mortality rate is at least 20% if hepatic failure develops. However, in those patients who recover there are no long-term sequelae.

Treatment

The hepatotoxicity of paracetamol can be prevented if treatment is started early.

257

Paracetamol causes liver damage because one of its metabolites is potentially toxic, though in normal therapeutic doses it is rendered harmless by preferential conjugation with glutathione within the hepatocyte. In overdose the hepatic glutathione rapidly is depleted and toxic liver cell damage occurs. The rationale of treatment is to prevent glutathione depletion, or inhibit selectively, the oxidation of paracetamol to its toxic metabolite.

Acetylcysteine (Parvolex) acts in both these ways. Acetylcysteine must be given within 15 hours of ingestion in those patients whose plasma paracetamol levels indicate a high risk of hepatic damage. It should not be administered later than this because the damaged liver will be unable to metabolize it and hepatic coma may ensue. This danger may have been overestimated (Smith *et al.*, 1978).

Acetylcysteine (Parvolex) is given as follows:

Initial dose   150 mg/kg in 200 ml 5% dextrose over 15 mins
Next 4 hours   50 mg/kg in 500 ml 5% dextrose
Next 16 hours   100 mg/kg in 1 litre 5% dextrose

This gives a total dose of 300 mg/kg over 20 hours. The volume of fluid infused should be reduced in children.

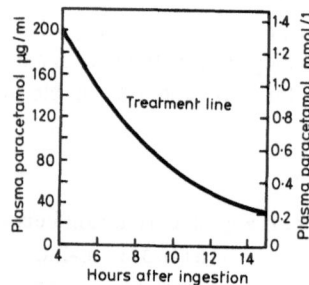

Fig. 16.1 Plasma paracetamol levels in patients.

DEXTROPROPOXYPHENE POISONING

This analgesic drug is a component of various proprietary analgesics such as Distalgesic, Depronal and Doloxene Compound, often with other analgesics such as paracetamol. In combination with alcohol it is particularly dangerous. The clinical features include delerium, convulsions, coma and respiratory and cardiac depression. Pulmonary oedema also occurs.

Treatment

Naloxone is a specific antidote for the respiratory depression, it has been suggested that this drug might also antagonise the cardiac toxicity. The aspirin or paracetamol content of several of these analgesic cocktails may have equally lethal effects and require specific therapy.

POISONING BY ANTIDEPRESSANT DRUGS

Mono-amine oxidase inhibitors

The importance of the drug is the hypertensive reaction that may be precipitated by tyramine-containing foods. In addition the group potentiate the action of many drugs including sympathomimetic amines, barbiturates and opiates. Particularly dangerous is the concomitant ingestion of tricyclic antidepressants and mono-amine oxidase inhibitors.

The *clinical picture* is mixed depending upon what particular combination of drugs is involved. The hypertensive or 'cheese' reaction is the commonest and characterized by restlessness, headaches, hallucinations, convulsions, high fever, tachycardia and sweating. Generally the blood pressure is raised, but it may be low, especially if the actions of barbiturates, opiates or other centrally acting depressive drugs are being potentiated.

The *treatment* is along the general lines outlined above. If the blood pressure is very high a short-acting alpha-blocker—phentolanine (Rogitine) 5 mg i.v. can be given. If hypotension is present pressor agents must *never* be given.

Tricyclic agents

The tricyclic group of antidepressants, which includes imipramine (Tofranil) and amitriptyline (Tryptizole), is popular and frequently taken in overdosage in conjunction with a benzodiazepine sedative such as diazepam (Valium).

Combination capsules including representatives from the two groups are widely prescribed, e.g. Limbritol (chlordiazepoxide and amitriptyline). More recently quadricyclic antidepressants have been introduced (e.g. maprotiline-Ludiomil). The effects and treatment of overdose are the same as for tricyclics.

Clinical picture

The patient is unconscious with depressed respiration, the pupils will often be fixed and dilated, reflexes are brisk, plantars extensor, convulsions may occur. An important feature is cardiac dysrhythmias and all patients should therefore be monitored. Multifocal ventricular ectopic beats, bundle branch block, ventricular tachycardia and ventricular fibrillation may occur. The blood pressure is low.

This group of drugs is rapidly absorbed and metabolized, so that the toxic effects do not usually last for more than 24 hours. However, a state of hypomania may last for several days and there is also a risk of death from cardiac dysrhythmia for up to 72 hours.

Treatment

The cardiac dysrhythmias are potentially lethal. Ectopic beats can be treated with intravenous lignocaine infusions, or beta-blockers such as propranolol. Rarely, temporary pacing may be necessary (see Chapter 9). Physostigmine salicylate has been suggested for the treatment of the anticholinergic effects of tricyclic overdose, but the drug is toxic and may itself precipitate fits.

Convulsions are treated with barbiturates or diazepam (but with caution, and with IPPV available because respiration is already depressed).

Dialysis and forced diuresis are not indicated.

Lithium

Lithium salts are used in the treatment of manic-depressive psychosis and the margin between therapeutic and toxic levels is a narrow one. Side-effects begin to appear at levels of about 2.0 mmol/l. Severe toxic side-effects can be expected if levels rise above 3.0 mmol/l. (The therapeutic range is 0.6–1.5 mmol/l.)

Clinical picture

Diarrhoea, vomiting, thirst, polyuria and tremor are the initial symptoms. These symptoms are followed by vertigo, dysarthria, ataxia, muscular twitching, convulsions and coma leading to death.

Treatment

(1) Osmotic diuresis with 20% mannitol. Diuretics must not be used.

(2) Alkalinisation of urine with sodium bicarbonate.

(3) If serial lithium levels do not fall, or the clinical condition deteriorates peritoneal or haemodialysis should be carried out until there is no lithium in the blood or dialysis fluid.

(4) It is important to check lithium levels for several days as a rebound rise may occur as a result of diffusion from body tissues.

OPIATES (Morphine, Heroin, Pethidine, Dihydrocodeine.)

Opiate poisoning will most commonly be seen in drug addicts, but may also require urgent treatment where, in hospital, a high dose has inadvertently been given, or perhaps injudiciously given to a patient with respiratory insufficiency.

The principal pharmacological effects are depressive, particularly of respiration. Coma, depressed respiration and pin-point pupils are a characteristic triad of findings, to which may be added, in the addict, the finding of needle marks and evidence of thrombophlebitis.

Treatment

Opiate poisoning is one of the rare situations in which a specific antidote is available. Naloxone (Narcan) is an opiate antagonist which differs from earlier similar drugs such as nalorphine in not producing respiratory depression itself.

In *adults* the initial dose of naloxone is 0.4 mg i.v. or i.m. This dose can be repeated to a total of three doses within a few minutes.

Children. 0.005–0.01 mg/kg body weight repeated as above.

We have also used naloxone in the treatment of overdose of pentazocine

(Fortral), dextropropoxyphene (which is part of the formulation of Distalgesic and doloxene, and is a respiratory depressant when taken in overdose—it should also be remembered that Distalgesic contains 325 mg of paracetamol in each tablet) and diphenoxylate (Lomotil).

It should be remembered that acute withdrawal symptoms may develop in narcotic addicts when an antidote is given.

Respiratory function should be monitored and mechanical ventilation commenced if necessary, particularly in patients who have diminished respiratory function due to pre-existing disease.

NON-BARBITURATE SEDATIVES AND HYPNOTICS

Benzodiazepines

This group embraces some of the most widely prescribed tranquillizers, and is therefore a particularly common cause of drug overdose. It includes diazepam (Valium), chlordiazepoxide (Librium), lorazepam (Ativan), nitrazepam (Mogadon), oxazepam (Serenid) and potassium clonazepate (Tranxene).

They are safe drugs and in overdose do not usually cause significant respiratory depression. Drowsiness, light coma, nystagmus and dysarthria are features. The blood pressure is seldom seriously reduced.

Treatment
On the general lines above.

Meprobamate (Equanil, Miltown.)

This drug has been eclipsed in popularity by the benzodiazepines. If serious overdose occurs forced osmotic diuresis is helpful (as in barbiturate poisoning—above). Hypothermia and hypotension are features of meprobamate poisoning and convulsions may occur during the recovery phase.

Phenothiazines

The phenothiazines and their derivatives characteristically cause an acute Parkinsonian-like syndrome when taken in overdose; although a similar syndrome is seen at therapeutic levels in susceptible patients, particularly children.

Drugs in this group include:
Trifluoperazine (Stelazine)
Promethazine (Phenergan)
Chlorpromazine (Largactil)
Promazine (Sparine)
Prochlorperazine (Stemetil)

Clinical picture
Coma with hypothermia and hypotension. Cardiac dysrhythmias may occur. A

261

characteristic finding is dyskinetic movements of a Parkinsonian type, sometimes with torticollis and convulsions. This type of dyskinesia is also found in poisoning with haloperidol (Serenace) or metoclopramide (Maxolon).

Treatment

The extrapyramidal manifestations of acute phenothiazine toxicity respond to 1-2 mg i.v. benztropine (Cogentin). Respiratory depression is unusual and general management is routine for unconscious patients with drug poisoning.

Glutethamide (Doriden.)

Prolonged unconsciousness is a feature of overdose with this drug, as it becomes bound to body fat. Severe intoxication (levels of over 3 mg%, or ingestion of over 10 g) may produce papilloedema, cerebral oedema and episodes of apnoea. If this occurs treatment with intravenous 20% mannitol is indicated. Dexamethasone can also be used to reduce cerebral oedema.

Respiratory depression is frequent and may be recurrent as more of the drug is released from fat stores. This is particularly likely to happen if haemodialysis, which may be indicated, lowers blood levels rapidly.

Mandrax (Methaqualone and Diphenhydramine.)

This non-barbiturate hypnotic is now less in use than previously. It was, and may still be, widely abused by drug addicts. The dangerous effects of overdose are due to the methaqualone component of the drug.

Prolonged deep coma, with convulsions, restlessness, extensor plantars and hyperreflexia are characteristic features. Papilloedema and acute pulmonary oedema may occur. However, respiratory depression is rare. Cardiac arrythmias are often a problem.

Treatment

Is supportive and symptomatic. Forced diuresis is contraindicated. Severe cases may justify haemodialysis.

Alcohol

Alcohol, ingested in large amounts, can itself cause lethal poisoning; it is frequently taken as part of a suicidal cocktail when the effects of other drugs, notably the barbiturates, will be potentiated. Severe accidental alcohol poisoning may be seen in children, in whom it is particularly dangerous causing hypoglycaemia. This can also occur in adults, but rarely. The physical findings are those of central nervous system depression. Levels over 350 mg% indicate severe poisoning and fatalities occur at, and above, this level.

Treatment

Alcohol is rapidly absorbed but gastric lavage will usually be indicated. Hypoglycaemia should always be looked for and i.v. glucose or dextrose given. Blood alcohol levels above 500 mg% are an indication for haemodialysis (peritoneal dialysis is also effective).

Methyl alcohol

Poisoning with methyl alcohol is not commonly seen, but may occur in alcoholics who cannot afford ethyl alcohol, or it may be taken by mistake if it is introduced into such drinks as fruit punches in a mistaken belief that commercial alcohol is a cheap and satisfactory substitute for ethanol.

The fatal dose of methyl alcohol is 60–250 ml.

It has profound metabolic and CNS effects. Severe acidosis occurs (due to the metabolite, formic acid); leading to rapid respiration with cyanosis and hypotension. Coma follows a period of headache and vertigo, during which time acute visual disturbances due to optic neuritis occur. Hypoglycaemia also is common.

Treatment

(1) Gastric lavage

(2) Treatment of acidosis with i.v. sodium bicarbonate.

(3) Ethyl alcohol i.v. appears to give some protection against the serious effects of methyl alcohol poisoning by reducing its metabolism to formaldehyde and formic acid.

The dose is 1.0–1.5 mg/kg% of 50% ethyl alcohol orally (diluted to a 5% solution) followed by 0.5–1.0 ml/kg 2–4 hourly either by mouth or i.v., aiming to maintain a blood ethanol level between 100–200 mg%. This treatment should be continued for 2–4 days.

(4) Haemodialysis is indicated with blood levels above 50 mg%.

Ethylene glycol

Ethylene glycol (antifreeze) initially causes symptoms similar to acute alcoholic intoxication, this is rapidly followed by coma, tetany (due to hypocalcaemia), respiratory and renal failure. Acidosis is due to metabolism to oxalic acid.

Treatment

(1) Ethyl alcohol (as above)

(2) Calcium gluconate i.v. (10 ml of 10% solution i.v.).

(3) Correct acidosis

(4) Early treatment for renal failure.

Other alcohols

Butyl or isopropyl alcohol are present in such items as after-shave lotions, floor polish and industrial solvents. Treatment is as with ethyl alcohol poisoning with particular attention to correction of acidosis and haemodialysis if severe poisoning is present. These alcohols are twice as toxic as ethyl alcohol.

OTHER DRUGS

Almost any therapeutic agent may be taken deliberately or accidentally (especially in children) in massive overdose. No attempt will be made here to cover the entire range of therapeutic substances. However features of two drug poisonings that may be seen, especially in children, must be described.

Digoxin

Poisoning with cardiac glycosides is most often seen in children. Toxicity is frequently seen in adults, especially in elderly patients, but this aspect of therapy will not be discussed.

The principal effect of digoxin poisoning is bradycardia, with prolongation of the P-R interval, missed beats and eventually asystole. In adults trachyarrythmias leading to ventricular fibrillation are common.

The treatment of bradycardia is with i.m. atropine 0.6 mg. Ventricular tachyarrythmias may respond to beta-blocking therapy such as propranolol, but it is often safer to insert a cardiac pacemaker.

It is essential that potassium levels are monitored carefully, as digoxin toxicity is much more likely to occur in the presence of hypokalaemia.

Iron

Poisoning with proprietary iron preparations is seen in children who mistake the brightly coloured tablets, or multicoloured capsules, for sweets.

Symptoms

Vomiting, diarrhoea and shock are the cardinal features. The child may complain of severe abdominal pain and gastro-intestinal bleeding frequently results from the irritant effect of iron salts on the gastric mucosa. Coma occurs in severe cases. Levels of over 500 $\mu g\%$ carry a high mortality rate.

Treatment

There is a specific antidote for iron poisoning—the cholating agent desferri-oxamine (Desferal). This agent is given as follows, and it must be emphasized that speed is essential:

(1) 2 g in 10 ml sterile water i.m.

(2) Gastric lavage, and 10 g of desferrioxamine in 50 ml of water is left in the stomach (1 g chelates approximately 85 mg Fe^+, which means that 5 g should cholate the iron contained in 10 tablets of ferrous sulphate or gluconate).

(3) i.v. infusion, rate not more than 15 mg/kg/hr, to a maximum dose in 24 h of 80 mg/kg. Desferrioxamine can be added to normal saline, dextrose or dextrose saline.

(4) Serum iron levels are monitored and the 2 g dose of i.m. desferrioxamine can be repeated 12 hourly if necessary.

General management is as described at the beginning of this chapter.

OTHER POISONINGS FOR WHICH THERE ARE SPECIFIC ANTIDOTES

Heavy metals

Lead

Acute lead poisoning, resulting in an acute encephalopathy with abdominal pains, diarrhoea and vomiting, is likely to be seen as a result of an industrial accident involving one of the organic compounds such as tetraethyl lead.

The *diagnosis* is made by finding a urine coproporphyrin above 0.5 mg/l, or a blood lead level above 0.1 mg%.

Treatment. (1) Calcium disodium edetate 15–25 mg/kg by slow (1 h) i.v. infusion twice daily, given as 0.5–3% solution in 5% dextrose (maximum dose 75 mg/kg/day). This treatment is continued for 3–4 days.

(2) Cerebral oedema is treated with 20% mannitol.

(3) D-Penicillinamine 20–40 mg/kg orally is given daily to patients who have a history of previous exposure to lead.

(Note—Calcium edetate can also be used for poisoning with copper, nickel, zinc, cadmium and cobalt).

Mercury

Acute mercury poisoning may result from environmental contamination as a result of industrial processes. Volatile mercury compounds may be used as fungicides and mercury is a component of many industrial waste products. The *clinical picture* is of intense thirst, vomiting, diarrhoea followed by acute renal failure. If volatile compounds are inhaled pneumonia, ataxia, convulsions and coma occur.

Treatment. (1) Dimercaprol (BAL) 2.5 mg/kg every 4–6 hours i.m. for 48 hours, reducing to 2 injections per day for 24 hours, and then once daily for 7 days.

(2) *D*-penicillamine 1.5 g/day orally is used in less severe cases.

(Note—Dimercaprol is also used in other heavy metal poisonings such as gold and antimony.)

Cyanide

Cyanides are widely used in industry; hydrogen cyanide as a fumigant, cyanamide as a fertilizer, and other salts in metal cleaning and ore extraction processes. Poisoning usually occurs when hydrocyanic acid gas (prussic acid) is released as a result of a strong acid reacting on cyanide salts.

Cyanide is a cellular poison, acting by inhibiting the cytochrome oxidase system for oxygen utilisation, and death from respiratory paralysis occurs very rapidly. Coma and death follow within a few seconds of ingestion or inhalation of large amounts.

Therefore speed is absolutely essential if survival is to occur.

Treatment

(1) Cobalt tetracemate (Kelocyanor) is given immediately. 0.6 mg in 40 ml (i.e. 2 ampoules) intravenously by rapid injection followed (using the same needle) immediately with 50 ml of 50% dextrose. If necessary a third ampoule of cobalt tetracemate followed by a further 50 ml of 50% dextrose can be given.

(2) An alternative treatment is sodium nitrite 3% 10 ml i.v. over 3 minutes followed by sodium thiosulphate 50% 25 ml i.v. An ampoule of sodium nitrite should be inhaled while the intravenous injection is prepared.

Mechanized ventilation will nearly always be necessary from the outset and high concentrations of oxygen should be administered.

It should be emphasized that there is no time to acquire these antidotes from the Pharmacy and the drugs must always be available in the Casualty Department.

WEEDKILLERS AND INSECTICIDES

Paraquat

This lethal substance is available in granular form for domestic use as the weed-killer 'Weedol' and in a far more dangerous liquid concentrate (Gramoxone) where professional farming or horticulture occurs. Paraquat is also known by different trade names in other countries. The liquid is attractively coloured and can readily be mistaken by children as lemonade. Tragedies have also occurred where the concentrate has been stored in containers subsequently used for drinking liquids.

Symptoms

The substance initially causes local irritation to the mouth and upper gastro-intestinal tract, this, in severe cases may be followed by tremor and convulsions. Hepatic and renal failure follow. These are potentially reversible, but the lethal consequences are due to the effect of paraquat on the lungs, where it causes a progressive pulmonary fibrosis. Dyspnoea, cyanosis and death from respiratory failure develop some days after ingestion.

Diagnosis

There is a quick test for determining the presence of paraquat in the urine. Two 25 ml samples of urine are taken and one pellet of sodium hydroxide is added to each. After shaking to dissolvé the pellets a medium spatula full of sodium di-thionite is added to one and a blue-green discolouration, as compared to the control, indicates the presence of paraquat.

Blood and urine samples should always be retained and used for quantitative analysis (laboratories capable of this can be contacted through the Poisons Information Service, see page 252).

Treatment

The object of treatment is to reduce blood levels, and thereby prevent the irreversible pulmonary fibrosis. The first assault must therefore be on the gastro-intestinal tract which acts as a reservoir, and secondly direct measures on the blood.

(1) to prevent further absorption from the gastro-intestinal tract:

(a) Stomach washout

(b) Give 1 litre of absorbent suspension (30% Fullers earth or 7% bentonite in N/Saline) orally.

(c) Give sodium or magnesium sulphate cathartic separately

(d) Repeat administration of 200–500 ml of absorbent (as in b above) every 2 hours for 24 hours and then 4 hourly for a further 24 hours. Each dose of absorbent should be followed by cathartic to ensure throughput of absorbent.

(2) If more than 1 g of paraquat has been taken (i.e. more than half a packet of the granular preparation, or any amount of liquid concentrate) haemoperfusion through a charcoal column or haemodialysis should be considered. These procedures will require transfer to a special unit. Haemodialysis will usually be necessary because, although the kidneys excrete paraquat well, early renal failure occurs in the majority of cases.

Oxygen should *not* be administered as there is evidence to suggest that it potentiates the pulmonary toxicity of paraquat.

Treatment of the pulmonary changes, if the above regime has been unsuccessful, is unsatisfactory although high dose steroids, azothioprine, d-Propanolol and potassium aminobenzoate have been used. Lung transplants have also been attempted.

ORGANOPHOSPHATE ANTICHOLINESTERASE INSECTICIDES (Parathion, Malathion, Endosulfan, Disulfoton and many others.)

There are very many insecticides of this group available for domestic and agricultural use. They are extremely dangerous as they act as cholinesterase inhibitors. Exposure is often through skin absorption, or inhalation.

Symptoms

These develop within 30 minutes of exposure and progress for 2–8 hours. The initial symptoms will be headache, dizziness, diarrhoea and miosis with impairment of visual acuity. As parasympathetic overactivity develops abdominal pain, vomiting, sweating and bradycardia with hypotension follow. In severe cases muscular fasciculation, weakness, respiratory distress, convulsions and coma are terminal events.

Treatment

(1) *Atropine* is lifesaving and must be given in full doses. The initial dose is

2 mg i.v. followed by 1 mg every 10-15 minutes until the bradycardia and miosis are corrected. Up to 12 mg may need to be given in the first 2 hours, and premature cessation of atropine therapy may be rapidly followed by acute respiratory failure.

(2) Specific antidote—*pralidoxime* which is a cholinesterase reactivator and must only be used when an organophosphate cholinesterase inhibitor has been taken. (It may be harmful under other circumstances, particularly if a carbamate insecticide has been taken. This group of insecticides are also cholinesterase inhibitors, where toxic effects are similar. If there is doubt as to the nature of the toxic agent concerned the Poisons Information Centre should be contacted. Atropine must, of course, be used in this group.)

The dose of pralidoxime is 30 mg/kg in 5 ml sterile water by slow i.v. injection repeated in 1 hour.

Mechanical ventilation should always be available and it should be remembered that barbiturates, phenothiazines and opiates potentiate the effect of these poisons. Suxamethonium must never be used under these circumstances.

OTHER CHEMICALS USED IN AGRICULTURE

DDT

Symptoms from toxic doses of DDT may be delayed for a few hours. Vomiting, apprehension, tremors, convulsions and coma occur. There is no specific treatment.

In common with many agricultural poisons skin absorption is an important route of entry and after removal of clothes the skin must be scrubbed. Gastric lavage and cathartics should be used if oral ingestion has occurred.

Dinitro compounds

These derivatives of phenol and cresol are used as insecticides and herbicides. The principal manifestation of poisoning with these pounds is hyperpyrexia. The patient should be put at complete rest, clothing removed, the skin thoroughly washed and hyperpyrexia treated with tepid sponging and chlorpromazine. Dehydration is frequent and careful electrolyte monitoring essential.

Arsenic

Arsenic compounds are used in some insecticides and weedkillers. Arsine gas may be released if acids act on metals in the presence of arsenic.

The symptoms of arsenic poisoning are acute, violent diarrhoea and vomiting followed by circulatory failure, convulsions and coma. Arsine gas exposure produces acute pulmonary symptoms followed by haemolytic anaemia, and renal failure. Routine measures (lavage, correction of dehydration are particularly important) are supplemented by dimercaprol (see page 265). Haemodialysis and exchange transfusion may be necessary in arsine gas poisoning.

Chlorate

Sodium chlorate is in wide use as a herbicide; it is also used industrially for the manufacture of some explosives.

Vomiting and cyanosis due to the formation of methaemoglobin are early symptoms, followed by acute renal and hepatic failure. Activated charcoal followed by gastric lavage is initial treatment followed by sodium thiosulphate 2-5 g in 200 ml 5% sodium bicarbonate by mouth. Ascorbic acid 1 g intravenously may help reverse methaemoglobinaemia and haemodialysis will be necessary if renal failure develops.

HOUSEHOLD SUBSTANCES

Solvents

Carbon tetrachloride is a highly toxic solvent used in many dry-cleaning liquids. Immediate symptoms are abdominal pain and vomiting, followed by confusion, coma, respiratory depression and hypotension. If these effects are survived liver and renal failure develop 2-4 days later. There is no specific therapy.

Other halogenated hydrocarbons are in widespread use in domestic cleaning substances, paint cleaners and plastic cements. The most dangerous is tetrachlorethane. Management is supportive only.

Bleaches etc

Household bleaches and some disinfectants contain sodium hypochlorite. If ingested sodium thiosulphate 5 g in 200 ml water should be given orally and calcium gluconate 10% 10 ml i.v. if the bleach contains oxalic acid.

Disinfectants

Phenol and Cresol are not widely used domestically now but may be available on industrial premises. They are locally corrosive and produce vomiting, collapse and coma; renal and hepatic failure ensue. Gastric lavage with water may rarely be carried out with great care and 60 ml of castor oil left in the stomach followed by a saline cathartic. If acidosis develops treat as for aspirin poisoning (page 255).

INHALATION OF POISONOUS GASES

The hazards of fires in general will not be discussed, but it should be remembered that firemen are exposed to risks of inhalation of poisonous gases, especially when dealing with fires in industrial premises. For example, isocyanate poisoning may occur if synthetic foam, such as used in mattresses, is ignited. Asphyxia and pulmonary irritation and heat damage are common to all smoke hazards.

Carbon monoxide

Self-poisoning with carbon monoxide is less common now that coal gas has been replaced with natural gas over most of the United Kingdom. However, car

269

exhausts are a potent source of carbon monoxide and there are increasingly frequent tragedies due to inefficient ventilation of small rooms, such as caravans or boat cabins, where natural gas or paraffin heaters are in use. The gas is produced by the incomplete combustion of carbon or carbonaceous materials.

The *clinical effects* of carbon monoxide poisoning are due to the great affinity that haemoglobin has for it—some 300 times greater than that for oxygen. The resulting carboxy haemoglobin is incapable of carrying oxygen and tissue hypoxia results. It is perhaps worth noting that the inhalation of smoke from one cigarette produces the same amount (8%) of tissue hypoxia as going from sea level to 4000 ft.

The patient will be dyspnoeic and may be bright red in colour due to the colour of carboxyhaemoglobin. In severe cases coma is present, sometimes with papilloedema and cerebral oedema. Milder cases will complain of headache, restlessness and dizziness, but it is important to remember that the clinical picture can deteriorate rapidly. The effects of carbon monoxide poisoning are due to cerebral hypoxia.

Treatment

The patient must be removed from the polluted atmosphere immediately and oxygen therapy commenced. Oxygen should always be given at a concentration of 100%. Assisted respiration may be indicated when the patient arrives at hospital, but it is the *urgent* removal from the gas and administration of oxygen that is the key to successful resuscitation from carbon monoxide poisoning, and this will generally be the responsibility of the ambulance crew.

Shock and cerebral oedema are treated as has been described previously. If coma is prolonged permanent brain damage may result; characteristically a Parkinsonian type of tremor is seen as a long-term sequel.

Hydrogen sulphide

Workers in sewage works, oil refineries and mines may be exposed to this gas. Its immediate effect is irritation of the eyes with cough, headache and dizziness. Exposure to high concentrations causes coma and respiratory depression.

Treatment

(1) remove from exposure

(2) oxygen therapy

(3) Nitrite therapy as described under the treatment of cyanide poisoning (page 265).

(4) assisted respiration and treatment of pulmonary oedema if necessary.

POISONING BY ANIMALS AND PLANTS

Snake bite

The only poisonous snake indigenous to the British Isles is the *adder* (*Vipera berus*). Its bite, though painful, is rarely serious in healthy adults, but fatalities do occur in children. The bites of poisonous snakes are differentiated from non-poisonous ones by the presence of fang marks. Intense pain, swelling and discolouration occur at the puncture site and the swelling can extend proximally. Systemic symptoms are unusual but hypotension and transient neurological signs (drowsiness, ptosis and diplopia) may develop. Vomiting, abdominal pain and diarrhoea may also be present.

The *treatment* of adder bite is largely symptomatic with local applications to relieve pain. Corticosteroids are often given but are not indicated unless systemic disturbance develops. The use of antivenin should be reserved for cases in whom there is evidence of cardiovascular or neurological involvement because they are antigenic and hypersensitivity reactions are common and can be serious.

Prophylaxis against tetanus should always be given. Venomous snakes in other countries are a far more serious problem, and bites from these creatures may be encountered in the employees of zoological institutes or private pet lovers.

Local features of snakebite are pain, swelling and tissue necrosis.

Systemic features depend upon the snake.

(1) *Neurotoxic* venoms (cobras, rattlesnakes, vipers) cause widespread muscular paralysis, sensation being unaffected. The sea-snakes cause severe muscle damage which may produce electrolyte disturbances and renal failure associated with myoglobinuria.

(2) Some snakes produce a venom which interferes with coagulation mechanisms, producing a syndrome of diffuse intravascular coagulation with consequent haemorrhagic diathesis.

Treatment

Treatment of these serious snake bites depends upon the prompt use of specific antivenins when there is evidence of systemic disturbance and preferably if the snake can be identified. Polyvalent sera are not as effective as specific sera and are particularly likely to produce allergic reactions. The principal indication for steroid therapy is to control these reactions.

The neurotoxic and cardiovascular aspects of snake-bite will require supportive therapy as described above.

The traditional manoeuvres of tourniquets and sucking the wound are of dubious value and should not replace specific therapy.

PLANT POISONS

Children may eat poisonous berries and some varieties of toadstool may be mistaken for edible mushrooms.

'Mushrooms' poisoning

There are two types of poisoning depending on which toxic fungus has been eaten:

271

(1) *Rapid-onset* poisoning is due to the cholinergic alkaloid muscarine which is present in *Amanita muscaria* (fly agaric).

The symptoms are those of cholinergic poisoning and develop 2–6 hours after ingestion—salivation, abdominal pain, miosis, circulatory insufficiency, vomiting and diarrhoea. *Treatment* with atropine 1 mg i.v. at 15–20 min intervals is effective.

(2) *Delayed onset* poisoning occurs when *Amanita phalloides* (death cap) or *A. verna* (fool's mushroom) are eaten—the onset of symptoms being between 10–20 hours later. The symptoms are similar to those described in rapid onset poisoning and are due to alkaloids similar to muscarine which are heat-stable and therefore survive cooking. The prognosis in this form of poisoning is much worse, there is a high incidence of hepatic and renal failure. Apart from atropine in the cholinergic phase there is no specific therapy. Antiphallinic serum is available but has to be given within 1 hour of ingestion—it is useless by the time symptoms have developed.

Other plants

(1) Deadly nightshade, Henbane, Thorn apple

The fruits or berries of these plants contain a variety of alkaloids including atropine and hyoscine. Nausea, vomiting, mydriasis, tachycardia, dryness of the mouth and convulsions occur. The antidote is neostigmine 0.5 mg i.m. repeated to control symptoms.

(2) Aconite

The roots of which may be eaten in mistake for horseradish produce a cholinergic poisoning picture leading eventually to paraesthesiae and convulsions. Atropine is helpful for the cholinergic features.

(3) Yew, Laburnum, Privet

All produce severe gastro-intestinal upset and in severe cases convulsions and coma. There is no specific therapy.

FURTHER READING

Alpert, J. J. (1969), Removing ingested poison. *Lancet*, 1, 728.

Cooke, N. J., Flenly, D. C. and Matthew, M. (1973), Paraquat poisoning serial studies of lung function. *Quart. J. Med.*, 168, 683.

Craft, A. W. and Sibert, J. R. (1977), Accidental Poisoning in children. *Brit. J. Hosp. Med.*, 17, 469.

Dreisbach, R. M. (1977), *Handbook of poisoning: diagnosis and treatment* 9th Edn. Lange Medical, Los Altos.

Lawson, A. A., Proudfoot, A. T., Brown, S. S., MacDonald, R. H., Fraser, A. G., Cameron, J. C. and Matthew, H. (1969), Forced Diuresis in the treatment of acute salicylate poisoning in adults. *Quart. J. Med.*, 38, 31.

Matthew, M. and Lawson, A. A. (1979), *Treatment of common acute poisonings.* 4th Edn. Churchill-Livingstone, Edinburgh.

North, P. M. (1967), *Poisonous plants and fungi.* Blandford Press, London.

Paracetamol Hepatotoxicity (1975), Leader. *Lancet*, ii, 1189.

Prescott, L. F., Park, J., Sutherland, G. R., Smith, I. J. and Proudfoot, A. T. (1976), Cysteamine, methionine, and pencillamine in the treatment of paracetamol poisoning. *Lancet*, ii, 109.

Proudfoot, A. T. and Brown, S. S. (1969), Acidaemia and salicylate poisoning in adults. *Br. Med. J.*, 2, 547.

Proudfoot, A. T. and Park, J. (1978), Changing pattern of drugs used for self-poisoning. *Brit. med. J.*, 1, 190.

Raeburn, J. A., Cameron, J. C. and Matthew, M. (1969), Severe Barbiturate poisoning. Contrasts in management. *Clin. Toxicol.*, 3, 133.

Schon, M., Amdisen, A. and Baartrup, P. C. (1971), The Practical Management of lithium treatment. *Br. J. Hosp. Med.*, 6, 53.

Smith, J. M., Roberts, W. O., Hall, S. M., White, T. A. and Gilbertson, A. A. (1978), Late treatment of paracetamol poisoning with mercaptamine. *Brit. med. J.*, 1, 331.

Snyder, R. (1962), Snake bites. *Am. Jl. Dis. Childh.*, 103, 85.

The treatment of Paraquat Poisoning–A Guide for Doctors. Imperial Chemical Industries, October 1974 and April 1976.

Wilkinson, S. P., McHugh, P., Henley, S. Tubbs, H., Lewis, M., Thould, A., Winterton, M., Parsons, V. and Williams, R. (1975), Arsine Toxicity aboard the Asia freighter. *Brit. med. J.*, 3, 559.

Wright, N. (1980), Common errors in the management of poisoning. *J. Roy. Coll. Phys.*, 14, 114.

SEVENTEEN

Liver disease

JAUNDICE

The spectrum of cases in the ITU is such that jaundice will frequently be a diagnostic challenge. In many cases the development of jaundice post-operatively is due to a combination of factors and accurate assessment of the clinical situation will depend on consideration of many points in the history, with an appreciation of the significance and limitation of biochemical and other tests of liver function.

Table 17.1 Aetiological considerations in diagnosis of jaundice in the ITU.

Pre-operative liver function
Drug history, including anaesthetic agents
Nature and site of operative procedure
Co-existing medical conditions, e.g. heart failure or haemolysis
Amount and age of transfused blood
History of hypoxia, shock or septicaemia

Investigation of jaundice

Biochemical tests of liver function

(1) *Bilirubin.* Jaundice cannot be detected clinically unless the serum bilirubin levels exceeds 25 μmol/l, and levels above this may be difficult to detect in poor lighting conditions. As the bile pigments become strongly bound to tissues clinical jaundice may not be apparent as the serum bilirubin rises rapidly and will persist as the blood level falls.

The serum bilirubin usually refers to the total serum bilirubin, which is the sum of conjugated and unconjugated bilirubin ('direct' and 'indirect' bilirubin using the Van den Bergh method). In clinical practice separate estimation of conjugated and unconjugated bilirubin is not as helpful as physiology might suggest. However, conjugated hyperbilirubinaemia occurs predominantly in obstructive jaundice, and in this condition the urine is dark due to excretion of the bilirubin (which is water soluble) by glomerular filtration. Unconjugated bilirubin, which does not cross the renal glomerulus, is present in excess when either an excess of pigment is produced due, for example, to haemolysis, or if the liver is unable to take up or conjugate bilirubin in the blood. Hepato-cellular disorders will produce a predominance of unconjugated bilirubin in the blood.

However, it is unwise to rely on an estimation of conjugated and unconjugated bilirubin to differentiate between the different types of jaundice. Total serum bilirubin estimations provide a fairly crude indication of the course of the pathological process causing jaundice.

(2) *Enzyme tests*

Alkaline phosphatase. Levels over 300 international units (30 King-Armstrong units) are very suggestive of obstructive jaundice, either in the liver as cholestasis, or extra-hepatic obstruction. Rises are also seen with metastases in the liver, without jaundice. If there is difficulty in deciding whether the rise in serum alkaline phosphatase arises from the liver or bone the serum 5-nucleotidase can be estimated.

Transaminases. Levels of SGOT (aspartate amino transferase) or SGPT (alanine amino transferase) are a sensitive indicator of hepato-cellular disease. However a modest increase often occurs in obstructive jaundice. Levels of over 10 times normal are very suggestive of hepato-cellular damage.

Lactic dehydrogenase (LDH) is a relatively insensitive indicator of liver damage as the enzyme is widely distributed in other tissues.

(3) *Plasma proteins.* A low plasma albumin occurs in chronic liver disease, but in the ITU this is not a very useful indicator of hepatic function as hypoproteinaemia is so often present for other reasons. Likewise a rise in gamma-globulin is not very specific in the context of patients suffering from severe disease.

(4) *Prothrombin time.* The prothrombin time is frequently elevated in jaundiced patients and must always be monitored. Correction with Vitamin K suggests extra-hepatic obstruction.

Radiology

Routine radiology is often unhelpful. Oral cholecystograms are unlikely to show any concentration of the dye in the jaundiced patient. Intravenous cholangiogram may be of some help in the presence of mild jaundice. However endoscopic examination of the biliary tract with retrograde cholangiography (ERCP) is of great value in the diagnosis of obstructive jaundice and is less hazardous than percutaneous cholangiography (Cotton *et al.*, 1972). Ultrasound imaging is non-invasive and may be helpful.

Radioactive scans

A radioactive liver scan may give some useful information as to the size of the liver. High splenic uptake suggests cirrhosis of the liver. Filling defects might indicate the presence of metastases. Combined scanning of the liver and lungs is sometimes useful in confirming the presence of subphrenic abscess. Radioactive rose-bengal scans can give information regarding obstructive jaundice that cannot be observed using technetium (Winston and Blahd, 1972).

Liver biopsy

Liver biopsy should not be undertaken if the prothrombin time is 3 seconds increased over the control or if the platelet count is below 80 000. Caution should also be exercised in the presence of very deep jaundice or if there is a possibility of cholangitis because of the risks of biliary leak and septicaemia.

Interpretation of liver function tests

Serial changes in the alkaline phosphatase and transaminase levels will often provide all the information required to decide the cause of the jaundice. Patience should be exercised before exposing the patient to the risks of invasive procedures. In those patients where jaundice is often a complication of other serious disease it is a potential disaster to advise surgical exploration for jaundice unless extra-hepatic obstruction is present. On the other hand, particularly after upper abdominal surgery, it is obstructive jaundice that must always be excluded as further surgery will then be mandatory. If there is doubt as to the nature of the jaundice a definite investigation such as retrograde cholangiography using an endoscope should be performed before exposing the patient to surgery. Surgery carries a high mortality if performed for hepato-cellular jaundice (Harville and Summerskill, 1963).

Differential diagnosis of jaundice

Some of the important aetiological factors are given in Table 17.1.

Drugs (including anaesthetic agents)

The list of drugs which can cause jaundice is very large. Any case who develops jaundice in the ITU must be carefully asked for a full drug history and prescription sheets scrutinized. The mechanisms of drug-induced jaundice are several and the abnormalities of liver function tests will depend on the predominant mechanisms.

(1) *Haemolysis.* Drug-induced haemolytic anaemia will show no abnormalities in the hepatic enzyme studies but the level of unconjugated bilirubin will be raised (rarely exceeding a total serum bilirubin level of 85 μmol/l unless there is pre-existing liver disease). The Direct Coombes test is positive and there is an increased reticulocyte count.

(2) *Hepatotoxicity.* This may be predictable and dose related, or due to a hypersensitivity reaction. The transaminases are considerably elevated, indicating liver cell damage; the alkaline phosphatase generally shows only a modest increase. Fever and eosinophilia may occur (see below—halothane).

Table 17.2 Common drugs associated with jaundice

| Haemolysis | Hepatotoxic | | Cholestasis | Mixed picture |
	Predictable	Hypersensitivity		
Methyldopa	Carbon tetrachloride	Monoamine oxidase inhibitors	Anabolic and androgenic steroids	Phenothiazines (incl. Chlorpromazine)
Phenacetin	Paracetamol	Methyldopa	Oral contraceptives	Chlordiazepoxide
	Tetracycline (in high dose i.v.)	Halothane		Tri-cyclic antidepressants
	Methotrexate	Isoniazid		
	Ferrous sulphate (in overdose in children)			Phenylbutazone
				Rifampicin and other antituberculous drugs
				Sulphonamides (incl. Co-Trimoxazole (Septrin))
				Erythromycin estolate
				Chlorpropamide

277

(3) *Intrahepatic cholestasis.* The characteristic feature of intrahepatic cholestasis is the considerable elevation of the serum alkaline phosphatase as the bilirubin (conjugated) rises, with slight or no abnormalities in the transaminases.

(4) *Mixed hepatitis-like and cholestasis.* This is a common hypersensitivity reaction to drugs in susceptible patients, and the group in whom the liver function studies are difficult to interpret because of the mixed picture of hepato-cellular involvement with elevation of the alkaline phosphatase.

Common drugs associated with the above different types of jaundice are given in Table 17.2.

Halothane and jaundice (Simpson *et al.*, 1971; Inman and Mushin, 1974; Sherlock, 1971; Simpson *et al.*, 1975; Editorial, 1980.)

Halothane is a valuable and safe anaesthetic agent which is used in up to 75–80% of all anaesthetic procedures. It is a volatile halogenated hydrocarbon metabolized by the liver. The association between halothane and jaundice is the subject of occasionally acrimonious discussion between anaesthetists and physicians. The incidence of jaundice after exposure to halothane is uncertain.

Clinical features. Halothane associated jaundice should be suspected if jaundice occurs after an anaesthetic procedure including halothane. Scrutiny of previous records may show an otherwise inexplicable fever, leucocytosis or a rise of hepatic enzymes after previous exposure to halothane. The clinical features of an acute hepato-cellular disturbance develop on the second or third post-operative day. A rise in bilirubin or hepatic enzymes is frequently accompanied by fever and eosinophilia. The disturbance can be mild but progression to acute hepatic necrosis occurs in a minority of cases.

It may be that the hepatotoxic effects of halothane are caused by metabolites which arise as a result of reductive pathways of halothane metabolism. Such metabolites are likely to be present in large amounts in the presence of enzyme induction which may in turn be caused by the stress of serious illness, especially in the presence of hypoxaemia. There may be a greater incidence of halothane-associated hepatitis in patients treated in an ICU than in others.

Wherever possible halothane should not be used for repeated anaesthesia, particularly in patients with disease of the biliary tract. Halothane should never be used if a previous halothane exposure has been followed by fever, jaundice or enzyme abnormalities.

Blood transfusion

(1) *Haemolysis.* 500 ml of transfused blood will release 250 mg of bilirubin for excretion by the liver if 10–15% undergoes haemolysis. This is likely to occur if the blood has been stored for 14 days. The rise in bilirubin is modest, not usually more than 5 mg%, if liver function is normal. Other liver function tests are normal; the bilirubin is largely unconjugated.

It should also be remembered that *absorption* of large haematomata, or of free blood in the thoracic or peritoneal cavity will cause a small increase in the serum bilirubin, without other biochemical evidence of hepatic dysfunction.

(2) *Hepatitis.* Viral hepatitis is potentially a dangerous problem in the ITU because of the risk of transmission of the disease to medical, nursing and technical staff. *All blood specimens from patients with suspected viral hepatitis (particularly type B) must be handled with great caution.* It should be remembered that the virus may be transmitted in saliva—particularly important in patients on ventilators, or as when mouth to mouth resuscitation may be employed.

Type A. Viral hepatitis ('infectious hepatitis, 'short-incubation hepatitis') can cause confusion because although the incubation period is from 15–50 days, laparotomy may have been performed for severe abdominal pain preceding the onset of jaundice.

Type B. Serum hepatitis may be transmitted by blood transfusion. On suspicion of serum hepatitis blood should be taken from the jaundiced patient for Australia antigen testing. The incubation period is from 15–180 days. The liver function tests show the abnormalities of hepatocellular dysfunction, i.e. considerable elevation of the transaminases and a modest increase in alkaline phosphatase. Some cases of serum hepatitis progress to hepatic necrosis. Other viruses producing jaundice may be transmitted by blood transfusion, notably the Epstein–Barr virus and cytomegalovirus (Leading article, *Brit. med. J.*, 1975).

Post-operative obstructive jaundice

The recognition of obstructive jaundice post-operatively is of great importance because it is this form of jaundice which constitutes the only indication for further surgery, which might be life-saving.

Any upper abdominal operative procedure can be complicated by jaundice if traumatic damage to the bile ducts has occurred. Occasionally pancreatitis in the post-operative period causes jaundice.

The liver function tests show considerable increase in alkaline phosphatase, a modest increase in transaminases and the progressive rise in serum bilirubin is predominantly of the conjugated type.

The diagnosis is best confirmed by fibre-optic retrograde cholangiography; if this technique is not available transhepatic cholangiography should be attempted.

(If the hepatic pedicle, bile ducts and hepatic blood vessels, are ligated at surgery, the liver infarcts, with a dramatic rise in bilirubin and enzyme tests, and fatal liver failure rapidly ensues.)

Hypoxia, circulatory failure and sepsis

In seriously ill patients subjected to surgery post-operative jaundice is frequently due to hypoxia and hypotension. The liver is very vulnerable to these factors, and the risk is considerably increased if vasopressor drugs have been used.

Therefore the assessment of post-operative jaundice must include careful attention to records of blood pressure and urine output both before, during and immediately after the surgical procedure. Patients with pre-existing liver disease, e.g. cirrhosis, are particularly vulnerable to these factors.

The liver function tests may suggest cholestasis with considerable increase in bilirubin and alkaline phosphatase, the transaminases show a moderate rise (600–1000 units).

It is in this group of patients that a mistaken diagnosis leading to further surgery will frequently have lethal consequences.

Sepsis. Most frequently a septicaemia with gram-negative organisms can cause severe jaundice. The liver function tests again suggest a cholestatic picture, and the hepatic damage is multifactorial in origin with infection, shock and hypoxia all contributing.

Treatment of post-operative jaundice

The only condition for which there is specific treatment is extrahepatic obstructive jaundice, for which surgery is mandatory.

Hepatotoxic drugs should be withdrawn, and general patient care with attention to circulatory status, hypoxia and the treatment of infection will be necessary in all cases.

There is no specific treatment for viral hepatitis. There is no place for the use of steroids for diagnosis or therapy under these circumstances.

ACUTE LIVER FAILURE

Acute liver failure is defined as the clinical syndrome associated with massive necrosis of the liver cells or with sudden severe impairment of hepatic function (Trey, 1973). This may arise in a previously normal liver or in cases with chronic liver disease, such as cirrhosis, when an acute deterioration in hepatic function occurs as a consequence of another event, e.g. massive gastro-intestinal haemorrhage or electrolyte disturbance consequent upon the misuse of diuretics.

Table 17.3 Aetiology of acute liver failure

Liver previously normal	Pre-existing liver disease
Viral hepatitis (Type A or B)	Gastro-intestinal haemorrhage
Drugs – paracetamol	Infection
halothane	Electrolyte disturbances (over-diuresis)
Unknown (probable hepatitis)	Surgery, anaesthesia
	Paracentesis
	Alcohol
	Misuse of sedatives or narcotics

Clinical features

The cardinal features of acute hepatic failure are
(1) neuropsychiatric disturbance
(2) jaundice
(3) bleeding disorders

The clinical picture may evolve very rapidly with confusion progressing to deep coma, deepening jaundice and haemorrhagic manifestations.

(1) Central nervous system manifestations

Beware of the patient with hepatitis or chronic liver disease who becomes sleepy, confused, irritable or aggressive.

The severity of hepatic encephalopathy provides a good guide to the prognosis of acute liver failure. The first symptoms are often subtle, and easily missed. Minor changes in behaviour might lead to the prescription of a sedative which could be lethal. As the encephalopathy progresses the characteristic flapping tremor of hepatic failure is observed. Signs in the nervous system are variable, including ataxia, extrapyramidal signs, spasticity with extensor plantars and convulsions.

The EEG is invaluable in the detection and monitoring of hepatic encephalopathy.

If there is any suspicion of hepatic encephalopathy an EEG should be performed. The initial change is slowing of normal frequency with increased amplitude, this is followed by characteristic triphasic waves, this progresses, in fatal cases, to a progressive decrease in amplitude until the record is flat (Kennedy *et al.*, 1973).

The precise metabolic abnormality that produces hepatic encephalopathy is unknown, but there is clearly an association between encephalopathy and the inability of the damaged liver to detoxicate nitrogenous substances derived from gastro-intestinal protein breakdown. However there is not a constant or good correlation between blood ammonia levels and the severity or prognosis of encephalopathy. Consequently blood ammonia level is a useless monitoring investigation in this condition. Other factors responsible for the clinical features of encephalopathy may include cerebral oedema (although high dose dexamethasone does not improve the outcome), acid-base balance disorders, depletion of neurochemical transmitters (dopamine and nor-adrenaline), or increased levels of short chain fatty acids (Sherlock, 1977; Knell *et al.*, 1974).

Table 17.4 Grading of hepatic encephalopathy

Grade 1	Mood change and confusion
Grade 2	Drowsy, inappropriate behaviour
Grade 3	Stupor, rousable
Grade 4	Unrousable with minimal or no response to painful stimuli

(2) Jaundice

Jaundice often lags behind the encephalopathy as acute liver failure develops. It is therefore unwise to rely on clinical observation or serum bilirubin levels as an indicator of the severity of the syndrome. However as progressive liver failure occurs the serum bilirubin steadily rises and the transaminase levels are very high.

(3) Haemorrhagic manifestations

Gastro-intestinal haemorrhage is a frequent cause of acute deterioration in hepatic function in patients with pre-existing liver disease and the bleeding tendency that invariably accompanies hepatic failure may compound the problem.

   (1) decreased clotting factors

   (2) thrombocytopenia

   (3) intravascular coagulation (possibly due to tissue thromboplastins released from necrotic liver cells)

   (4) abnormal blood vessel fragility

Haemorrhage is a serious problem in liver failure and bleeding leading to hypotension will inevitably have a further adverse effect on both hepatic and renal function. Bleeding is usually from the gastro-intestinal tract; purpura and subcutaneous bruising is very common.

(4) Other clinical features

(a) *Foetor hepaticus*: the characteristic rather sweet, faecal odour of liver failure disappears if antibiotics are given, which suggests that it originates in the intestinal tract, the flora of which is modified by antibiotic therapy.

(b) *Features of pre-existing liver disease*: where acute hepatic failure develops in patients with pre-existing liver disease there may be clinical indications of chronic liver disease such as:

   clubbing
   spider-naevi and palmar erythema
   leuconychia
   splenomegaly
   ascites

(5) Metabolic changes

Complex metabolic and biochemical changes occur, the management of which is discussed below:

   (a) hypoglycaemia

   (b) renal failure

   (c) electrolyte disturbances, in particular hypokalaemia

   (d) acid-base disturbances, which are often difficult to assess because (1) hypokalaemia is associated with a metabolic alkalosis (2) hyperventilation will lead to respiratory alkalosis (3) metabolic acidosis tends to occur as a result of tissue necrosis and (4) lactic acidosis is common (Wilkinson *et al.*, 1974; Malhausen *et al.*, 1967).

The overall metabolic effect, however, is probably a predominant metabolic acidosis, particularly after correction of hypokalaemia.

Treatment of acute liver failure

Table 17.5 Outline of treatment of acute hepatic failure

Control of nitrogenous intoxication
    Protein restriction
    Enemas
    Neomycin
    Lactulose
	no sedatives or opiates

Correction of biochemical changes
    Treatment of hypokalaemia; acid-base balance
    Correction of hypoglycaemia
    Treatment of renal failure – dialysis

Control of haemorrhagic manifestations
    Vitamin K
    ? Fresh frozen plasma
    ? Heparin
    Cimetidine

Temporary hepatic support
    Extracorporeal liver perfusion
    Haemoperfusion over actuated charcoal   } in a specialized
    (Liver transplant)   liver unit

Treatment of complications – Renal failure : Pancreatitis
    Respiratory failure : Infection : Cerebral Oedema

The object of treatment is to provide support in the hope that hepatic regeneration will occur.

(1) General measures: correction of precipitating factors

If there is an obvious precipitating factor, in a patient with chronic liver disease, such as haemorrhage, infection or electrolyte disturbance, this must be corrected. The failing liver is vulnerable to hypovolaemia and a central venous pressure line will be essential in these cases. (The management of haemorrhage from oesophageal varices is discussed below.) If blood transfusions are required the blood should be as fresh as possible.

(2) Hepatic encephalopathy: control of nitrogenous intoxication

(a) *Diet.* No protein should be given. Approximately 1500–2000 calories daily are provided as glucose orally, or 20% glucose through a gastric tube, or as intra-venous dextrose.

(b) *Antibiotics.* To reduce intestinal bacterial flora and thus reduce the absorp-tion of nitrogenous substances that result from bacterial degradation within the bowel.

Neomycin is the drug of choice. It can be given orally in the form of tablets or syrup. Rectal administration is also possible. The dose is 6 g daily given in divided doses 4 hourly.

(c) *Enemas or purgation.* Again to reduce bacterial activity. Magnesium sulphate is commonly used to induce purgation (but may be unnecessary when lactulose is used).

(d) *Oral lactulose* (Duphalac). This synthetic disaccharide is neither digested nor absorbed in man and it acts as an osmotic laxative in the colon after it has been split into lactic and acetic acid by bacterial action.

Its beneficial action in hepatic encephalopathy may be due entirely to its laxative properties, but it has also been suggested that ammonia trapping by the acidic stools is a factor; it has also been postulated that by promoting the growth of lactae fermenting organisms in the colon, urease producing organisms such as bacteroides are suppressed. The dose of lactulose is 30–50 ml three times daily, the dose being adjusted so that 2–3 semi-solid stools are passed daily.

These measures are conventional for the control of chronic hepatic encephalo-pathy, where they are helpful, but their value in acute hepatic failure is more uncertain. However, no serious adverse effects can arise from them and therefore the regime outlined above should be instituted in all cases.

It should be emphasised that sedative or narcotic agents are highly dangerous in patients with hepatic failure. If the patient is very confused and difficult to control small doses of diazepam (Valium) can be given.

(3) Metabolic disturbances

(a) *Hypoglycaemia* is a constant finding in acute liver failure, because of reduced glycogen stores in the liver and gross impairment of hepatic gluconeogenesis.

The blood sugar should be monitored at least 12-hourly. Very large amounts of glucose may need to be given (Felig *et al.*, 1970); Samson *et al.*, 1967).

(b) *Hypokalaemia.* Potassium deficiency is of great importance. Frequently it is a provocative factor, produced by the misuse of diuretics, and the effect of hypokalaemia with its associated alkalosis is to increase the blood ammonia levels (Baertl *et al.*, 1963).

Diuretics are potentially very dangerous in hepatic failure. Frequent electro-lyte estimation is essential.

(c) *Sodium.* The serum sodium may rise or fall as the condition advances. Hypo-natraemia should not be treated with intravenous saline (but with fluid restriction). Hypernatraemia most commonly results from osmotic diuresis resulting from hypertonic dextrose solutions (Wilkinson *et al.*, 1974).

(d) *Acid-base balance.* As has been described above, the acid-base changes are complex and multifactorial. After potassium depletion has been corrected cautious administration of intravenous bicarbonate may be indicated (James *et al.*, 1969).

(e) *Renal failure.* Renal failure is common. It can be subdivided into two groups, one with acute tubular necrosis and the other with 'functional renal failure' (with low urine sodium concentration).

Uraemia contributes towards coma, aggravates the bleeding tendency and increases the risk of infection. Treatment with mannitol may lead to hyper-natraemia. High dose frusemide therapy has not been helpful. Although increasing urine output, renal function does not benefit.

Peritoneal dialysis is the treatment of choice.

(4) Haemorrhagic manifestations

Bleeding in hepatic failure is often a lethal complication, producing acute hypovolaemia and thereby further damage to the liver and kidneys. The control of haemorrhagic disorder is as vital as the treatment of encephalopathy.

(a) Parenteral vitamin K (Konakion) in a dose of 10–20 mg daily should always be given, but in the presence of severe hepatic dysfunction it is unlikely that the prothrombin time will return to normal.

(b) Impaired synthesis of coagulation factors II, V, VII, IX and X contributes to the bleeding and fresh-frozen plasma will be helpful. It should be noted that this preparation contains a great deal of sodium, which may cause problems in patients with hypernatraemia or renal failure.

(c) Thrombocytopaenia may be part of DIC (see below), but there is some evidence that platelet function may be abnormal, and platelet transfusions should always be considered when the count is very low (less than 50 000 cm).

(d) *Intravascular coagulation.* The significance of this in hepatic failure is controversial. The use of heparin (see Chapter 18) is potentially lethal–it should only be attempted if full laboratory control, preferably including the technique of plasma protamine dilution, is available (Williams, 1975). It would obviously be very unwise to treat a patient bleeding from varices or a peptic ulcer with heparin.

The indications for the use of heparin, with fresh-frozen plasma, are not clearly defined. A high level of fibrin degradation products (FDP) in the blood, hypofibrinoginaemia and a low platelet count are indicators of DIC.

If it is decided to use heparin, the dosage will be that required to give a heparin equivalent of 0.5 mg% as measured by the plasma protamine dilution technique. This estimation must be made every 4–5 hours. The usual dose of heparin is between 20 000–30 000 units daily (Rake *et al.*, 1970; Hillenbrand *et al.*, 1974).

This treatment is best carried out in a specialized liver unit.

(e) *Gastro-intestinal haemorrhage.* Cimetidine should invariably be given, even if there is no clinical evidence of haemorrhage.

(5) Temporary liver support

These techniques are the province of highly specialized units. Patients should be transferred to such units when encephalopathy progresses to grade III, IV (see Table 17.4) or when a severe bleeding tendency develops.

(1) Exchange blood transfusion

(2) extracorporeal liver perfusion using animal, human cadaver liver or cross-circulation with a volunteer (this techique cannot, of course, be used if the patient has viral hepatitis).

(3) Haemoperfusion using actuated charcoal

(4) liver transplant

(6) Steroids

Steroid therapy plays no part in the treatment of acute liver failure.

Causes of death in acute hepatic failure

It has been estimated that only a minority of patients die of liver cell necrosis alone. Most of the mortality relates to complications such as renal failure, infection, haemorrhage, cerebral oedema, respiratory failure or pancreatitis.

Unfortunately the overall mortality rate is 80–90% once grade IV coma is reached.

The treatment of the complications is discussed in the relevant chapters.

GASTRO-INTESTINAL BLEEDING – OESOPHAGEAL VARICES

Massive upper gastro-intestinal bleeding is one of the commonest major emergencies in clinical practice. In liver disease it is a frequent complication and important cause of death. Between 2–4% of patients with massive haematemesis are suffering from chronic liver disease and bleeding varices; although it must also be remembered that the incidence of peptic ulcer is increased also in this group of patients. The importance of bleeding from varices or peptic ulcer is compounded by the bleeding diathesis that accompanies chronic liver disease.

Differential diagnosis

The *history* is often unreliable and many patients with known peptic ulcers have been shown to be bleeding from sources other than the known ulcer. However, a known duodenal ulcer is more likely to be the cause of bleeding than a known gastric ulcer. Absence of a dyspeptic history does not rule out the presence of a

Table 17.6 Causes of massive upper GI tract haemorrhage

Peptic ulcer
Hiatus hernia with oesophagitis
Oesophageal varices
Acute erosions due to drugs
   (e.g. aspirin, steroids, butazolidine, indomethacin)
Acute erosions secondary to severe stress
   (major trauma, major surgery, severe sepsis, diabetic ketosis)
Mallory–Weiss syndrome

peptic ulcer. A history of salicylate or other analgesic ingestion should always be asked for, but it is very unwise to assume that the drug is the cause of bleeding and thereby anticipate a benign course.

Bleeding from *oesophageal varices* is often catastrophic and it is important to search for clinical clues to chronic liver disease.

Table 17.7 Stigmata of chronic liver disease

Jaundice
Hepato-splenomegaly
Ascites
Spider naevi
Leuconychia
Palmar erythema

Even if a patient is known to have varices, these are not necessarily the source of the haemorrhage and proper investigation of all cases must be carried out (Cotton *et al.*, 1973).

Investigation—radiology or endoscopy?

The investigation of upper gastro-intestinal tract bleeding has been revolutionized by the development of fibre-optic endoscopy. Routine radiology often is unreliable and occasionally actively misleading. Barium should always be used in preference to gastrografin if endoscopic examination is not available. Acute erosions cannot be diagnosed radiologically and a barium meal may show potential causes of bleeding such as peptic ulcer, hiatus hernia or varices but can never demonstrate the actual area of haemorrhage. Blood clot may obscure the site of bleeding.

Endoscopy is the investigation of choice. If this procedure is accompanied by saline lavage to clear blood clot a firm diagnosis should be possible in 90% of patients (Lightdale *et al.*, 1974).

MANAGEMENT OF HAEMORRHAGE FROM OESOPHAGEAL VARICES

General measures

Bleeding from varices is a common precipitating cause of hepatic encephalopathy because of hypoxic damage to the liver and the large protein load delivered to the lower gastric-intestinal tract.

Every effort must therefore be made to maintain the pulse, blood pressure and central venous pressure by adequate blood transfusion. A deep central line will nearly always be necessary as large amounts of blood may need to be given very rapidly. The transfused blood should be as fresh as possible (see Chapter 3 for complications of massive blood transfusion). A nasogastric tube should be passed in all cases, but gravity drainage is preferable to aspiration because of the risk of damaging the gastric mucosa.

Pending results of biochemical tests an intravenous dose of Konakion 10 mg should be given (see page 285 for further details of management of the haemorrhagic aspects of liver disease).

Specific measures to control haemorrhage

Cimetidine

A recent development in gastroenterology has been the introduction of H_2-receptor antagonists. This group of drugs are potent inhibitors of histamine stimulated gastric acid secretion. Cimetidine (Tagamet) is available for oral and intravenous use. In hepatic disease the drug appears to be effective in both the prophylaxis and treatment of upper gastrointestinal bleeding (MacDougall *et al.*, 1977). The intravenous dose is 150 mg given as often as is necessary to maintain the intragastric pH above 5. (Usually about 6 hrly.) The oral dose is 1 g/24 h.

The drug appears to be free of serious side effects and should be given routinely to all patients with hepatic failure whether bleeding or not.

In other causes of upper GI tract haemorrhage cimetidine has been widely used, but it is very unlikely that bleeding from a chronic lesion will be helped; however in acute erosions lowering gastric acid may be beneficial and as these are so often the cause of haemorrhage it should be used in the majority of cases.

The use of cimetidine does not absolve the clinician from making an anatomical diagnosis as soon as possible.

Pitressin

Pitressin reduces portal pressure by producing vasoconstriction of the splanchnic arterioles. It will also produce colicky abdominal pain (sometimes severe) with the passage of the melaena stool (which is desirable to prevent an excess protein load). It should be used with caution if ischaemic heart disease is present as it also causes coronary vasoconstriction. By lowering portal pressure, bleeding from varices is reduced.

Technique 20 units of vasopressin in 200 ml of 5% dextrose is given intra-venously over 20 minutes. If the drug is inactive, or out-of-date, no colic or diarrhoea will occur and a different pack should be used.

The effect of this lasts up to 4 hours. If further bleeding occurs the dose can be repeated, but with repetition it has less effect.

This drug causes an undesirable reduction in hepatic blood flow, which can be obviated by using intra-arterial infusion of vasopressin into the superior mesen-teric artery via a catheter introduced into the femoral artery (Nusbaum *et al.*, 1968). However, this specialized technique has a high complication rate. Vaso-pressin should be regarded as the first line of treatment in bleeding varices.

Sengstaken-Blakemore tube

When repeated doses of vasopressin have failed to control haemorrhage the Sengstaken tube should be used (Sengstaken and Blakemore, 1950). The principal of the tube is to inflate an elongated balloon in apposition to the varices at the lower end of the oesophagus. This is achieved by inflating a balloon in the stomach which is then pulled up by gentle traction to the cardia so that the oesophageal balloon is adjacent to the varices and can then be inflated. The tube has three lumens, two for the balloons, and the third, which is open, protrudes into the stomach for aspiration.

Before using the tube it is essential to check the integrity of the balloons by inflation with air or water. The well lubricated tube is passed into the stomach with the balloons deflated. At this stage the stomach balloon is inflated with water to which some gastrografin has been added. The balloon should be inflated to its maximum capacity, and the amount of fluid necessary to achieve this should have been determined before the tube was passed. The patient is now screened and under X-ray control the inflated balloon is pulled up to the fundus and cardia of the stomach. The tube is now fixed in position by the use of surgical tape on the face; occasionally gentle traction is necessary if, on the X-ray screen, the inflated balloon is seen to fall away from the cardia.

The elongated oesophageal tube is now inflated with the same fluid, and its position checked radiologically. The pressure required in the oesophageal balloon is 40 mm Hg. The pressure is checked using a blood pressure machine and a three-way tap. It is essential that the pressure is checked every hour.

While the tube is *in situ* continuous pharyngeal suction is necessary to prevent aspiration of saliva (Boyce, 1962). The tube should not be left *in situ* inflated for over 24 hours. At the end of this time the oesophageal balloon should be deflated and only re-inflated if gastric aspiration shows further bleeding. If the balloon is kept inflated for longer periods there is a serious risk of oesophageal ulceration.

Repeated passage of the Sengstaken tube should be avoided because the risk of oesophageal and pharyngeal trauma is greatly increased.

The tube can however be left *in situ* deflated so that further bleeding can rapidly be controlled. It is, however, extremely uncomfortable for the patient.

289

Surgery

If the above measures have failed to control bleeding surgery will have to be considered. However heroic procedures are unlikely to be successful if liver function is considerably reduced, and it should be remembered that these patients withstand surgery very badly.

Surgery for bleeding varices is probably best carried out in a specialised unit. The Sengstaken tube should be left in position during transfer, but can be deflated if the haemorrhage has been temporarily arrested.

Emergency procedures (Johnston and Rodgers, 1973; Orloff *et al.*, 1967)

(1) injection of varices

(2) transeosophageal ligation

These procedures are all that are indicated in the presence of hepatic failure as shunt procedures will inevitably lead to further deterioration in liver function.

It should always be remembered that portal hypertension leading to haemorrhage from varices can occasionally be due to extra-hepatic lesions and in these cases definitive shunt procedures are always indicated.

If there is any doubt as to the suitability of a patient for a shunt procedure he should be transferred to a specialized unit for full assessment. It should be noted that emergency shunt procedures carry an operative mortality of at least 50%.

FLUID AND ELECTROLYTES IN CHRONIC LIVER DISEASE

The problems of electrolyte balance, especially after the use of diuretics has been referred to above in relation to the pathogenesis of acute liver failure.

Patients with cirrhosis are at grave risk if diuretics are used injudiciously, and it should be remembered that the dangers of diuretics may exceed those of ascites and fluid retention.

Electrolytes and renal function in cirrhosis

Fluid and sodium retention

Retention of fluid and ascites in cirrhosis of the liver is associated with sodium retention, reduction of plasma proteins and possibly as yet uncertain mechanisms involving hepato-renal function.

The tendency to sodium retention may be associated with reduced glomerular filtrate and therefore increased sodium re-absorption by the tubules. The reduction in GFR may be partly due to a reduction in effective blood volume because of portal hypertension leading to vascular pooling in the sphlancic bed; but there are probably other mechanisms.

Secondary hyperaldosteronism will also lead to sodium retention and this occurs in patients with cirrhosis, but 'escape' occurs to some extent, with a resumption in sodium excretion.

Other factors leading to salt and water retention in chronic liver disease are controversial and, as yet, not fully worked out. Possible explanations include (Blendis, 1975)

(1) change in physical factors in the kidney following expansion of extra-cellular volume (ECV) leading to failure of salt diuresis secondary to a drop in renal vascular perfusion.

(2) redistribution of blood flow within the kidney

(3) a substance which normally promotes a salt diuresis, secondary to expansion of ECV, and which may be absent in cirrhosis.

Renal function (Wilkinson *et al.*, 1974; Summerskill, 1966)

Two types of renal insufficiency are seen in chronic liver disease.

(1) *'Functional' renal failure* (Shear *et al.*, 1965) occurs with a fall in renal perfusion, this may be precipitated by over-enthusiastic diuretic therapy, para-centesis, vomiting, or insidiously, without apparent cause. The blood urea rises steadily, but urinary output remains normal. Terminally, hyponatraemia may occur, but the urinary excretion of sodium is very low—often less than 1 mmol/24 h—during the phase of normal urinary output with a rising blood urea.

(2) *Acute renal failure*

(a) *Acute tubular necrosis* is a common complication of fulminant hepatic failure, and is often precipitated by acute hypotension secondary to haemor-rhage. Oligurea and a rising blood urea occurs, and the urine contains casts. Urine sodium excretion is not reduced.

(b) *Renal failure with obstructive jaundice.* There is a close association between the depth of jaundice in obstructive hepatic disease and the incidence of renal failure after surgery, particularly if hypotension occurs.

Control of fluid retention in chronic liver disease

It should be remembered that the presence of oedema and ascites does not constitute an automatic indication for intensive diuretic therapy. There is, however, an indication for treatment if abdominal distension is marked, because a large amount of ascites may cause gastro-intestinal haemorrhage by raising intrabdominal pressure, and there is also a risk of infection of the ascitic fluid.

The cardinal rule for the control of fluid retention in cirrhosis is to proceed slowly, gauging therapy so that weight loss does not exceed 0.5 kg/day.

(a) *Sodium restriction.* The normal diet in the United Kingdom contains approximately 100 mmol of sodium, by omitting salt from cooking and food this can be reduced to 50 mmol/day; further reduction to 20 mmol is achieved by avoidance of sodium-containing food, but the diet is then very unpalatable.

Generally, reduction of sodium intake to 50 mmol is indicated and only in resistant cases will more stringent dieting be necessary.

(b) *Diuretic therapy.* The complications of diuretic therapy are described below; intensive diuretic therapy must always be monitored by frequent electrolyte estimations.

Table 17.8 Diuretics used in the control of fluid retention in cirrhosis

(i) Potassium losing diuretics	(ii) Potassium sparing diuretics
Frusemide	Amiloride
Thiazides	Spironolactone
Ethacrynic acid	Triamterene
Bumetanide	
Metolazone	

The choice of diuretic, or combination of diuretics, will depend upon the electrolyte status, in particular the levels of urinary sodium excretion.

Thus if sodium excretion figures are low initial therapy should be with a diuretic that acts on the distal renal tubules (potassium-sparing).

Amiloride (15–30 mg/day) is the agent of choice. Generally a diuretic that acts on the proximal tubule or loop of Henle (potassium-losing) is used in conjunction with a distal acting agent.

Frusemide is the drug of choice, but care must be taken not to use too high a dose initially as too rapid a diuresis must always be avoided. The initial dose is 80 mg/day, this can be cautiously increased to 200 mg/day.

Combination preparations (e.g. Moduretic) are best avoided in these circumstances as it is not possible to alter the dose of the two agents independently of each other.

Complications

Hypokalaemia. Body potassium is reduced in patients with cirrhosis. The use of diuretics, even potassium-sparing ones, exposes the patient to the risk of serious hypokalaemia. Serum potassium levels must be monitored frequently and potassium supplements prescribed if the serum potassium is less than 4 mmol/litre.

Hypochloraemic alkalosis is particularly associated with the injudicious use of ethacrynic acid. This electrolyte disturbance carries a grave risk of the induction of hepatic encephalopathy.

Hyponatraemia can occur during diuretic therapy and is treated by restricting fluid intake to 1–1.5 l/day. If associated with other electrolyte abnormalities the prognosis is very poor.

Renal failure. A rise in blood urea is particularly likely to occur in patients with resistant ascites where the dose of diuretics has been increased too high. This is associated with reduced renal perfusion. Diuretic therapy should be reduced and attempts made to increase perfusion. However many agents have been tried with varying success. These include mannitol, high dose steroids, angiotensin, dopamine, and alpha adrenergic drugs with L-Dopa.

Encephalopathy is frequently provoked by electrolyte abnormalities secondary to diuretic therapy.

LIVER TRAUMA

Injury to the liver occurs in up to half of patients with blunt abdominal injuries. The diagnosis may be difficult to establish using conventional investigating techniques, even needling the four quadrants of the abdomen or peritoneal lavage may give negative results, particularly when an intrahepatic haematoma is present. Symptoms and signs may be minimal or absent, although upper abdominal pain, especially if referred to the shoulder area, and persistent shock should alert suspicions as to hepatic damage. Liver scan and selective coeliac axis angiography may be helpful, but a negative result does not exclude hepatic trauma and there should be no hesitation in proceeding to exploratory laparotomy if suspicion persists because mortality and morbidity increase the longer definitive treatment is delayed.

The surgical procedure will depend on the nature and extent of the injuries. In stab wounds suture ligation and drainage will be all that is necessary; if there is extensive damage partial lobectomy and debridement of devitalised tissue is performed, and in some severe cases hepatic artery ligation with debridement will be necessary. Gauze packing of large destructive wounds is dangerous and is no longer used. Adequate drainage of the peritoneal cavity; and biliary tree with a T-tube will be necessary in all except the most minor cases.

In the post-operative phase particular attention to infection and electrolyte status, particularly hypoglycaemia, is essential. Hypoalbuminaemia is an indication for albumin infusion (25–75 g/day).

Drug prescribing in liver disease

Many drugs are metabolised in the liver and caution must be exercised in prescribing when either active liver disease or hepatic decompensation is present. The pattern of altered drug metabolism, however, is not constant, and this may be because of the phenomenon of enzyme induction. Many drugs including phenobarbitone, steroids and spironolactone have the property of stimulating the microsomal enzymes in the hepatocytes to increased activity.

There are certain groups of drugs which must never be used in patients with hepatic failure. The most important of these are narcotics and sedatives, which, even in low dose may precipitate encephalopathy. Mono-amine oxidase inhibitors are also contra-indicated.

Drug dosage in liver disease should always be kept low, and wherever possible, blood levels should be monitored.

Anticoagulant drugs are potentially very dangerous in liver disease because

293

clotting factors may already be deficient and bleeding from such lesions as oesophageal varices or associated peptic ulceration can readily be provoked.

REFERENCES

Baertl, J. M., Sancetta, S. M. and Gab, G. J. (1963), Relation of acute potassium depletion to renal ammonia metabolism in patients with cirrhosis. *J. Clin. Invest.*, **42**, 696.

Blendis, L. M. (1975), Fluid retention in liver disease. *Brit. J. Hosp. Medicine*, **13**, 47.

Boyce, H. W. (1962), Modification of the Sengstaken–Blakemore balloon tube. *N. E. J. Med.*, **267**, 195.

Cotton, P. B., Salmon, P. R., Blumgart, L. H., Burwood, R. J., Davies, G. T., Pierce, J. W. and Read, A. E. (1972), Cannulation of papilla of Vater via fibre-duodenoscope. *Lancet*, i, 53.

Cotton, P. B., Rosenberg, M. T., Waldram, R. P. and Axon, A. T. (1973), Early endoscopy of oesophagus, stomach and duodenum in patients with haematemesis and melaena. *Brit. med. J.*, ii, 505.

Editorial (1980), *Brit. med. J.*, **280**, 1197.

Felig, P., Brown, N. V. and Levine, R. A. (1970), Glucose homeostasis in viral hepatitis. *New Eng. J. Med.*, **283**, 1436.

Harville, D. D. and Summerskill, W. H. (1963), Surgery in acute hepatitis. *J.A.M.A.*, **184**, 257.

Hillenbrand, P., Parbhoo, S. P., Jadrychowski, A. and Sherlock, S. (1974), Significance of intravascular coagulation and fibrinolysis in acute hepatic failure. *Gut*, **15**, 83.

Inman, W. H. and Mushin, W. W. (1974), Jaundice after repeated exposure to halothane: an analysis of reports to the Committee on Safety of Medicines. *Brit. med. J.*, **1**, 5.

James, I. M., Nashat, S., Sampson, D., Williams, H. S. and Garassini, M. (1969), Effect of induced metabolic acidosis in hepatic encephalopathy. *Lancet*, ii, 1106.

Johnston, G. W. and Rodgers, H. W. (1973), A review of 15 years experience in the use of sclerotherapy in the control of acute haemorrhage from oesophageal varices. *Brit. J. Surgery*, **60**, 797.

Kennedy, J., Parbhoo, S. P., MacGillivray, B. and Sherlock, S. (1973), Effect of extracorporeal liver perfusion on the electro-encephalogram of patients in coma due to Acute Liver Failure. *Quart. J. Med*, **42**, 549.

Knell, A. J., Davidson, A. R., Williams, R., Kantamanoni, B. and Curzon, G. (1974), Dopamine and Serotonin Metabolism in Hepatic Encephalopathy. *Brit. med. J.*, **1**, 549.

Lightdale, C. J., Kurty, R. C., Boyle, C. C., Sherlock, P. and Winawer, S. J. (1974), Aggressive endoscopy in critically ill patients with upper gastrointestinal bleeding and cancer. *Gastrointest. Endos.*, **20**, 152.

MacDougall, B. R., Bailey, R. J. and Williams, R. (1977), H_2 receptor antagonists and antacids in the prevention of acute gastro-intestinal haemorrhage in fulminant liver failure. *Lancet*, i, 617.

Mulhausen, R., Eichenholz, A. and Blumentals, A. (1967), Acid-base disturbances in patients with cirrhosis of the liver. *Medicine* (Baltimore), **46**, 185.

Nusbaum, M., Baum, S., Kuroda, K. and Blakemore, W. S. (1968), Control of portal hypertension by selective mesenteric arterial drug infusion. *Archs. Surg.*, **97**, 1005.

Orloff, M. J., Halasz, N. A., Lipman, C., Schuabe, A. D., Thompson, J. C. and Weidner, W. A. (1967), The complications of cirrhosis of the liver. *Am. Int. Med.*, **66**, 165.

Rake, M. O., Flute, P. T., Pannell, G. and Williams, R. (1970), Intravascular coagulation in acute hepatic necrosis. *Lancet*, i, 533.

Samson, R. I., Trey, C., Timme, A. H. and Saunders, S. T. (1967), Fulminating hepatitis with recurrent hypoglycaemia and haemorrhage. *Gastroenterology*, **53**, 291.

Sengstaken, R. W. and Blakemore, A. H. (1950), Balloon temponage for the control of haemorrhage from oesophageal varices. *Am. Surg.*, **131**, 780.

Shear, L., Hall, P. W. and Gab, G. J. (1965), Renal failure in patients with cirrhosis of the liver. *Am. J. Medicine*, **39**, 199.

Sherlock, S. (1971), Progress report: halothane hepatitis. *Gut*, **12**, 324.

Sherlock, S. (1977), Hepatic encephalopathy. *Brit. J. Hosp. Med.*, **17**, 144.

Simpson, B. R., Strunin, L. and Walton, B. (1971), The halothane dilemma: a case for the defence. *Brit. med. J.*, **4**, 96.

Simpson, B. R., Strunin, L. and Walton, B. (1975), Halothane and Jaundice. *Brit. J. Hosp. Med.*, **13**, 433.

Summerskill, W. M. (1966), Hepatic failure and the kidney. *Gastroenterology*, **51**, 94.

The several viruses of Post-transfusion Hepatitis (1975), Leading article. *Brit. med. J.*, **3**, 663.

Trey, C. (1973), The fulminant hepatic failure surveillance study. In *Liver*, pp. 120–121. Eds. Saunders, S. J. and Terblanche, S. J. Pitman Medical, London.

Wilkinson, S. P., Blendis, L. M. and Williams, R. (1974), Frequency and Type of Renal and Electrolyte Disorders in Fulminant Hepatic Failure. *Brit. med. J.*, **1**, 186.

Williams, R. (1975), Management of liver failure. In *Intensive Care*, pp. 166–170. Churchill-Livingstone, London.

Winston, M. and Blahd, W. (1972), I^{131} rose-bengal imaging techniques and the differential diagnosis of jaundiced patients. *Sem. Nucl. Med.*, **2**, 167.

EIGHTEEN

Haematological problems

DIFFUSE INTRAVASCULAR COAGULATION

Many conditions described elsewhere in this book are complicated by diffuse intravascular coagulation (DIC). It is necessary therefore to give a short account of this condition and its treatment. The term 'diffuse intravascular coagulation' indicates clearly the thrombotic element but the cardinal feature of the syndrome is the paradoxical situation of thrombosis and bleeding occuring simultaneously. Other terms employed for this condition include 'consumption coagulopathy' and 'defibrination syndrome'. Its manifestation in clinical practice is an acutely acquired bleeding diathesis.

Pathophysiology

In the normal subject coagulation and fibrinolysis are in a state of dynamic equilibrium. In both systems an inactive precursor is converted into the active substance, inhibitors being present to prevent excessive activity. This equilibrium is shown in simplified form in Fig. 18.1.

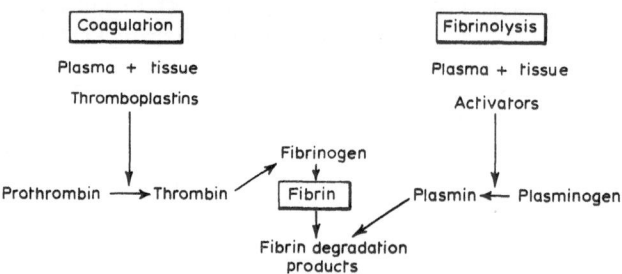

Fig. 18.1 Equilibrium of coagulation and fibrinolysis.

The initial phase of DIC occurs when pathological activation of the normal coagulation mechanism is stimulated. It should be noted that the coagulation mechanism has two components—intrinsic and extrinsic (plasma and tissue).

Stimulation of either the intrinsic or extrinsic clotting mechanisms may precipitate DIC. If collagen is exposed as a result of injury to endothelial cells the Hageman factor (XII) will initiate the intrinsic clotting mechanism—this process is characteristically caused by septicaemic states. Actuation of the extrinsic clotting system occurs when large amounts of tissue factors (thromboplastins) are released into the circulation—this phenomena occurs in obstetric disasters such as amniotic fluid embolism or intra-uterine death; some malignant tumours also produce large amounts of thromboplastins.

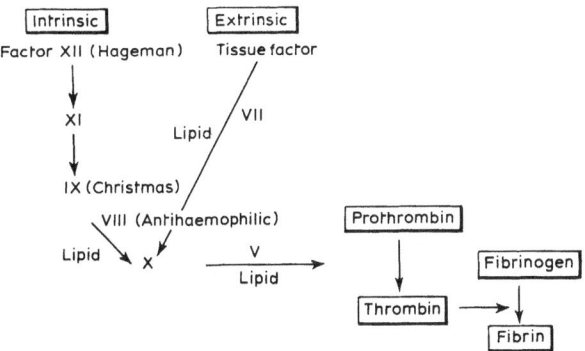

Fig. 18.2 Normal coagulation.

As this cascade of clotting occurs the usual equilibrium is disturbed and the fibrinolytic system is actuated. The end result of this dual process is that thrombin and plasmin are simultaneously active at the site of fibrin formation. Fibrin degradation products (FDP) have, themselves, important actions in haemostasis by interfering with platelet function and also have a direct anticoagulant effect. This becomes important as the excess clotting will consume the coagulation factors and the net result is a haemorrhagic diathesis. A variable thrombocytopenia develops as this process occurs.

In the patient, therefore, the manifestations of DIC will depend upon several factors; in most bleeding will be the dominant feature; in others clot formation with the risk of micro-emboli; and variable combinations of co-existent bleeding and clotting in others.

The development of the DIC syndrome is outlined in Fig. 18.3

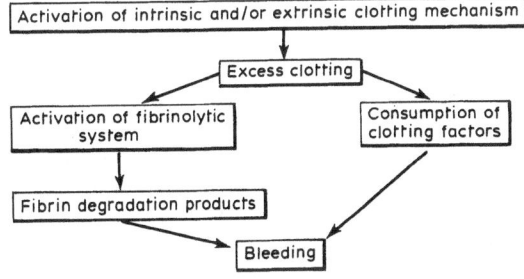

Fig. 18.3 The pathophysiology of diffuse intravascular coagulation.

Causes of DIC

The acute conditions associated with DIC are described in other chapters and the reader is referred to these chapters for details of the clinical conditions listed in Table 18.1.

Table 18.1 Causes of diffuse intravascular coagulation

Tissue injury	
Obstetric conditions	Amniotic embolisms
	Intra-uterine death
	Abruptio placentae
	Toxaemia
Surgery	Extensive surgery (particularly lungs, carcinoma of prostate and cardio-pulmonary bypass)
Neoplastic	Disseminated malignancy
	Leukaemia (particularly in association with the onset of chemotherapy).
Heat stroke	
Endothelial injury	
Septicaemia	
Prolonged shock	Tissue hypoxia. Lactic acidosis.
Acute viral infections, e.g. rubella, varicella, vaccinia.	
Platelet or red cell injury	
Acute haemolysis	Mismatched blood transfusion
	Drowning
	Malaria
Snake bite	
Liver disease	
Fulminant hepatitis	
Cirrhosis	

Clinical features

The usual clinical manifestation of DIC is bleeding. This may be confined to the skin in the form of a purpuric rash (occasionally a purpuric rash will be associated with large areas of superficial cutaneous gangrene). Other sites include gastro-intestinal bleeding, bleeding from a surgical wound or from the urinary tract. An important feature of DIC is pulmonary haemorrhage; this is particularly seen in severe shock states. The haemorrhage is usually acute in onset, but more insidious bleeding can occur. Thrombotic manifestations are not so clinically obvious, although thrombosis of major arteries or veins can occur. Progressive renal failure with micro-angiopathic haemolyte anaemia (haemolytic uraemic syndrome) is usually considered to be a manifestation of DIC, although the mechanism is obscure. Acrocyanosis is often observed.

Diagnosis

There is no single confirmatory test for DIC. However if an acute bleeding diathesis develops, or major vascular thrombosis occurs in a patient who might be considered as susceptible to DIC (see Fig. 18.3) simple investigations will provide considerable information.

Table 18.2 Diagnosis of DIC

Thrombin clotting time	↑
Fibrinogen level	↓
FDP estimation	↑
Platelet count	↓

The *thrombin clotting time* is more specific for DIC than the prothrombin time which is abnormal in many other conditions. The *fibrinogen level* must be interpreted with caution because the significant point is a relative, not an absolute, reduction in levels. It should be remembered that after surgery and in late pregnancy fibrinogen levels are markedly increased to as much as 800–900 mg per 100 ml, a 'normal' figure of 250 mg per 100 ml in these circumstances can therefore indicate a very severe real drop in fibrinogen levels. However a figure of less than 160 mg per 100 ml must be considered as highly significant if there are clinical grounds for suspecting the occurrence of DIC. The same criteria apply to the *platelet count* which may also be above the usually accepted normal values in the immediate post operative phase, and is characteristically elevated in many neoplastic states. Unfortunately estimation of *fibrin degradation products* (FDP) is not in the routine repertoire of many biochemistry departments, however the level is raised almost invariably in DIC and although it takes longer than the three investigations above, this estimation should be made in all suspected cases. It is important to emphasize that treatment must be instituted as soon as possible and sophisticated and time-consuming investigations of clotting factors etc., although of academic interest, are of no value in the acute clinical situation.

Treatment

General measures

Treatment of the underlying condition is essential. Thus attention to hypoxia, tissue perfusion and acidosis in the shocked patient, antibiotics in septicaemia states, and surgical drainage of abscesses is vital.

Specific therapy

As has been described above pathological activation of the clotting mechanism is the prime pathophysiological event in DIC. Treatment of the other side of the equilibrium, i.e. the fibrinolytic mechanism, may be considered of secondary importance, and sometimes fraught with grave risks.

Not all cases of DIC require heparin therapy. If the process is low grade the risks of treatment outweigh possible advantages and treatment of underlying disease, e.g. neoplasm, should be the prime objective.

The decision to use potentially dangerous anticoagulant therapy in a patient who is already bleeding must be undertaken after consideration of the clinical situation and laboratory findings. In general seriously ill patients with septicaemic states, in particular meningococeal septicaemia, and in cases where severe shock and oliguria are present should be considered for treatment with heparin.

The usual dose of heparin is 100 units/kg body weight given intravenously as a bolus, followed by 10–15 units/kg/h. If organic bleeding sites such as a peptic ulcer are present heparin should be given by infusion, using a mechanical syringe pump, to avoid high peaks of heparin activity. If liver disease is present Vitamin K must also be given,, and particular attention paid to the possibility of the presence of bleeding oesophageal varices. It has been suggested that, in liver disease, fresh frozen plasma should be given in addition (see Chapter 17). Plasma heparin levels can be monitored by plasma protamine dilution, the level should be a heparin equivalent of 0.5 mg %.

Response to therapy can be monitored on clinical grounds by assessing bleeding. Laboratory investigations into clotting mechanisms will be interfered with by heparin (thrombin time, prothrombin time). Although there may be a time lag, the fibrinogen level, platelet count and FDP level will give an indication of the efficacy of therapy. A second attack of DIC may occur if heparin therapy is terminated too rapidly and the original provocative cause still present. Under these circumstances the dose of heparin can be reduced while treatment for the underlying lesion continues.

The use of antifibrinolytic agents. Fibrinogen is used only when a very acute cause of DIC is known to be present, and in the knowledge that normal haemostasis will return when the provoking agent is relieved. Such a combination of circumstances is seen in abruptio placentae. If acute haemorrhage occurs in this condition i.v. fibrinogen can be given as normal haemostasis rapidly occurs when the fetus is delivered. This emergency must be treated, therefore, with fibrinogen, blood and fresh frozen plasma if necessary.

The dose of fibrinogen is 2.0 g, reconstituted with 200 ml of sterile water and infused over 2–3 hours. It should be remembered that there is a risk of transmitting serum hepatitis with reconstituted fibrinogen.

The use of fresh frozen plasma to replenish clotting factors after heparin therapy has been used has been suggested. Each unit of fresh frozen plasma can be expected to cause a rise in fibrinogen of 25 mg/100 ml.

Inhibitors of fibrinolysis such as tranexamic acid (Cyklokapron) should not be used in DIC because of the risk of inducing multiple intravascular thrombi;

although used topically for bladder haemorrhage there may be an indication for its use.

HAEMORRHAGIC DISORDERS

It would not be appropriate to discuss in detail all the haemorrhagic disorders. If a patient is suspected of having a bleeding diathesis there is no single investigation that will indicate its nature. It is very important to note that if there is a suspicion of such a problem blood must be sent to the haematology laboratory for investigation *before* blood transfusions are given. Full investigation requires many laboratory tests many of which are invalidated if blood has been given. It it also important to emphasize that bleeding and clotting times by themselves are not reliable tests and no conclusions can be drawn from them. If possible, a family history should be obtained and details of bleeding in childhood asked for. In general, the distinction is between congenital disorders such as haemophilia, and acquired, such as platelet deficiency, liver disease (see Chapter 17) and anti-coagulant overdosage.

Haemophilia

This hereditary bleeding disorder is confined to males. It is due to deficiency of factor VIII (see Fig. 18.2). The treatment of bleeding in haemophiliacs is discussed here as the patients may be involved in traumatic episodes in common with normal males, but additionally trivial injuries may be followed by severe haemorrhage requiring resuscitation. Such haemorrhage may be intracerebral, intrathoracic, intraabdominal or into joints or muscles. The only treatment for bleeding in haemophiliacs is the i.v. infusion of the deficient factor VIII.

Table 18.3 Treatment of haemophilia – material available

	Average factor VIII (units/ml)	Effect on patients blood (% normal)
Fresh whole blood	0.3	4–6
Fresh frozen plasma	0.6	15–20
Cryoprecipitate	3.5	100+
Freeze dried human AHG	3.5	100+

The use of fresh whole blood and fresh frozen plasma has been superseded by concentrated preparations of antihaemophiliac globulin (AHG). The concentration in cryoprecipitate may vary, whereas dried AHG concentrate has the potency of each batch assayed. If antibodies to human AHG develop an animal AHG concentrate is available.

Major surgery and serious trauma will require large doses of cryoprecipitate or AHG. The aim of therapy is to raise the patients factor VIII level to 80–120% of normal and the dose of AHG required will be 50–100 units/kg body weight. It should be noted that the half life of transfused factor VIII is about 12 hours.

Whole blood will, of course, be required as indicated by the clinical state of the patient, but no reliance should be placed on the presence of factor VIII in transfused blood.

Ideally emergencies in the haemophiliac should be managed in the special centres that have been established throughout the UK. Catastrophes will occur if inexperienced clinicians attempt to treat haemorrhage using obsolete therapeutic materials.

Christmas disease. Due to factor IX deficiency is clinically identical to haemophilia and management is along similar lines. A dried factor IX concentrate is available from the blood transfusion service. Cryoprecipitate is not of use in Christmas disease. Fresh frozen plasma can be used in mild cases.

Thrombocytopenia

Bleeding from platelet deficiency is not usually a severe problem until the count falls below 20 000/ml, less severe haemorrhage may occur with counts of under 60 000/ml.

Thrombocytopenia is usually seen as part of an aplastic picture, most commonly drug induced, or in association with acute leukaemia. A fall in platelet count occurs in DIC (see above). The treatment of bleeding due to thrombocytopenia will depend upon the underlying condition. Platelet transfusions can be given. Stored blood is not rich in platelets, and if red cells and plasma are required fresh whole blood should be given. If red cells are not required, platelet rich plasma or platelet concentrate are available.

The other problem in patients with aplastic states is infection secondary to neutropenia. This is discussed in Chapter 25.

Anticoagulants

(a) Oral anticoagulants

Bleeding from an unsuspected peptic ulcer is the commonest severe haemorrhagic complication with the coumarin and indanedione type of anticoagulant. The risk of haemorrhage is greatest in elderly and very ill patients, and the effect of anticoagulants can be potentiated by other drugs such as phenylbutazone and aspirin (both of which may also independently provoke gastric haemorrhage), clofibrate and broad spectrum antibiotics. Patients in the Intensive Therapy Unit who are often receiving a multitude of different drugs must have their anticoagulant control checked by daily prothrombin times.

The effects of oral anticoagulants can be reversed by Vitamin K (phytomenadione–Konakion) 25–50 mg intravenously.

(b) Heparin

Haemorrhage is an unusual complication of heparin therapy. However if it occurs the effects of heparin can be neutralized by protamine which combines with heparin to form a stable inactive complex. 1 mg of protamine neutralizes 110 units of heparin, this dose can be reduced if the last dose of heparin had been given more than 15 minutes previously. It should be given by slow i.v. injection (over 10 minutes).

SICKLE CELL CRISIS

Sickle cell disease may cause problems in the Intensive Therapy Units. The basic pathology is a molecular abnormality of the haemoglobin molecule which leads to distortion of the red cell. Low-grade haemolysis and anaemia are constant features of sickle cell disease. An important constituent of the clinical picture is the increase in blood viscosity due to the abnormal shape of the red cell which leads to occlusion of small vessels and consequent tissue damage. This phenomenon is seen at its worst during a 'crisis'.

Sickle cell crisis can be precipitated by hypoxia, general anaesthesia, infection, shock and acidosis. The presentation may be with severe abdominal pain, mimicing an acute surgical emergency; or with severe pain in the limbs and back associated with fever and collapse. An acute exacerbation of haemolysis may occur with sudden drop in Hb concentration; acute marrow aplasia may follow. If vessel occlusion occurs tissue damage to the brain, lungs or abdominal organs will result.

The diagnosis of sickle cell crisis should be made readily from examination of the blood film; and should be suspected in patients from Africa, the Mediterranean area and the West Indies who present with severe abdominal pain and collapse. Patients with a sickle cell crisis will invariably be anaemic. (Rarely a minor form of crisis may be precipitated by hypoxia or anaesthesia in patients who have the sickle cell trait without sickling under normal circumstances.)

Treatment of sickle cell crisis is unsatisfactory. General principles include adequate oxygenation, analgesia and control of infection. Blood transfusion should not be given unless very severe anaemia is present, as blood viscosity may be further increased. However a technique of exchange transfusion has been used successfully. A reduction in viscosity can be achieved by the infusion of a plasma volume expander such as low molecular weight dextran. Treatment with intravenous urea and low dose cyanate has been suggested but these procedures are of doubtful value. It should be noted that intravenous urea will cause an osmotic diuresis which would further increase viscosity unless large amounts of intravenous fluid are given. Recent work has suggested that hypotonic saline will rapidly improve pain in sickle cell crisis and reduce the risk of vascular occlusion by reducing viscosity and improving perfusion. The initial dose is 5.0 ml/kg body weight/h of 0.45% saline, if necessary this dose can be doubled. Osmolality should be monitored during this form of therapy.

If an aplastic crisis develops packed red cells should be given in small frequent infusions to raise the Hb level to the patients *usual* level. If too much is given erythropoiesis will be depressed. Packed red cells should also be given if there is evidence of acute haemolysis.

MISMATCHED BLOOD TRANSFUSION

The management of acute renal failure due to mismatched blood transfusion is discussed in Chapter 13. The problems of massive blood transfusions are described in Chapter 3.

A febrile reaction may occur due to pyrogens or leucocyte antibodies. If the temperature rises above 37.8°C (100°F) and is accompanied by rigors the transfusion should be stopped.

Minor degrees of haemolysis will occur if out-dated blood is used or if the transfused blood has been frozen or overheated.

The principal serious complication of blood transfusion is incompatibility due to mismatching of the ABO and Rhesus blood groups. Group O blood should not be given, before cross-matching, except in grave clinical situations since severe haemolytic reactions can sometimes be induced in patients of group AB, A or B as antibodies against these groups are sometimes present. There are, however, clinical situations where it is justifiable to use O Rhesus negative blood pending adequate cross-matching.

The majority of incompatible blood transfusions result, not from mismatching in the laboratory, but from errors in the clinical situation. Patients name tags, record numbers, and serum taken for cross-matching purposes must be exhaustively checked by responsible personnel; and no blood given until it is quite certain that the bottle presented for transfusion has indeed been cross-matched for the particular patient in question.

Serious incompatibility usually manifests itself by an acute rise in temperature, followed by rigors. This is rapidly followed by hypotension, chest pain, dyspnoea and lumbar pain; jaundice will not develop for several hours. It should be noted that the symptoms of mismatched blood transfusion will not be present in the unconscious or anaesthetized patient.

If there is any clinical indication of an incompatible blood transfusion the transfusion must be stopped immediately and donor blood, patients blood and urine retained for examination by the pathologist, and Blood Transfusion Service.

If renal failure develops this must be treated as described in Chapter 13. It should be noted that DIC (see above) may develop as a result of mismatched blood transfusion.

PLASMA EXCHANGE

The term plasma exchange is used in preference to plasmapheresis which implies the removal of plasma and its replacement by a crystallized solution. It is a technique that is unlikely to be available outside specialist units but there should be some awareness of its potentialities in auto-immune-disease.

Basically it is an extension of the exchange transfusion technique used for the treatment of severe rhesus disease in neonates. Plasma, containing antibodies, is removed and replaced with a colloid solution such as PPF or fresh-frozen plasma. This crude explanation is, of course, an oversimplification, and account should also be taken of the removal of some of the humoral components of the inflammatory response which might actually reduce tissue damage due to an antibody.

If plasma exchange is performed on patients on steroids or other immuno-suppressive agents, as will often be the case, the incidental removal of immuno-globulins will greatly increase the risk of infection.

The table below gives a test of some of the conditions in which these techniques have been used (Pinching, 1978).

Table 18.4 Plasma exchange

Antibody mediated disease	Goodpastures syndrome
	Myasthenia gravis
	Herpes gestationis
	Idiopathic thrombocytopenic purpura
	Hypogammaglobulinaemia
	Rhesus iso-immunisation
Immune complex disease	Rapidly progressive nephritis
	SLE
	Tumours
	Some cutaneous vasculitis
Diseases of excess plasma factors	Paraproteinaemias
	Homogygous familial hypercholesterol-aemia
Miscellaneous	Renal transplantation
	Raynaud's disease
	Thrombotic thrombocytopenic purpura
	Drug overdose

REFERENCE

Pinching, A. J. (1978), Plasma Exchange. *Brit. J. Hosp. Med.*, **20**, 552.

FURTHER READING

Biggs, R. (1969), The treatment of haemophilia. *J. Roy. Coll. Physns Lond.*, **3**, 151.

Cerami, A. (1972), Cyanate as an inhibitor of red-cell sickling. *N. E. J. Med.*, **287**, 807.

Colman, R. W., Robboy, S. J. and Minna, J. D. (1972), Disseminated intra-vascular coagulation (DIC): an approach. *Am. J. Medicine*, **52**, 679.

Deykin, D. (1970), Clinical challenge of disseminated intravascular coagulation. *N. E. J. Med.*, **283**, 636.

Grey, R. B. and Rothenberg, S. P. (1973), Sickle cell crisis. *Med. Clin. N. Am.*, **57**, 1591.

Lerner, R. G. and Goldstein, R. (1973), Tests of coagulation use and interpreta-tion. *Med. Clin. N. Am.*, **57**, 1609.

Sherman, L. A. (1973), Therapeutic Problems of disseminated intravascular coagulation. *Arch. Int. Med.*, **132**, 446.

NINETEEN

Neurological problems

Intensive care of neurological cases is demanding, but, ultimately, in many cases, very rewarding as many of the conditions discussed in the following sections carry an excellent prognosis.

Meticulous nursing, care of ventilators and physiotherapy are all essential as, in this field, prolonged periods of immobility on assisted ventilation are frequent.

Table 19.1 Impaired respiration

Muscular	*Neuropathy*	*Spasmodic disorders*	*Central*
Myasthenia gravis	Guillain-Barré	Status epilepticus	Raised IC tension
Polymyositis	Porphyria	Tetanus	Meningitis
		Rabies	Encephalitis
			Poliomyelitis
			Transection cervical cord

Assessment of ventilatory insufficiency

This is fully discussed in Chapter 4. The need for mechanical assistance of respiration is the indication for the admission of many neurological conditions to the Intensive Care Unit. It is preferable for such patients to be admitted to the unit prophylactically in order that serial observations of respiratory function can be made and, if necessary, assisted respiration instituted as soon as it becomes indicated.

Clinical observations of respiratory rate, tachycardia, sweating, and increasing restlessness may be helpful but serial measurements of tidal volume and vital capacity using simple apparatus such as a Wright's anemometer will give a more accurate assessment of the clinical condition. Changes in these parameters are of great importance and it is essential that the figures are accurately and regularly charted.

A progressive fall in tidal volume and vital capacity may be an indication for blood gas analysis, where a fall in P_aO_2 and a rise in P_aCO_2 will indicate a need for assisted respiration. Serial changes are more important than absolute figures, but in general a tidal volume of less than 300 ml, P_aO_2 less than 50, P_aCO_2 greater than 60 indicates respiratory dysfunction that might be helped by IPPV.

MYASTHENIA GRAVIS

Patients with myasthenia gravis are at risk of respiratory insufficiency due to an acute exacerbation of weakness, principally affecting the bulbar and respiratory muscles. The risk is of both ventilatory insufficiency and inhalation, leading to infection. An acute myasthenic crisis can be precipitated by infection, surgery, childbirth, emotional stress and certain drugs which affect neuromuscular transmission (see Table 19.2).

Table 19.2 Drugs contra-indicated – or used with caution in myasthenia gravis

Neuromuscular blocking drugs	
Aminoglycosides	Streptomycin
	Gentamicin
	Kanamycin
	Colistin
	Tobramycin
Anti-dysrhythmic agents	Lignocaine
	Beta-blockers
	Procaineamide
	Quinidine
	Quinine
CNS depressants	Chlorpromazine
	Morphine
	Barbiturates

Myasthenia gravis is due to a defect in the synthesis or storage of acetylcholine at the nerve ending. This is almost certainly due to antibodies directed at the acetylcholine receptors, such antibodies can be detected in most patients with acute myasthenia and it is postulated that they interfere with acetylcholine reception at the motor end plate. The treatment is with drugs which inhibit the enzyme cholinesterase, thereby preventing the normal action of this enzyme and enhancing the efficacy of what acetylcholine is produced at the nerve ending. However these drugs may themselves, if used in overdosage, aggravate the weakness by occupying the acetylcholine receptors and preventing normal neuromuscular transmission at the distal end of the transmitting process.

Table 19.3 Anticholinesterase drugs in myasthenia gravis

Neostigmine 15 mg 4 hourly
    (Parenteral dose 0.5 mg ≡ 15 mg orally)

Pyridostigmine (Mestinon) 60 mg 2–4 hourly

Ambenonium chloride (Mytelase)
    6 mg ≡ 60 mg Pyridostigmine
    (long-acting, but cumulative action, not in general use)

Parasympathetic side effects (abdominal pain, diarrhoea, excessive salivation, nausea and sweating) often are an indication for prescribing atropine.

Myasthenic crisis: cholinergic crisis

Acute exacerbation of myasthenic weakness may therefore be due to an exacerbation of the disease, or due to overdose with anticholinesterase drugs. Patients with deteriorating respiration or swallowing must be treated in a unit where assisted ventilation is rapidly available.

The determination of the type of crisis is often difficult and the safest way to deal with this emergency is to with-hold all medication, institute assisted ventilation and recommence anticholinesterase agents after 72 hours (Havard, 1975).

Tensilon test may be useful in differentiating between an acute exacerbation of myasthenia and poisoning by anticholinesterase drugs. 5 mg of Tensilon (edrophonium chloride) solution is injected (slowly) intravenously. This drug is a short-acting anticholinesterase agent and if paralysis is due to an exacerbation of the disease, transient improvement will occur. When the test is performed a parameter such as vital capacity should be measured, and attention concentrated on the respiratory and bulbar muscles to assess any increase in function. Conversely, if the patient's condition is due to a cholinergic crisis, transient deterioration will occur, and this test must therefore always be carried out with facilities for intubation and assisted ventilation immediately available (Osserman and Genkins, 1966). Clinically the differentiation between the two sorts of crisis may be helped by a history of infection, or exposure to the drugs listed in Table 19.2. There may be a history of injudicious increase in anticholinesterase drugs because of increasing weakness (under these circumstances a mixture of myasthenic and cholinergic crisis affecting different muscle groups may be present) (Osserman and Genkins, 1971).

Generally signs of parasympathetic activity are an unreliable indication of cholinergic crisis. A pupil size of less than 2 mm in normal room lighting may indicate impending cholinergic crisis (Simpson, 1969). It should be noted that atropine will mask these signs,, and this drug is of no value in the treatment of cholinergic crisis. However, it may be valuable to give atropine before a dose of Tensilon to avoid excessive parasympathetic stimulation (e.g. bradycardia).

Management of myasthenic and cholinergic crisis

(1) The patient must be in a unit where mechanical support for ventilation is available.

(2) A very cautious tensilon test may give a clear indication as to the nature of the crisis, but often will not.

(3) Drug medication is discontinued, assisted respiration instituted and anticholinesterase agents cautiously recommenced after 48–72 hours. The dose being gradually increased to a point of maximum effect.

Steroids in myasthenia gravis

Steroid therapy either by mouth, or in the form of ACTH injections has a place in the treatment of myasthenia gravis. However an initial deterioration occurs in many patients, and this form of therapy should always be instituted in hospital where Intensive Care facilities are available. The period of risk is from the first to tenth day of therapy, thereafter about 50% of patients improve, and it is important to remember that the dose of anticholinesterase drugs will need to be reduced to avoid the risk of cholinergic crisis. The usual dose is 30-60 mg prednisolone daily, and alternate daily dosage has been advised once improvement has occurred (Jenkins, 1972).

(It should also be remembered that patients with established and well-controlled myasthenia have the same risk of deterioration if steroids are prescribed for some other unrelated condition. Under these circumstances the institution of steroid therapy should always be undertaken in hospital.)

Thymectomy

There is increasing evidence that thymectomy is of benefit to patients with myasthenia gravis. There is a trend to performing the operation early in the course of the disease. Improvement rates of up to 90% have been claimed, even in patients without thymomas.

Thymectomy should only be performed where ITU facilities are available and such patients' postoperative care must be in an ITU. The postoperative management depends upon regular assessment of vital capacity and by using the Tensilon test, the time for re-introduction of anticholinesterase drugs is readily assessed. The dosage required will usually be 50% of the pre-operative dose. Myasthenic crisis is common in the immediate postoperative period. Steroid therapy should follow, and not precede thymectomy. The reduction in mortality in thymectomy is due to improved techniques of assisted respiration, anaesthesia and the better understanding of myasthenia and cholinergic crisis (Havard, 1973; Genkins *et al.*, 1975).

Plasma exchange

Recently this technique has been applied to myasthenia. It may be of great value in myasthenic crisis, cholinergic crisis or when thymectomy is performed. The response is relatively rapid and by its means long periods of assisted ventilation might be avoided (Newsom-Davis *et al.*, 1978).

Neonatal myasthenia

The incidence of neonatal myasthenia in children born to mothers with myasthenia is about 15%. The babies develop symptoms within 72 hours of birth. Respiratory insufficiency is common, and is associated with general hypotonia, feeding difficulties and a weak cry. The condition lasts for 3-6 weeks and responds rapidly to neostigmine (Millichap and Dodge, 1960; Namba *et al.*, 1970).

Myasthenic syndromes

The myasthenic syndromes associated with bronchial carcinoma are of great

309

importance to the anaesthetist because these patients show great sensitivity to curare. There is poor response to anticholinesterase drugs but Guanidine hydrochloride (20–50 mg/kg body weight orally in 24 hours, given 8 hourly) is effective. Severe respiratory problems are rare in this syndrome.

POLYMYOSITIS

Polymyositis may be associated with underlying malignant disease, collagen diseases or recent viral infection. Skin rashes are frequently associated (dermatomyositis). The weakness is generally predominant in the proximal and trunk muscles. A characteristic feature is often weakness of the anterior and posterior neck muscles, so that the patient has difficulty in holding his head upright; under these circumstances maintenance of the airway can cause problems. Pain and tenderness in the muscles is a good clinical indication of the primarily muscular nature of the condition. The tendon jerks are often preserved.

The diagnosis is made clinically by the course of the disease, with characteristic proximal weakness. The ESR is often elevated, but the gross elevation of creatine-kinase (CPK) indicates diffuse muscle disease. Electromyography gives a characteristic appearance and muscle biopsy will show muscle necrosis with an inflammatory infiltrate (however an isolated biopsy specimen may be negative and it is unwise to place too much reliance on biopsy).

The spectrum of weakness is broad and many cases show no respiratory embarrassment, however the disease can be fulminant and routine, regular assessment of respiratory function should be carried out in all cases.

Treatment is steroid therapy, occasional cases resistant to steroids may improve with immunosuppressive drugs. The usual dose of prednisolone is 60 mg/day in divided doses, reducing as clinical improvement occurs. Improvement can be monitored by serial CPK measurements. Management of respiratory insufficiency will be as described in Chapter 4, and monitored by regular measurements of tidal volume and vital capacity.

Prognosis is good, particularly in 'idiopathic' cases, probably secondary to viral infection; where the condition is associated with collagen diseases outlook will depend upon the other organs involved. However cases associated with underlying malignant disease, in general, respond less well to steroid therapy. In some patients with underlying carcinoma there is a myasthenic element to the muscle weakness (De Vere and Bradly, 1975).

POLYNEUROPATHY

Guillain-Barré syndrome

This important condition will almost always justify admission to the ITU as respiratory involvement is frequent and may be prolonged.

Clinical features

The picture is of an acute (or unusually subacute) mixed motor and sensory polyneuropathy. The onset may be after an unspecified viral or febrile illness, often with a latent period of several days. More specific associations are with infective mononucleosis (glandular fever), measles, psittacosis or mycoplasma infections. Motor symptoms usually predominate over sensory, but distal paraesthesiae are common. Weakness often starts distally and advances centrally rapidly with severe disorders of respiration and swallowing, leading to grave risk of inhalation and infection. Cranial nerve involvement is common. An important feature of the syndrome is associated *autonomic disturbances* (Edmonds and Sturrock, 1979). This may produce bladder atony leading to retention, wide fluctuations in the pulse rate and blood pressure and constipation.

Diagnosis
Lumbar puncture shows elevation of the protein, which may be very high (though sometimes the rise is delayed). The CSF cell count is normal or only slightly raised. SCPK levels are normal. Peripheral nerve conduction velocities may be abnormal. However the diagnosis is usually evident from the clinical features and high CSF protein.

Treatment
(1) IPPV will frequently be indicated (Hewer *et al.*, 1968). The indications as described above (and see Chapter 4). It may be required for a considerable period of time and elective tracheostomy will be indicated in all but the mildest cases. There is a particular risk of cardiac arrest, especially after tracheal aspiration (Newsom-Davis, 1974).

(2) Drug therapy is controversial. Conventionally, steroids in the form of ACTH or prednisolone are prescribed, but evidence as to their efficiency is not conclusive (Goodall *et al.*, 1974) and the risks of high dose steroid therapy with prolonged IPPV, leading to infection are considerable. Immunosuppressive therapy has also been used, but the same risk of infection is present.

(3) Physiotherapy to the limbs is essential to prevent wasting and contractures. Patients are also particularly grateful for frequent full range passive movements of the limbs to relieve pain.

Prognosis
Recovery is often incomplete in cases severe enough to have required assisted ventilation. Mortality is about 25% in this group. Milder cases can be expected to make a full recovery.

Porphyria
See Chapter 14.

STATUS EPILEPTICUS
Continued grand-mal seizures without intervening periods of recovery constitute a grave risk to life. The principal risk is airway obstruction leading to hypoxia

with consequent cerebral damage or cardiac arrhythmia. Therefore an adequate airway, preferably a cuffed endotracheal tube (which will also prevent aspiration of vomit or saliva), and oxygen should be given.

Table 19.4 Treatment of status epilepticus

Secure airway
Protect patient from injury
Drug therapy
Maintenance of fluid and electrolytes

The drug therapy of status epilepticus

(1) *Diazepam* (Valium). Intravenous diazepam is the first line of treatment and should be administered immediately. The dose is 10 mg in adults; children over 7 should receive 5 mg; under this age 2.5 mg. In infants the dose is 0.25 mg/kg body weight. The injection may need to be repeated after 15 minutes, but there is some evidence to suggest that it becomes less effective with repeated doses. However a continuous infusion may be successful if repeated bolus injections fail.

50 mg of diazepam in 500 ml normal saline is given at a dose rate of 1 mg/min (i.e. 10 ml a minute) and the effect assessed after each 10 mg has been administered. During the administration of large amounts of diazepam respiratory function must be monitored carefully. It should also be noted that intravenous diazepam can cause local pain and is irritant to the veins.

It is important to note that the infusion should be continued (at a rate of approximately 10 mg/h) for 12 hours after the last fit.

(2) *Paraldehyde* is given by deep intramuscular injection. It must *not* be used in plastic syringes. The dose is 0.1 mg/kg body weight. Intravenous infusions of paraldehyde emulsion (30 ml in 500 ml *N*/Saline) must be given through all glass infusion sets.

(3) *Phenytoin* (Epanutin). Epanutin injection should be given by infusion not exceeding 50 mg/minute in adults. If an initial dose of 250 mg is not successful a further 150 mg can be given after 30 minutes. However this drug is invariably more effective when given by mouth or via a naso-gastric tube as the chemical structure of the intravenous preparation is such as to cause uncertain blood levels. For this reason the intravenous benzodiazepines or chlormethiazole are usually preferable.

(4) *Clonazepam* (Rivotril). This benzodiazepine is given by slow intravenous injection at a rate of 1 mg in 30 seconds (half this dose in children). This may be followed by a slow intravenous infusion, 3 mg in 250 ml of 5% dextrose hourly.

(5) *Phenobarbitone* 200 mg, i.m.

(6) *Chlormethiazole* (Heminevrin). This drug is given by intravenous infusion. The solution is 0.8% and the total dose is between 200–1500 ml given at a maximum rate of 80 drops/minute. Higher infusion rates carry a risk of hypotension.

Choice of drug

Intravenous diazepam is the drug of choice and if this fails, either paraldehyde or chlormethiazole should be used. Clonzepam has not been in clinical use long enough for its value to be fully assessed, but may be a useful stand-by drug when other remedies have failed. The barbiturate drugs are best avoided because of the risk of respiratory depression. Sodium valproate (Epilim) is a useful drug for the oral control of resistant cases of epilepsy, but is not available for parenteral use.

Other measures

(1) EEG monitoring may be necessary if the patient is heavily sedated, as clinical signs of continuing epileptic activity may not be obvious.

(2) If drug therapy fails to control the fits, anaesthesia may be necessary with thiopentone. This must only be done with full respiratory resuscitation measures available.

(3) Modern anticonvulsant therapy makes the paralysing of the patient with a muscle relaxant and maintaining IPPV, a rare necessity.

(4) Dehydration can occur readily in an unconscious patient who may be febrile and sweating profusely in association with exaggerated muscular activity. Cooling by means of a fan or tepid sponging is advisable under these circumstances. The intravenous line (which should preferably be a deep line, and thoroughly secured) is therefore used for maintenance of fluid balance as well as the vehicle for anticonvulsant drugs.

Investigation of status epilepticus

It must be remembered that status epilepticus may be the presenting symptom of intracranial disease. A history of preceding infection, trauma, exposure to toxic chemicals, headaches or visual disturbances should be obtained from relatives.

Table 19.5 Causes of symptomatic status epilepticus

Intracranial tumour (often frontal lobe)
Cerebral abscess
Encephalitis, meningitis
Cerebral trauma
Metabolic causes, e.g. hypoglycaemia

If there is any doubt about the underlying pathology, a lumbar puncture and isotope scan can be carried out as soon as the fits are under control. Lumbar puncture is indicated immediately if there is any suggestion of infection (especially in children), and contraindicated in the presence of papilloedema.

Transfer to maintenance therapy

Many patients, who are known to have epilepsy, will present with status epilepticus because of failure to take prescribed drugs. Alternatively a change in medication may result in this complication. Rarely intercurrent infection or emotional trauma will precipitate status.

When the acute emergency is over and the fits controlled by intravenous therapy routine drug therapy can be reintroduced, possibly with EEG monitoring.

It should be remembered that numbers of different drugs should be avoided in the management of epilepsy, and this applies also to the control of status.

When oral therapy is recommenced serum levels should be assayed regularly to achieve therapeutic rather than toxic levels. Interactions between drugs can affect accurate assay levels, particularly when phenytoin and sodium valproate are being given together.

TETANUS

The mortality rate of tetanus is 30%. The treatment involves many disciplines and should be in a designated centre of which there are several in the UK (Editorial, *Lancet*, 1967). Although uncommon in urban areas, and unlikely to occur as a consequence of major trauma because of general awareness and availability of tetanus prophylaxis, the condition is not rare in rural areas, often as a consequence of relatively minor trauma, with wounds contaminated with soil. There is also evidence to suggest an increasing incidence in drug addicts. In underdeveloped countries tetanus neonatorum is an important problem.

Clinical course

The disease is due to the toxin produced by *clostridium tetani*. The organism is anaerobic and the spores are widely distributed in soil, dust and the general environment. Contamination of a wound does not necessarily result in clinical tetanus, it flourishes only under anaerobic conditions. The neurotoxin, tetano-spasmin, is produced as the organism multiplies and attacks the central nervous system after an incubation period of 7–10 days.

The first symptom is usually pain and spasm of the jaw muscles, trismus, and this is accompanied by pain and stiffness in the back and neck. By this time the wound, that has been the portal of entry, may be insignificant. The organism does not have any local effect and therefore wound healing is not affected.

Local spasm in the jaw area is followed by more severe pain and stiffness in the trunk muscles, pain often aggravated by movement. At this stage the characteristic facial spasm of risus sardonicus may be seen. Severe spasms

Table 19.6 Severity of tetanus		Table 19.7 Course of tetanus	
Factor	*Score*	*Factor*	*Score*
Incubation time		Severity of spasms	
less than 48 h	5	Opisthotonus	5
2–5 days	4	whole body spasm	4
5–10 days	3	limited spasms	3
10–14 days	2	generalized stiffness	2
over 14 days	1	trismus only	1
Site of infection		Frequency of spasms	
internal & umbilical	5	3 + spontaneously in	5
head, neck, body wall	4	15 min	
peripheral proximal	3	less than 3 spontaneous in	4
peripheral distal	2	15 min	
unknown	1	occasional spontaneous	3
		with stimuli only	2
State of protection		less than 6 in 12 h	1
None	10		
possibly some or	8	Body temperature	
neonates mother		Under 36.8 or over 38.9	10
immunized		38.3–38.8	8
protected more than	4	37.8–28.2	4
10 years ago		37.2–37.7	2
protected less than	2	36.7–37.1	0
10 years ago			
'complete' protection	0	Respiration	
		Tracheostomy	10
Complicating factors		apnoea after all spasms	8
Injury or illness	10	apnoea after occasional	4
hazarding life		spasm	
or neonate		apnoea during spasms only	2
Severe injury or	8	minimal interference	0
illness not im-			
mediately a hazard			
to life			
Injury or illness not	4		
hazarding life			
Minor injury or illness	2		

Table 19.8 Treatment of tetanus

Immunotherapy
Control of spasms
Maintenance of respiratory function
General management

follow this within a period of hours or days depending upon the severity of the infection.

At this stage there is severe risk to life because of apnoea associated with the spasms. At first infrequent, and precipitated by minor stimuli such as knocking the bed, the spasms become more frequent until they are almost continuous. Every muscle goes into tonic spasm, the back and limbs arch and respiration ceases. The spasm may last a few seconds or several minutes.

Clinical examination is, formally, unhelpful. Reflexes are intact and between spasms muscle power is normal although some rigidity usually persists. The differential diagnosis from other causes of stiffness of the back and neck, such as meningitis, is made from the intermittent nature of the muscle spasms. The CSF is normal.

Depending upon the severity of the infection the clinical picture may evolve within a few hours to several days of the onset of symptoms. If treatment is successful the spasms improve over a period of 10–20 days and full recovery occurs.

Prognosis

By use of the tables below the disease can be graded and an assessment made of the prognosis (Phillips, 1967).

The scores from each of the four sections (Tables 19.6 and 19.7) is added together. A total below 10 indicates a spontaneous recovery; 10–14 should survive; 15–23 indicates severe tetanus which will require the utmost in care and a score in excess of this implies very severe disease with a likely fatal outcome.

Immunotherapy

Wound debridement should be carried out. In fulminating cases the portal of entry is often obvious, and the wound should be thoroughly cleaned and necrotic tissue excised. Irrigation with hydrogen peroxide is recommended and infiltration of the wound with immuno globulin has been suggested. Debridement should not be carried out before antitoxin has been given.

Antibiotic therapy, the organism is sensitive to penicillin, and Crystalline Penicillin 10 000 000 units i.m. daily should be given—not to influence the course of the disease, which is due to the neurotoxin, but to prevent further production of toxin by any organisms that have escaped surgical toilet.

Serum therapy is an important adjunct to treatment, especially where the original wound cannot be identified or treated. Although the toxin is fixed in the central nervous system by the time clinical tetanus has developed any circulating toxin can be neutralized by antitoxin.

Human antitetanus immunoglobulin should be given in a dose of 30–300 IU/kg body weight intramuscularly.

Equine tetanus antitoxin can also be used if the human preparation is not available, but carries risk of anaphylactic reactions. The dose is 10 000 units/i.m.

Active immunization with tetanus toxoid must be instituted. 0.5 ml of alum precipitated tetanus toxoid is given i.m. (at a site different to that used for the immunoglobulin injection). A complete course of active immunization should always be completed as the immunity conferred by the disease itself is often poor and short lived.

Control of spasms: maintenance of respiration

In all but the very mildest of cases, and it is difficult to prognosticate as to subsequent clinical events at the time of diagnosis, a *tracheostomy* should be performed (Chapter 5). Respiration is affected by inhalation of secretions because the normal swallowing mechanism is affected by oropharyngeal muscle spasm, and by tetanic convulsions which fix the chest in either expiration or inspiration.

Many regimes for the control of spasms have been suggested, intravenous diazepam in the dosage suggested for the treatment of status epilepticus (page 312) is probably the drug of choice (Bacon, 1968).

If drug therapy is not successful the patient will need to be paralysed with muscle relaxants and maintained on IPPV (for detailed description of tracheostomy care, the maintenance of mechanical ventilation and its complications, and muscle relaxant technique see Chapter 6).

General management

Sympathetic nervous system overactivity (Prys-Roberts *et al.*, 1969)

There are many reports of cardiac dysrhythmia, sudden death and extreme lability of the blood pressure, often occurring in the second or third week of tetanus (Heurick *et al.*, 1973; Corbett *et al.*, 1973). It is now considered that these complications are due to overactivity to the sympathetic nervous system. Other manifestations may be fever, sweating and peripheral vasoconstriction.

It has been suggested that it would be logical to block the sympathetic nervous system in the same way that neuro-muscular blocking agents are used to prevent muscle spasms.

Beta-adrenergic blocking agents are indicated if there is a consistent tachycardia over 120/min, in a normothermic patient with normal blood gases. The dose of propranolol is that necessary to reduce the pulse rate to 100—about 10 mg 8 hourly (orally).

Intravenous propranolol should be used with great caution, if necessary by small incremental doses of 0.2 mg under direct monitoring of the ECG and pulse rate.

Alpha adrenergic blocking is more difficult, because of the lack of a predictable drug with a reasonably short period of action. The cautious use of thymoxamine (Opilon) may be justified. Bethanidine in small doses (5-10 mg/8 hourly/intragastrically) has been suggested when hypertension develops and persists after control of tachycardia by beta-adrenergic blocking agents.

If hypotension persists, simple measures such as head-down tilt, or increasing

317

arterial carbon dioxide by temporarily adding a dead space to the airway, are preferable to catecholamine infusion, which would be highly dangerous if the hypotension suddenly changes, as it sometimes does, to hypertension (Sheeby and Roba, 1967). Sudden attacks of hypotension may follow stimuli such as tracheal aspiration.

Metabolic problems

Parenteral nutrition (see Chapter 15) will be necessary in most cases. Caloric requirements of 7000 calories daily are often necessary (Parsa *et al.*, 1972).

Metabolic alkalosis, occurring in the 3–4 week of treatment has been reported. This is reversible with spironolactone, and this therapy will prevent hypokalaemia, that will further weaken affected muscles (Heurick *et al.*, 1973).

Hyperthermia is consequent upon severe tetanic spasms, and infection. If effective drug therapy is preventing muscle spasm hyperthermia should not be a serious problem. It should be remembered that a raised temperature is not an indication for antibiotic therapy unless a clinically significant infection is present (see Chapter 25).

Fluid balance must take into account the profuse perspiration that results from muscular spasms and sympathetic overactivity.

Tetanus neonatorum

The disease is fulminating in neonates, where the portal of entry is the umbilical cord. Management is along the same general principles as described above. IPPV with muscle relaxants is used from the onset. Positive end expiratory pressure of 5 cm water has been suggested. Also topical antibiotic therapy, instilled down the tracheostomy tube is indicated (0.25 ml of sterile penicillin 500 U with Colistin 500 U 4 hourly for the first 48 hours) (Smythe *et al.*, 1974; Voss, 1973).

R A B I E S (Editorial, *Brit. med. J.*, 1975; Bhatt *et al.*, 1974)

Rabies, at present, is not endemic in the British Isles, but the disease occurs on the continent of Europe and there is every possibility of its introduction across the English Channel. Elsewhere in the world it is endemic in the animal population.

The disease is transmitted from the infected saliva of a rabid animal, by being bitten or even by licking of a superficial skin abrasion. The incubation period varies from 2 weeks to 2 months, but can be longer. Once the virus has reached the central nervous system mortality rates are virtually 100%. During the incubation period, however, immunization can prevent the development of rabies.

The disease is characterized by hydrophobia—a terrible fear of water—accompanied by severe spasms of the laryngeal and respiratory muscles.

Generalized muscular convulsions develop before the encephalitic phase of the illness leads to coma. Before lapsing into coma the patient may develop acute confusional states of an often violent nature.

Risk to ventilatory function is present during the spasmodic phase, when secretion may be inhaled and when coma supervenes respiration is almost invariably depressed.

Occasionally the disease may mimic the Guillain-Barré syndrome with a picture of paralysis ascending from the site of the bite (dumb rabies).

It is important to remember that tetanus can result from animal bites. The incubation period, however, is shorter. Hydrophobia does not occur in tetanus, nor does violent alteration in behaviour.

Diagnosis is made from the history of contact with a rabid animal (if known). Frozen skin biopsy, brain biopsy, fluorescent serum antibody and specific fluorescence in corneal impression smears are useful laboratory confirmatory tests, but not always reliable. The diagnosis is essentially clinical.

Treatment

(1) Control of spasms with intravenous diazepam as in tetanus

(2) Tracheostomy with IPPV, and muscle relaxants

(3) Heavy sedation

(4) Treatment of raised intracranial pressure in the encephalitic phase (though steroids are not generally helpful, dexamethasone 4 mg 6 hourly may reduce intracranial pressure)

(5) Immunotherapy—human hyperimmune gammaglobulin rabies antiserum

Despite these measures there are reports of only two patients who have survived the disease (Hattwick *et al.*, 1972).

Protection of staff

It is very important to remember that staff dealing with a case of rabies must wear protective clothing gloves and goggles. Barrier nursing is essential.

DIFFERENTIAL DIAGNOSIS OF COMA

The differential diagnosis of coma depends upon meticulous attention to history, physical signs, and laboratory investigations. Often important aspects of the history, which will narrow the spectrum of possible causes, can be obtained from relatives.

Focal or lateralizing signs must always be looked for. Reaction to painful stimuli will not only enable the depth of coma to be assessed but may also indicate a monoparesis or hemiparesis. Pupillary inequalities are an important observation, and serial changes in pupil size and reactivity must be charted. The presence of papilloedema suggests a rise in intracranial pressure (and also occurs in some drug overdose and carbon dioxide narcosis); and may therefore indicate caution as to the wisdom of performing a lumbar puncture. Neck stiffness is

Table 19.9 Differential diagnosis of coma

Without focal signs			With focal signs	
Intracranial disease	Metabolic	Poisons	Intracranial	Metabolic
Head injury	Hypoglycaemia	Alcohol	Head injury	Hypoglycaemia
Meningitis	Uraemia	Drugs	Meningitis	
Encephalitis	Respiratory failure		Encephalitis	
Subarachnoid haemorrhage	Diabetes		Cerebrovascular accident	
Epilepsy	Hepatic failure		Subarachnoid haemorrhage	
Cerebral malaria	Myxoedema		Cerebral tumour	
	Hypothermia			
Cerebral oedema	Anoxia			

usually apparent, even in deeply unconscious patients. The scalp must always be examined for evidence of injury.

Treatment of the unconscious patient

Regardless of cause, immediate treatment must ensure that an adequate airway is present and that the patient is positioned on his side to reduce the risk of inhalation of vomit. If ventilatory insufficiency is present, or seems likely to develop, a cuffed endotracheal tube should be passed. IPPV can be instituted if indicated clinically or as a result of simple bedside measurements such as tidal volume. Although blood gas estimations may be important, valuable time can be wasted in performing them and waiting for results. It is preferable to ventilate a patient unnecessarily than to allow progressive hypoxia to develop.

If there is any reason to suppose hypoglycaemia to be the cause of coma an immediate intravenous injection of 50 ml 50% dextrose should be given. This will not do any harm in other causes of coma, even diabetic coma.

Investigation of the unconscious patient

Blood must be taken for urea, electrolytes, blood sugar and liver function tests. Unless the cause of coma is obvious the blood should also be examined for barbiturates and salicylates (although most modern suicide attempts involve drugs that are not rapidly identifiable in blood specimens). If there is reason to suppose drug poisoning urine and blood should be retained for full toxological investigation. Blood gas estimations will only confirm clinical judgement in most cases but serial measurements may be a useful monitor in assessing the efficiency of treatment. Haemoglobin and white cell count may be helpful in assessing the likelihood of bacterial infection.

Specific neurological investigations

(1) Skull X-ray will show a fracture if present, but the opinion of an experienced radiologist is more valuable than that of a casual observer of X-rays. Shift of midline structures may be identified as pineal shift, but it is often difficult to produce a properly centred film in a confused patient.

(2) Lumbar Puncture should be done if there is any reason (fever, skin rash, neck stiffness, focal neurological signs) to suspect infection of the CNS, or subarachnoid haemorrhage. Generally, papilloedema is a contraindication to lumbar puncture unless full neurosurgical facilities are at hand.

(3) Echo-encephalography is a useful non-invasive technique to detect mid line shift.

(4) EEG will give quite specific information in hepatic failure or encephalitis and may be helpful in suggesting the presence of supratentorial mass.

(5) Isotope imaging is non-invasive and only a relatively short period of immobilization is necessary in the restless patient. A supratentorial mass, or haematoma, and midline shift can be identified.

(6) Neuroradiology. Angiography will be necessary to identify subdural

haematomata, space occupying lesions and cerebral aneurysms. It will also demonstrate occlusion of major vessels. Cerebral angiography is indicated if there is clinical indication of, or other investigations suggest, a space occupying lesion.

(7) Computer assisted tomography (CAT Scan), if available, is non-invasive, and may give useful information.

MENINGITIS

Severe cases of bacterial meningitis are likely to be encountered in the ITU. Fulminating cases, at all age groups, may rapidly become comatose and respiratory insufficiency, with the risk of aspiration of vomit, will frequently be an indication for IPPV.

AETIOLOGY

Table 19.10 Aetiology of bacterial meningitis

	Neonate	Infant	Children and adults	Elderly
Meningococcus		+++	+++	+
Pneumococcus		+++	+++	++
H. influenzae		++		
Gram-negative organisms	+++			
Listeria	++	+	+	
Staphylococci ⎱ Streptococci ⎰	++			

Table 19.10 indicates the spectrum of bacteriological aetiology at different age groups. It should be noted that this is not intended to be a complete list of bacterial agents which can produce meningitis. In particular patients with compromised immunological systems (e.g. in malignant disease, leumaemia, cytotoxic therapy) are susceptible to infections with more unusual organisms, such as cryptococcus neoformans (see Chapter 25).

Diagnosis

The first indication as to the aetiological agent will be from a gram stain of the CSF.

Lumbar puncture is essential for this diagnosis, although in fulminant cases of meningococcal meningitis (see below) CSF examination in the earliest stages may not reveal any abnormality of cell count or protein.

CSF should be examined in every patient, in whom there are clinical grounds for suspecting infection of the central nervous system.

(1) Headache

(2) Fever

(3) Signs of meningism, i.e. stiffness of neck, Kernig's sign positive
(4) Alteration in level of consciousness
(5) Photophobia

Table 19.11 Cerebro-spinal fluid in meningitis

	Cells	Protein	Sugar
Acute bacterial	↑ polymorphs	↑	↓
Viral	↑ 25–50/cmm lymphocytes	slight increase	normal
Tuberculous	↑ 20–500 lymphocytes	↑ ++	↓
Acute polyneuritis	normal	↑ ++	normal
Poliomyelitis	↑	↑ moderate	normal

(1) *CSF sugar* is markedly reduced in pyogenic meningitis, but the diagnosis does not rest on this finding. In the differentiation between a benign viral meningitis and tuberculous meningitis, however, the CSF sugar estimation is important, and it should be noted that a blood sugar estimation must be performed simultaneously. (The CSF sugar is approximately 60% of the blood sugar.)

(2) *Other causes* of a raised cell count in the CSF include meningeal carcinomatosis, sarcoidosis of the CNS, recent cerebro-vascular accident. Particular mention must be made of the lymphocytosis that may occur in the CSF in association with a cerebral abscess.

(3) *Viral meningitis* is unlikely to be a problem in the ITU. The disease is usually mild; though headache may be severe, alteration in consciousness, respiratory insufficiency and focal signs do not occur.

Treatment

The appropriate chemotherapy will depend upon the organism, but, of course, treatment cannot be delayed until the results of CSF culture are available. Often a gram stain of the CSF will give useful information, but if the diagnosis of bacterial meningitis is suspected because of CSF findings and the clinical picture, a negative gram stain must not be a deterrent to antibiotic therapy pending culture reports. Many patients, especially children, will have received antibiotic therapy before admission to hospital. Under these circumstances bacteriological studies of the CSF may be negative (particularly in meningococcal infection).

Table 19.12 indicates antibiotic therapy for the three major pathogens (meningococcal meningitis is discussed below). However if the infecting

Table 19.12 Antibiotic therapy of bacterial meningitis in adults

	Drug	Route	Dose
Meningococcus		see below	
Pneumococcus	Penicillin G	i.v.	30 mega units/24 h
H. influenzae	Chloramphenicol	i.m.	50–75 mg/kg/24 h
	Ampicillin	i.v.	50 mg/kg/4 hourly

organism cannot immediately be identified blind antibiotic therapy must be started pending bacteriological confirmation; under these circumstances it is appropriate to commence treatment with a combination of penicillin G and chloramphenicol. Daily blood counts must be done because of the risk of aplastic anaemia with chloramphenicol. Chloramphenicol is a more effective drug than ampicillin in infection of the CNS as it crosses the blood-brain barrier more readily and effective levels are achieved in the CSF.

Intrathecal antibiotics are rarely necessary in meningitis due to the three commonest pathogens above. However, if at lumbar puncture, the fluid is obviously purulent, an intrathecal injection of penicillin can be given—*maximum* dose 20 000 units. (Note: Penicillin specially prepared for intrathecal use must always be used.)

Meningococcal meningitis

Meningococcal meningitis is the commonest cause of acute bacterial meningitis in the UK. The condition may be fulminating, causing coma, respiratory depression and death within a few hours. Meningococcaemia is always present and in these cases with overwhelming blood stream infection, signs of CNS involvement are often very slight at first. In the early stages the CSF is not diagnostic, as cultures will be positive, but cell count and gram stain negative. However, the commonest presentation is with symptoms and signs of meningeal irritation.

Special features of meningococcal meningitis:

(1) Rash—purpuric in nature. Occasionally sparse, and may be confined to the conjunctivae

(2) Disseminated intravascular coagulation (DIC)

(3) Waterhouse-Fridericksen syndrome—profound hypotension and extensive skin haemorrhages are associated with high mortality. At autopsy the adrenal glands show extensive haemorrhages. This syndrome is probably a manifestation of coagulation disturbances.

(4) arthritis

Diagnosis. The presence of signs of meningeal irritation with a purpuric rash is almost pathognomic of meningococcal meningitis. Blood should be taken for culture and CSF examined for organisms and sent for culture. A gram stain of the buffy coat may enable the bacteriologist to find gram negative intracellular diplococci after other methods have failed.

Management of meningococcal meningitis

The meningococcus is rapidly becoming resistant to the sulphonamides and this drug should therefore *not* be used alone for treatment of meningococcal meningitis.

Table 19.13 Antibiotic therapy in meningococcal meningitis

	Adults		Children	
Drug	*Loading*	*Total (24 h)*	*Loading*	*Total (24 h)*
Sulphadimidine	3–6 g	6–12 g	0.5–2.0 g	3–6 g
i.v. Penicillin g	20–30 mega units/24 h		0.5–1.0 mega units/ kg/24 h	
Chloramphenicol	50–75 mg/kg/24 h *NB: Neonates not more than 25 mg/kg/24 h*			
i.v. Ampicillin	150–250 mg/kg/24 h			

Treatment should be commenced with sulphadimidine and penicillin G in the doses above. This should be continued for 5 days. If the organism is sensitive to sulphonamides the penicillin can be discontinued. Oral treatment should be continued for a further 5 days after the i.v. regime has been completed.

Patients sensitive to penicillin can be treated witn cephaloridine 1 g 6 hourly i.v. in adults, this drug does not pass the blood-CSF barrier very effectively and it has been suggested that intrathecal doses of 50 mg should be given for 3 days.

Steroid therapy

Recommended as routine because of risk, the Waterhouse–Fridericksen syndrome causing acute hypo-adrenalism, and because of their role in the treatment of septicaemic shock, but treatment of DIC is more important. The recommended dose of hydrocortisone is 200 mg as a stat. dose followed by 500 mg 4–6 hourly (in adults). Steroids may also have a beneficial effect in reducing intracranial pressure.

Heparin

If there is profuse skin haemorrhage, a fulminating history, or hypotension, heparin should be given concurrently with the institution of antibiotic therapy. Bolus injections of heparin 10 000–15 000 units 4 hourly (in adults) should be given for 24–36 hours.

DIC should be monitored as described in Chapter 18.

Meningitis due to Gram-negative organisms (Smith, 1975; Rahal, 1972)

Meningitis due to organisms of the *E. coli, Klebsiella, Pseudomonas* and *Proteus*

325

groups are commonest in neonates, or in neurosurgical cases. Infection with this group of organisms can also occur in septicaemic states or as an opportunistic infection with an impaired immunological system. Treatment is difficult because antibiotics of the aminoglycoside group do not penetrate the CNS well and high dosage is necessary to achieve therapeutic levels in the CSF. Chloramphenicol might be helpful if the organism is sensitive.

It has been shown that antibiotics given intrathecally by the translumbar route do not travel to the ventricular system. In adults and older children (whose fontanelles are closed) it might be necessary to administer the drugs by the intraventricular route. Generally this will need to be done in a neurosurgical unit.

(1) In the majority of patients gentamicin or tobramycin should be given systemically with intrathecal injections of 5 mg every 18-24 h.

(2) If the organism is sensitive to chloramphenicol this drug should be given systemically in a dose of 75-100 mg/kg/day (dose reduction essential in neonates).

(3) In desperate clinical situations, with a moribund patient 5 mg of tobramycin or gentamicin should be given every 18-24 h by the intraventricular route with systemic therapy. This regime can also be adopted if there is relapse after intrathecal administration.

Neonatal meningitis

Meningitis is a particular problem in premature babies, and in babies with spina bifida. The usual organisms are the gram negative ones described above, in addition streptococcal or staphylococcal infection occurs, also infection with Listeria monocytogenes. Because of this broad spectrum of infecting agents full bacteriological studies must be performed on the blood and CSF.

Empirical treatment, pending results of cultures, will usually be gentamicin or tobramycin. Intrathecal or intraventricular dose is 1 mg/day. Systemic therapy should also be given—3-6 mg/kg/day in two doses and continued for 10-12 days.

When the organism has been identified, and sensitivities are available the antibiotic regime may need changing, especially if staphylococci, streptococci or listeria are incriminated as penicillin will then be indicated. Penicillinase resistant antibiotics may be necessary if the organism is penicillin resistant.

ENCEPHALITIS

There are many viral agents implicated in the aetiology of acute encephalitis. The condition may arise in a previously healthy person or after a known virus infection, e.g. the acute childhood illnesses such as measles, chicken pox or mumps. Encephalitis also occurs as a complication of vaccination procedures for smallpox or rabies.

Clinical picture is varied. Severe cases may lapse into coma rapidly and have signs mimicking a space occupying lesion. Generally the history is of fever, malaise, headaches and other symptoms of meningeal irritation, followed by alteration in levels of consciousness, accompanied by focal neurological signs or epileptic fits. Sometimes encephalitis presents as psychotic behaviour.

Diagnosis depends upon a previous history of viral illness or vaccination where applicable, otherwise it is largely by exclusion of other acute CNS syndromes including meningitis, cerebral abscess or other space occupying lesions. If focal signs are present an EEG, cerebral angiography and isotope brain scans will be necessary to exclude a local structural lesion.

The CSF will show an increase in cell count, predominantly lymphocytes, but there are no particular diagnostic features.

Treatment

Specific therapy is available only for meningoencephalitis due to herpes simplex, or herpes zoster. The EEG may be helpful in identifying herpes encephalitis, temporal abnormalities are often prominent. CSF should be sent for virological studies, but treatment should not be delayed until the result of these rather protracted investigations are available.

If herpes encephalitis is diagnosed Vidarabine should be given by slow daily intravenous infusion 10 mg/Kg/day for 5 days. Steroids should not be given to patients with herpes encephalitis (Smith, 1975).

Steroid therapy is conventional for other types of encephalitis, although there is no clear evidence that the course of the disease is influenced by their use. There can be no doubt, however, that raised intracranial tensions can be reduced by the use of dexamethasone 4–8 mg 6 hourly. The improvement in level of consciousness that occurs with the use of dexamethasone in encephalitis is probably due to reduction in cerebral oedema. There is no justification for long courses of steroid therapy.

General measures are those of general care of unconscious patients. Particular attention must be paid to the airway and maintenance of adequate respiratory function. Fits can be controlled as described on page 312. Recovery from encephalitis can be very protracted.

POLIOMYELITIS

Poliomyelitis is now very rare in the UK, but occurs in underdeveloped countries, or where there is no active programme of immunization. The disease is due to an enterovirus which invades the central nervous system. Clinically it is divided into two phases. In the first phase of viraemia there may be slight fever, general malaise, sore throat and minor gastro-intestinal upset. The second phase, a few days later, occurs when the virus invades the central nervous system. The symptoms are those of a viral meningitis accompanied by pain and paraesthesiae in muscles which may soon become paralysed.

The *paralytic phase* develops within 24–72 hours of the second phase of the illness. A lower motor neurone lesion may affect any muscle or group of muscles. Particularly dangerous is involvement of the bulbar muscles when aspiration

327

of secretions and respiratory insufficiency develop. Paralysis progresses for up to 72 hours.

Recovery may be very delayed, and is often incomplete.

Diagnosis

(1) CSF shows an initial rise in cell count, at first there is an excess of polymorphs but in later stages lymphocytes predominate. Rises in protein are moderate in the early stages.
(2) Viral studies on the CSF and stools.

Treatment

Respiratory function must be monitored carefully and IPPV instituted if indicated. During the phase of progression of the paralysis and patient must be kept on total rest, without physiotherapy, as paralysis is worse if affected muscles are exercised during this phase. Thereafter the importance of physiotherapy cannot be overemphasized.

There is no specific treatment for poliomyelitis.

SUBARACHNOID HAEMORRHAGE

The management of subarachnoid haemorrhage in the ITU of a general hospital usually poses more ethical than medical problems. The condition is essentially one for a specialist neurosurgical unit but many cases will be admitted to the ITU in the first instance.

If the onset is catastrophic with very rapid deterioration in respiratory function associated with deepening coma, IPPV will have been commenced before the diagnosis is established. It is this group of patients in whom the prognosis is virtually hopeless and difficult decisions will have to be made with regard to continuing assisted ventilation.

Medical measures include control of hypertension, dexamethasone to reduce intracranial pressure, and occasionally tranexamic acid (Cyklokapron).

Bad prognostic signs are
 (1) unremitting coma
 (2) focal neurological signs
 (3) hypertension
 (4) previous subarachnoid haemorrhage

If the level of consciousness improves following medical measures the patient should be transferred to a neurosurgical unit for cerebral angiography.

CEREBRAL MALARIA

As rapid air travel becomes more common, so it is becoming more likely for tropical illnesses to develop in temperate zones. Malaria can readily be contracted abroad, even at a stop-over at an airport in endemic zone, and the clinical picture develop on return home. If a comatose patient is admitted, febrile, and no other cause can be found, it is essential to enquire as to a history of travel to, or through, an area where malaria occurs. This enquiry should cover travel up to 6 months previously.

Cerebral malaria occurs in *malignant tertian malaria* (plasmodium falciparum). The symptoms are headache, drowsiness, coma, mental disturbances and convulsions.

Diagnosis

Depends on thinking of a possibility of cerebral malaria and finding the parasite in the peripheral blood.

Treatment

Chloroquine 200 mg (base) i.v. given in 500 ml N/saline over 30 minutes. Repeated 6-8 hourly. Oral treatment with chloroquine must follow this. Steroids (dexamethasone 10 mg initially, followed by 4 mg 6 hourly for 3-4 days).

CEREBRAL OEDEMA

Cerebral oedema has been mentioned in other chapters as, for example, a complication of the treatment of hyperosmotic non-ketotic diabetic coma, hyponatraemia of varying aetiology and, of course, in association with neurological illness. Cerebral oedema can be subdivided into several types according to aetiology.

Table 19.14 Types of cerebral oedema

Type	Cause
Vasogenic	Vascular damage
Cytotoxic	Hypoxic brain damage
Hydrostatic	High cerebro-vascular transmural pressure
Interstitial	Obstructive high pressure hydrocephalus
Hypo-osmotic	Low plasma colloid osmotic pressure

The diagnosis of cerebral oedema should be considered where the condition of the patient deteriorates under the circumstances described in the table. The level of consciousness will decline and focal signs of hemispheric disturbance might develop.

The diagnosis can be confirmed by CT-scan, where this is available, as increases in brain-tissue water content are shown as decreases in density.

Treatment (Miller, 1979)

The general measures will be to treat the underlying cause if this can be identified. Therefore severe hypoxaemia and carbon dioxide retention should be treated and the arterial perfusion maintained with a systolic blood pressure of 110–140 mm Hg.

Specific measures

(a) Hyperventilation (see Chapters 6, 12).

(b) Hypertonic Solution. 20% mannitol is the agent usually employed. It should be given rapidly in sufficient dosage, 1 g/kg body weight over 10 minutes. If mannitol has to be given more than every 3–4 hours serum osmolality should be monitored carefully. If it rises to greater than 320 mosmol/litre no further mannitol should be given.

(c) Steroids. Steroid therapy is most helpful in focal cerebral oedema, for example in association with a tumour or abscess. Although widely prescribed in head injury there is little convincing evidence to support their use.

Dexamethasone is generally used—initial dose 10 mg i.m. followed by 4 mg 6 hourly for up to 5 days.

Diuretics

(d) Diuretics. Frusemide and ethacrynic acid have been used but their effect is mild.

REFERENCES

Bacon, A. K. (1968), Diazepam in tetanus. *Brit. med. J.*, 2, 646.

Bhatt, D. R., Hattwick, M. A., Gerdsen, R., Emmons, R. W., and Johnson, H. M. (1974), Human rabies—diabetes, complications and management. *Am. J. Dis. Child.*, 527, 862.

Corbett, J. L., Spalding, J. M. and Harris, P. J. (1973), Hypotension in Tetanus. *Brit. med. J.*, 2, 423.

DeVere, R. and Bradly, W. G. (1975), Polymyositis: its presentation morbidity and mortality. *Brain*, 98, 637.

Diagnosis and treatment of human rabies (1975), Editorial. *Brit. med. J.*, 3, 721.

Edmonds, M. E. and Sturrock, R. D. (1979), Autonomic neuropathy in the Guillain-Barre syndrome. *Brit. med. J.*, 2, 668.

Genkins, G., Papatestas, A., Horowitz, S. H. and Kornfeld, P. (1975), Studies in myasthenia gravis: early thymectomy. Electrophysiologic and pathologic correlations. *Am. J. Med.*, 58, 517.

Goodall, J. A. D., Kosmidis, J. C. and Geddes, A. M. (1974), Effect of Corticosteroids on the course of Guillain-Barré Syndrome. *Lancet*, i, 524.

Hattwick, M. A., Weis, T. T., Stechschulte, C., George, M., Baer, D. A. M. and Gregg, M. B. (1972), Recovery from rabies—a case report. *Ann. Int. Med.*, 76, 931.

Havard, C. W. (1973), Progress in myasthenia gravis. *Brit. med. J.*, 3, 437.

Havard, C. W. (1975), Myasthenia Gravis. *Brit. med. J.*, 4, 152.

Heurick, A. E., Brust, J. C. and Richter, R. W. (1973), Management of urban tetanus. *Med. clin. N. Am.*, **57**:6, 1373.

Hewer, R. L., Hilton, P. J., Crampton-Smith, A. and Spalding, J. M. K. (1968), Acute Polyneuritis requiring artificial ventilation. *Q. Jl. Med.*, **37**, 479.

Jenkins, R. B. (1972), Treatment of myasthenia Gravis with prednisone. *Lancet*, i, 765.

Kaiser, A. B. and McGee, Z. A. (1975), Aminoglycoside Therapy of Gram Negative bacillary meningitis. *N. E. J. Med.*, **293**, 1215.

Lichtenfeld, P. (1971), Autonomic dysfunction in the Guillain–Barré syndrome. *Am. J. Med.*, **50**, 772.

Millichap, J. and Dodge, P. R. (1960), Diagnosis and treatment of myasthenia gravis in infancy, childhood and adolescence: a study of 51 patients. *Neurology*, **10**, 1007.

Miller, J. D. (1979), The management of cerebral oedema. *Brit. J. Hosp. Med.*, **21**, 152.

Namba, T., Brown, S. B. and Grob, D. (1970), Neonatal Myasthenia Gravis: report of two cases and review of the literature. *Paediatrics*, **45**, 488.

Newsom-Davis, J. (1974), Neurological Intensive Care. *Medicine*, **34**. 2008.

Newsom-Davis, J., Pinching, A. J., Vincent, A. and Wilson, S. (1978). *Neurology* (Minneapolis), **28**, 266.

Osserman, K. E. and Genkins, G. (1966), Critical reappraisal of the use of adrophonium (tensilon) chloride tests in myasthenia gravis and significance of clinical classification. *Am. N.Y. Acad. Sci.*, **135**, 312.

Osserman, K. E. and Genkins, G. (1971), Studies in myasthenia gravis: review of a 20 year experience in over 1200 patients. *Mt. Sinai J. Med.*, **38**, 497.

Parsa, M. D., Anderson, M. D. and Richter, R. W. (1972), Central venous nutrition in severe tetanus. *Arch. Surg.*, **105**, 420.

Phillips, L. A. (1967), A classification of tetanus. *Lancet*, i, 1216.

Prys-Roberts, C., Corbett, J. L., Kerr, J. H. and Spalding, J. M. K. (1969), Treatment of sympathetic over-activity in tetanus. *Lancet*, i, 542.

Rahal, J. J. (1972), Treatment of Gram Negative bacillary meningitis in adults. *Ann. Int. Med.*, **77**, 295.

Sheehy, T. W. and Roba, R. C. (1967), Complications of falciparum malaria and their treatment. *Ann. Int. Med.*, **66**, 807.

Simpson, J. A. (1969), Myasthenia Gravis and myasthenic syndrome; *Disorders of Voluntary Muscles*. Ed. J. N. Walton. Churchill, London.

Smith, C. C. (1975), Meningitis and encephalitis. *Brit. med. J.*, **4**, 335.

Smith, M. (1975), Bacterial Meningitis. *Medicine* (Series 2), **2**, 92.

Smythe, P. M., Bowie, M. D. and Voss, T. J. (1974), Treatment of tetanus neonatorum with muscle relaxants and I.P.P.V. *Brit. med. J.*, **1**, 223.

Tetanus in Britain (Editorial) (1967), *Lancet*, i, 886.

Voss, T. J. (1973), Ways of reducing atalectasis and improving oxygen uptake from the lungs. *S. A. med. J.*, **47**, 761.

TWENTY

Paediatric intensive care

Specialized paediatric intensive care units are viable only as Regional Centres and these will usually be associated with paediatric hospitals or university departments. Financial and manpower resources seldom permit the establishment of more than one unit for intensive care in the district general hospital and this has to serve all age groups. Despite the psychological and other objections to the management of children in adult units, serious problems are seldom encountered although it is important to have close co-operation between intensive care and paediatric staff. The district general hospital is not equipped to carry out specialized neonatal intensive care and some patients must be transferred to Regional Centres. Care must be taken when small babies are transported in ambulances to ensure that they arrive in as good a condition as possible and this may demand attention to the airway and ventilation as well as to heat regulation and nutrition.

Some of the disorders which require intensive care in paediatric practice are listed in Table 20.1. It is not, however, possible to consider all these in detail in this chapter.

Whenever a small baby needs therapy the medical staff must be aware of the differences between the physiology of adults and infants.

Neonatal physiology

The neonate is defined as an infant during the first 28 days of life.

(1) *Respiration.* The lungs of the newborn are less efficient than those of older children. The ribs are more horizontal and the diaphragm is elevated by the large liver. Physiological deadspace is increased. The respiratory pattern is variable but average figures for respiratory rate are 34 to 40 per min and average tidal volume is about 20 ml. The respiratory surface per unit weight is about one third that of adults. Respiratory reserve is diminished.

(2) *Cardiovascular.* Profound haemodynamic changes occur at birth with closure of the ductus arteriosus and the foramen orale. Ligation of the umbilical vessels produces a rise in systemic resistance while onset of lung function is accompanied by a profound fall in pulmonary vascular resistance. The blood pressure of the neonate is about 80/60 mm Hg and heart rate 120–140/min. The haemoglobin

Table 20.1 *Disorders requiring intensive care in*
paediatric practice

Respiratory disorders

Upper airway obstruction
  Acute epiglottitis
  Laryngotracheobronchitis
  Congenital subglottic stenosis
  Foreign bodies
  Vascular ring
  Burns

Lower airway obstruction
  Asthma
  Bronchopneumonia
  Cystic fibrosis
  Aspiration syndrome

Alveolar disorders
  Infection
  Pulmonary oedema
  Effects of trauma
  Oxygen toxicity
  Respiratory distress syndrome of the newborn

Extrapulmonary
  Pneumothorax
  Haemothorax
  Severe spinal malformations
  Diaphragmatic hernia

Neurological disorders
  Encephalitis
  Meningitis
  Poisoning
  Tetanus
  Poliomyelitis

Trauma
  Head injury
  Multiple injuries
  Postoperative care

Congenital
  Oesophageal atresia
  Duodenal atresia
  Diaphragmatic hernia
  Omphthalocoele
  Imperforate anus
  Cardiovascular abnormalities

Prematurity

content of the blood is high and more than half exists as fetal haemoglobin (HbF) which disappears almost completely during infancy.

(3) *Fluid requirements*. The infant has a large surface area relative to the adult, the head and neck accounting for 19% of the total (compared to 9% in the adult). The weight of the newborn infant is 80% water and more in small and premature babies. Babies requiring surgery for congenital abnormalities may have low weight. Renal function also differs in the neonate who may not be able to regulate fluids infused intravenously. The neonate kidney cannot excrete a high sodium load.

Blood volume is about 85 ml/kg in the first year of life (Mollison *et al.*, 1950) and this falls to 75 ml per kg by the age of 10 years.

The *daily water requirement* in the paediatric surgical patient has been given as follows:

Age	ml per kg
1 day	50
5 days	100
10 days	150
15 days	150–180
6 months	150
1 year	120
4 years	100
10 years	70

The basic requirement must be supplemented by addition of calculated deficits.

Electrolytes. The daily requirements for sodium and potassium are 3 mmol/kg/day in neonates and 2 mmol/kg/day in the older child. It may be necessary to provide calcium 2 and magnesium 1 mmol per kg per day when prolonged infusion is necessary.

Hydrogen ions. Specific therapy is usually indicated when the measured base deficit is greater than 10 mmol/l and the adult formula 0.3 X base deficit X body weight in kg is satisfactory in calculation of bicarbonate dose required for correction.

(4) *Metabolism*. The newborn can suffer depletion of carbohydrate reserves in liver and muscle with consequent hypoglycaemia and acidosis. This is likely to occur following asphyxia or hypothermia. Brown fat, which contains beta-adrenergic receptors, is an important source of energy. Heat loss occurs readily if the baby's skin is exposed to a cold environment and since the head is large in relation to the rest of the body radiant heat loss from the head can be important if it is not covered.

Asphyxia at birth can lead to acidosis and hypoglycaemia with blood sugar levels as low as 1.7 mmol/l. It may therefore be necessary to administer glucose by intravenous drip.

(5) *Temperature.* Heat loss occurs rapidly in the neonate who has a larger surface area relative to body mass than the older child. This particularly applies to the head which can be a significant source of heat loss unless protected by a stockinet cap. The heat regulating mechanisms of the neonate are unstable. Body heat is in part maintained by the metabolic activity of brown fat which is found around the kidneys and adrenals.

Iatrogenic hypothermia can occur as a result of undue exposure and the use of cold fluids for intravenous infusion. Temperature monitoring is mandatory during operative procedures when the oesophageal probe combining stethoscope, ECG leads and thermistor has been found useful (Inkster, 1966).

Intensive care of the neonate

General considerations

Specific therapy will be of little avail unless attention is paid to such factors as:
(1) Temperature regulation. Prevention of hypothermia.
(2) Acid base balance.
(3) Nutrition.
(4) Oxygenation.

Congenital abnormalities

Major abnormalities will require surgical correction in a specialized Regional Centre. Immediate care should be directed to keeping the baby warm while transport is expedited. It is generally unwise to delay transfer in the hope of improving the baby's general condition.

Exceptions to this rule include oesophageal atresia and diaphragmatic hernia. Such patients are likely to require preliminary tracheal intubation and the latter may need assisted ventilation. The stomach should be emptied when possible by nasogastric tube and in the case of oesophageal atresia a tube should be passed into the blind pouch to remove secretions.

The neonate who requires surgery should have estimations of haemoglobin, packed cell volume and serum electrolytes carried out. Blood sugar should also be determined. It is rare for dehydration or electrolyte imbalance to be manifest in the first 12 hours of life, but in older babies adequate correction of abnormalities may be life-saving. Glucose should be given by intravenous infusion when there is evidence of hypoglycaemia. Starvation may exacerbate acidosis.

Respiratory distress syndrome (RDS)

This is said to occur in 1% of live births but in one third of premature infants. Prematurity is the main predisposing factor but others include maternal diabetes, asphyxia during birth, and the condition is commoner in the second of a pair of twins.

Signs

The baby has obvious respiratory difficulty with a rise in respiratory rate, indrawing of intercostal and subcostal soft tissues during inspiration, use of the alae nasi and grunting respiration. There is central cyanosis, rise of heart rate, rales over the lung fields on auscultation. Chest x-rays show development of a characteristic reticulo-granular pattern or a uniform opacity of both lung fields. Death is likely if the condition deteriorates, but if recovery is to occur it is usually complete, the natural course taking about 5 days. Persistent lung pathology may have an iatrogenic basis.

Pathophysiology

There is a deficiency in lung surfactant (Avery and Mead, 1959) which is related to prematurity and leads to alveolar atelectasis and reduction of lung compliance. Ventilation-perfusion relationships are disturbed due to continued perfusion of poorly ventilated lung tissue with marked A-a gradients.

Prevention

Prevention of RDS can be achieved with some success by good antenatal care to identify those at risk and plan their delivery in centres where special facilities exist for monitoring of mother and baby before delivery (e.g. maternal oestriol, fetal pH) as well as special baby units for the management of RDS should it develop. Unnecessary premature delivery, especially by Caesarean section, is to be avoided.

Management

(1) *Administration of oxygen.* This should be given to achieve a PaO_2 of 6.5 kPa, but this may not be possible where shunts account for more than 40% of blood passing through the lungs. *Oxygen toxicity* to the lungs may occur with $F1O_2$ more than 60% but, *retrolental fibroplasia* as a complication can be discounted when arterial oxygen tensions remain low (Baum and Bulpitt, 1970).

(2) *IPPV.* Controversial, but may be indicated when situation deteriorating.

(3) *PEEP or CPAP.* The use of positive pressure in the expiratory phase has been advocated in the treatment of RDS whether the baby is breathing spontaneously in a head box (Gregory, 1971) with tracheal tube, or when IPPV is being used.

(4) *Correction of acid base imbalance.*

THE OLDER CHILD

Patients may need admission to an intensive care unit for a variety of reasons. Certain important conditions only will be considered here.

ACUTE LUNG INFECTIONS IN BABIES

Depending upon the severity of the condition the baby may require:
(1) Routine antibiotic treatment; observation.
(2) Tracheal intubation for the removal of secretions.
(3) IPPV.

Laryngo-tracheobronchitis

This condition may present as an acute infection of the upper respiratory tract with stridor. The mucosa of the larynx and trachea is inflamed with muco-purulent exudate. Obstruction to respiration is most likely to occur in the immediate subglottic region where the airway is narrowest. Children below the age of 6 years are most likely to become distressed and require a period of intensive care. Tracheal intubation may be necessary to allow removal of sec-retions by gentle suction and it is usually best achieved under careful general anaesthesia. Specimens of the aspirate should be sent for bacterial culture as although the condition is often viral in origin a superimposed bacterial infection is usually present. It is usually possible to remove the tracheal tube after a few hours, but re-intubation is sometimes necessary.

Stridor in small babies

This may have various causes. *Laryngomalacia* may cause obstruction as a result of weakness of the laryngeal cartilages; it usually improves as the baby grows. *Papilloma of the larynx* is a serious condition, likely to require tracheostomy for the duration of treatment. *Vascular ring* causes obstruction when an abnormal artery compresses the trachea. The stenosis is seen as a localized lesion at bronchoscopy. Thoracotomy and division of the offending vessel is required. *Foreign bodies* must be diagnosed and removed.

Acute epiglottitis

This is a potentially lethal condition which may cause death by respiratory obstruction. Although it can occur at any age, severe problems are most commonly seen when children are affected. The history is usually a short one in a previously healthy child. There is evidence of upper respiratory tract infection with pyrexia and the development of stridor. Within hours the child may be cyanosed, dyspnoeic, exhausted with the effort of breathing and on the point of collapse.

Such cases need to be managed by experts if tragic accidents are to be avoided. Attempts to inspect the throat and examine the child should be restricted to one quick look with the laryngoscope. Otherwise complete res-piratory obstruction can be precipitated. One glance of an oedematous inflamed epiglottis is sufficient to make the diagnosis. The following steps are then recommended:
(1) Administration of high concentration of oxygen.
(2) Administration of atropine intramuscularly.

(3) Preparation of theatre for tracheal intubation or tracheostomy. An experienced anaesthetist and ENT surgeon should be available.

(4) Transport to theatre under continuous medical supervision.

(5) Cautious induction of general anaesthesia with adequate assistance and the back-up of the whole theatre team. This should be carried out in the theatre on the operating table with an ENT surgeon standing by prepared to carry out emergency tracheostomy.

(6) Nasotracheal intubation with a suitable plastic tube.

(7) Careful fixation of such a tube. Under no circumstances must it be accidentally removed. The hands must be restrained and proper sedation given. Intravenous increments of dilute solutions of Thalamonal (droperidol and fentanyl) have been used by the authors with success.

(8) Postoperative care in an intensive therapy unit with continuous observation. An intravenous drip should be used to supply necessary fluids.

(9) Therapy is continued with ampicillin and hydrocortisone.

It is essential to keep the tube in place for 24 to 36 hours while the inflammation subsides. The child should be nursed in an oxygen tent with humidification and careful tracheal suction as required. Laryngoscopies and tracheal tubes should be immediately available for emergency use.

It is the authors experience that the tube can be removed after this period of time and that conventional nursing is all that is then required. It has been pointed out (Rapkin, 1973) that occasionally the inflammatory condition extends to involve the larynx so that tracheostomy is required. Others have suggested that tracheostomy is the safest form of first line treatment and this is certainly so if the facilities of a modern intensive therapy unit are not available.

Asthma

The asthmatic child may be managed in a manner similar to the adult (see Chapter 8). The indications for intensive care arise in the rare case where the condition is deteriorating or the child is becoming exhausted. Medical treatment may then be supplemented by tracheal intubation and IPPV.

TRACHEAL INTUBATION

Orotracheal. This route is preferred by many, especially in the neonate. Preoxygenation should always be carried out. Awake intubation is recommended for the neonate and for the exhausted older child. Otherwise general anaesthesia may be indicated. Secure fixation of the tube is essential to prevent dislodgement and it is preferable to attach tape to the relatively stable upper lip rather than to the mobile lower lip.

The *size* of tube required cannot be predicted accurately and the wise operator prepares a range of tubes. The tube finally chosen should not be tight in the childs larynx, and if there is doubt a smaller tube should be substituted. Various guides have been suggested for choice of tube size. The formula

$\dfrac{\text{age in years}}{4}$ + 4.5 has been recommended. Keep and Manford (1974) suggest choice according to Table 20.2.

Table 20.2 Size of tube (Keep and Manford, 1974).

Age	Weight	Size of tube (mm int diam)
neonate	<1 kg	2.5
neonate	1–2 kg	3.0
neonate	>2 kg	3.5
6–18 months	6–11 kg	4.0
9 months–2 years	8–13 kg	4.5
2–4 years	11–17 kg	5.0
3–6 years	15–22 kg	5.5
4–7 years	18–25 kg	6.0
6–9 years	20–30 kg	6.5
8–11 years	25–40 kg	7.0
10–14 years	31–50 kg	7.5
13–15 years	43–62 kg	8.0

Laryngoscope blades recommended include the Macintosh in older children and the Robertshaw or Shrivastiva in infants (Shrivastiva, 1965).

Nasotracheal. The advantage of the nasotracheal tube is that it is easier to fix securely than the oral tube. It may also be more comfortable for the child. The diameter recommended is 0.5 mm internal diameter less than for oral tubes. In Table 20.3 recommendations have been made for length.

Table 20.3 Length of tube

Age	Length in cm
3 months	11.8
4–7 months	12.6
8–11 months	13.6
1 year	14.5
2 years	15.2
3 years	15.6
4 years	16.5
5 years	16.8
6 years	17.1
7 years	17.8
8 years	18.3
9 years	18.8
10 and 11 years	19.1

Nasal intubation is best performed in children under direct laryngoscopic vision, perhaps preceded by orotracheal intubation to secure the airway. It is important to check after final fixation that the tube is in correct position and that the tip has not passed into a main bronchus. The lung fields should be auscultated to make sure there is air entry on both sides of the chest.

Fixation can be accomplished by use of a head harness. The Jackson Rees tube, deservedly popular, can be securely held beneath a head bandage. For further recommendations on tube fixation, see Jones and Owen Thomas (1971); Thomas *et al.* (1965); Rees and Owen Thomas (1966); Reid and Tunstall (1966); Inkster (1973).

IPPV in the infant and child

Paediatric ventilators are designed for the particular needs of small subjects. They must be able to supply small tidal volumes and rapid respiratory rates as compared to the adult. Apparatus which has been recommended include the Loosco, Sheffield, Penlon and Newcastle, and the subject has been reviewed by Inkster (1973 and 1976). Warm humidified gases must be supplied, and the inspired oxygen concentration should be accurately controlled. Nebulisers should not be used for humidifcation since over-hydration can result.

Detailed discussion of IPPV in paediatric practice is beyond the scope of this book. The reader is referred to the excellent reviews in the literature: (Jones and Owen-Thomas, 1971; Inkster, 1976). There is some evidence that a prolongation of peak inspiratory pressure improves the efficiency of ventilation (Reynolds and Taghizadeh, 1974). PEEP is indicated especially in conditions where loss of surfactant is found. This is the case in respiratory distress of the newborn (Vidyasagar and Chernik, 1971; Cumarasamy *et al.*, 1973). It is also used following open heart surgery (Hatch *et al.*, 1973). PEEP is not without disadvantages, however. Over-inflation of the lungs and even pneumothorax can occur and may be a particular hazard in the presence of fibrocystic disease. If cardiac output is reduced the net oxygen available to the tissues may be reduced even when PaO_2 has risen. The method of producing PEEP may also have a bearing on the overall effect (Kolft *et al.*, 1972). A simple resistance can be hazardous since its operation varies with respiratory volume and rate as well as with lung compliance; a spring-loaded check valve has advantages.

Oxygen therapy

Infants and small children tolerate oxygen masks and catheters badly. It is difficult to keep them in position and to maintain a good fit, while provision must be made for a safety blow off in case unduly high pressures develop. The head box may be used for infants up to 3 months and can achieve a high FlO_2. Oxygen tents are widely used but have disadvantages. The oxygen concentration within them rarely exceeds 40% and they form a barrier to communication with the patient.

The danger of retrolental fibroplasia is real in the neonate. PaO_2 must be kept below 33 kPa (Baum and Bulpitt, 1970). The problem is, however, remote in the presence of severe lung pathology when it is difficult to achieve a high

PaO$_2$ even when F1O$_2$ is high. The danger then is one of direct oxygen toxicity in the lung (Stern, 1973; Shanklin and Wolfson, 1967; Brewis, 1969).

REFERENCES

Avery, M. E. and Mead, J. (1959), Surface properties in relation to atelectasis and hyaline membrane disease. *Am. J. Dis. Child*, 97, 517.

Baum, J. D. and Bulpitt, C. J. (1970), Retinal vasoconstriction in premature infants with increased arterial oxygen tensions. *Arch. Dis. Child.*, 45, 350.

Brewis, R. A. L. (1969), Oxygen toxicity during artificial ventilation. *Thorax*, 24, 656.

Cumarasamy, N., Nussli, R., Vischer, D., Dangel, P. H. and Duc, G. V. (1973), Artificial ventilation in hyaline membrane disease = the use of positive end-expiratory pressure and continuous positive airway pressure. *Pediatrics*, 51, 629.

Gregory, G. A., Kitterman, J. A., Phibbs, R. H., Tooley, W. H. and Hamilton, W. K. (1971), Treatment of the idiopathic respiratory distress syndrome with continuous positive airway pressure. *N. E. J. Med.*, 284, 1333.

Hatch, D. J., Cogswell, J. J., Taylor, B. N., Battersby, E. F., Glover, W. J. and Kerr, A. A. (1973), Continuous positive airway pressure after open heart operations in infancy. *Lancet*, ii, 469.

Inkster, J. S. (1966), A monitoring probe for use in paediatric anaesthesia. *Anaesthesia*, 21, 111.

Inkster, J. S. (1973), Respiratory assistance for neonates and infants. *Anaesthesia*, 28, 653.

Inkster, J. S. (1976), Paediatric Anaesthesia and Intensive Care. In *Recent Advances in Anaesthesia and Analgesia—12* eds. Hewer, C. L. and Atkinson, R. S., Churchill-Livingstone, Edinburgh, London and New York.

Jones, R. S. and Owen-Thomas, J. B. (1971), *Care of the Critically Ill Child.* Arnold, London.

Keep, P. J. and Manford, M. L. M. (1974), Endotracheal tube sizes for children. *Anaesthesia*, 29, 181.

Kolft, J., Webb, J. A. and Loop, F. D. (1972), Electrical analogues of methods for continuous positive pressure ventilation. *J. Thorac. Cardiovasc. Surg.*, 64, 586.

Mollison, P. L., Veall, N. and Cutbush, M. (1950), Red cell and plasma volume in newborn infants. *Arch. Dis.*, 25, 242.

Rapkin, R. H. (1973), Tracheostomy in epiglottis. *Paediatrics*, 52, 426.

Rees, G. J. and Owen-Thomas, J. B. (1966), A technique of pulmonary ventilation with a nasotracheal tube. *Brit. J. Anaesth.*, 38, 901.

Reid, D. H. S. and Tunstall, M. E. (1966), The respiratory distress syndrome of the newborn. *Anaesthesia*, 21, 72.

Reynolds, E. O. R. and Taghizadeh, A. (1974), Improved prognosis of infants mechanically ventilated for hyaline membrane disease. *Arch. Dis. Child*, 49, 505.

Shanklin, D. R. and Wolfson, S. L. (1967), Therapeutic oxygen as a possible cause of pulmonary haemorrhage in premature infants. *N. E. J. Med.*, 27, 833.

Shrivastiva, R. K. (1965), A laryngoscope for infants and the newborn. *Anaesthesia*, 18, 532.

Stern, L. (1973), Therapy of the respiratory distress syndrome. *Ped. Clin. N. Am.*, 19, 221.

Thomas, D. V., Fletcher, G., Sunshine, P., Schafer, I. A. and Klaus, M. H. (1965), Prolonged respiratory use in pulmonary insufficiency of the newborn. *J. Am. med. Ass.*, 193, 183.

Vidyasagar, D. and Chernik, V. (1971), Continuous positive transpulmonary pressure in hyaline membrane disease. A simple device. *Pediatrics*, 48, 296.

TWENTY-ONE

Acute pancreatitis

Acute pancreatitis carries a mortality between 9-35% and if this figure is to be reduced a multi-disciplinary approach must be adopted. The condition justifies a special chapter because of its high mortality, and difficult and often controversial, management.

Aetiology
Acute pancreatitis is most often associated with gall bladder disease. Other associations are with alcoholism, hypercalcaemia (primary hyperparathyroidism), lipid abnormalities, virus infections and scorpion stings. However in many cases no predisposing cause is found. Drugs, including frusemide, thiazide diuretics, steroids and oral contraceptives have also been implicated in its aetiology.

Clinical features
Severe epigastric pain with radiation to the back is the cardinal symptom. The pain may be sudden in onset and mimic a perforated peptic ulcer. Nausea and vomiting occur invariably. In fulminating cases profound shock may develop rapidly. The patient is often restless, in contradistinction to the patient with perforated peptic ulcer, who tends to lie still. If retroperitoneal haemorrhage occurs a haemorrhagic discoloration may develop in the flanks, or at the umbilicus.

Diagnosis
The diagnosis of acute pancreatitis depends upon finding a raised serum amylase. The increase is often considerable, and a six-fold rise over normal invariably indicates acute pancreatitis. The serum amylase is also elevated, though to a lesser extent, in gall bladder disease, perforated duodenal ulcer, ruptured ectopic pregnancy, leaking abdominal aortic aneurysms and intestinal obstruction. The severity of the illness is not related to the level of the serum amylase. However it has recently been suggested that a truer indication of the severity of the condition may be derived from an estimation of the amylase: creatinine clearance ratio.

The calculation is made after estimating amylase and creatinine in a specimen of urine and blood using the following formula:

$$\frac{\text{urine amylase}}{\text{serum amylase}} \times \frac{\text{serum creatinine}}{\text{urine creatinine}} \times 100$$

A normal value is less than 3%. In most cases of acute pancreatitis the mean value is around 6% (Murray and Mackay, 1977). The serum calcium may be low, and the methaemalbumin raised. Serum lipase levels are also elevated.

Clinical course

Mild cases are often unrecognized and require no specific treatment. However, often the condition is fulminant and characterized by prolonged ileus, severe hypocalcaemia, hypomagnesaemia, disorders of carbohydrate tolerance, coagulation disturbances, a great susceptibility to gram negative infection, with septicaemia, circulatory collapse with profound shock leading to renal failure, hepatic failure and respiratory failure.

Later in the course of the disease pancreatic abscesses and pseudo-cysts may develop with a grave risk of haemorrhage.

Mortality increases with age.

TREATMENT OF ACUTE PANCREATITIS

General measures

(1) Fluid and electrolyte management

The patient will be hypovolaemic and shocked. Intravenous fluid and volume replacement must be commenced immediately. Naso-gastric suction is usually advised. Expansion of the extracellular fluid volume is best achieved under control of a central venous pressure line, aiming to maintain the CVP at 5–10 cm of water. The plasma volume may be depleted by 30–40%.

The nature of fluid and volume replacement will depend on the electrolytes and Hb. Solutions containing dextrose should be avoided as hyperglycaemia occurs early. Whole blood, plasma, or plasma substitutes can be given depending on the Hb. Metabolic acidosis may require small doses of bicarbonate.

(2) Analgesics

Caution applies to the use of analgesics, as some agents cause a rise in intraductal pressure. Pethidine should be used in the lowest dose that controls symptoms.

(3) Antispasmodics

Although it is traditional, to use an anticholinergic agent such as probanthin there is little evidence to support this regime. Use of anticholinergics may prolong ileus, or cause tachycardia and urinary retention.

(4) Calcium

Hypocalcaemia is a frequent sequel to acute pancreatitis. i.v. calcium gluconate

1 g in 8 hours should be given with frequent monitoring of the serum calcium level. The serum magnesium levels should also be checked daily and replacement therapy given if necessary.

(5) Insulin

Blood sugar levels must be monitored and soluble insulin given to keep levels below 11.0 mmol/l. It has been suggested that an insulin infusion (10 units/h— see Chapter 14) is the best way to achieve this.

(6) Antibiotics

Antibiotic therapy should be reserved for the treatment of infection, and not given in an attempt at prophylaxis. Gram-negative septicaemia is a frequent complication of pancreatitis, and probably this is associated with the indiscriminate use of broad-spectrum antibiotics prophylactically.

(7) Parenteral nutrition

If the ileus is prolonged parenteral nutrition will be necessary; hypercatabolism is a feature of acute pancreatitis in all but the mildest cases (see Chapter 15).

Specific therapy

This is the controversial aspect of the therapy of acute pancreatitis. Many authorities would insist that the general measures outlined above, with special attention to the early diagnosis and management of complications (see below), constitute the therapy for this condition.

(1) Trasylol

Aprotinin (Trasylol) is a broad spectrum protease inhibitor. Although available for several years doubt about its role in the management of acute pancreatitis remains. The results of recent trials suggest that pain is reduced but the evidence for reduction of mortality is less convincing (Trapnell *et al.*, 1974; *Lancet*, 1977).

The dose is 200 000 units stat. followed by 200 000 units 6 hourly by intravenous infusion for 5 days.

(2) Glucagon

The rationale for the use of glucagon in acute pancreatitis is in the substance's pharmacological actions, the principal ones being as follows:

(1) possible inhibition of flow of pancreatic juice
(2) relaxation of duodenal musculature
(3) increased blood flow in coeliac axis
(4) increase in cardiac contraction (Leader, *Brit. med. J.*, 1973).

Studies have shown a rapid decrease in pain and a rapid fall in serum amylase (Conden *et al.*, 1973). However, as has been described above, the serum amylase does not give a clear indication of either the severity or progress of the disease.

The dose of glucagon is 1 mg i.v. as a stat. dose, followed by 1 mg infusion over 5 hours.

(3) Peritoneal lavage

Peritoneal lavage, either in the form of peritoneal dialysis, or with tubes inserted at laparotomy has been used in some centres (Rosato *et al.*, 1973).

(4) Glucose/insulin infusion

Recent work has suggested that a glucose and insulin infusion may have a part to play in the treatment (Hallberg and Theve, 1974). The dose adopted is 20 units of soluble insulin per litre of 5.5% glucose and 80 mmol sodium given by intravenous infusion: 300–400 ml in the first hour with a total of 2 litres over 24 hours.

(5) Surgery

The role of surgery in acute pancreatitis has not yet been clearly defined. Some cases will deteriorate despite the measures described above—and blood may have been demonstrated by peritoneal lavage, indicating a severe haemorrhagic pancreatitis. Under these circumstances a heroic decision to perform laparotomy may be made, but the decision as to the correct surgical procedure will be difficult (Herman-Taylor, 1977). If a necrotising haemorrhagic mass is present excision of the pancreas (leaving the head *in situ*) may be possible.

If biliary tract disease is found it might sometimes be feasible to restore patency of the common bile duct.

Laparotomy should be considered as an opportunity to institute peritoneal lavage.

Treatment of complications

The complications of acute pancreatitis may involve many other systems and their diagnosis and treatment is described in other chapters
(1) Diffuse intravascular coagulation
(2) Gram negative septicaemia
(3) Renal failure
(4) Respiratory failure—a syndrome of pleural effusions, falling P_aO_2 and increasing respiratory insufficiency, similar to 'shock lung' has been described (Ranson *et al.*, 1974).
(5) Hepatic failure.

Clinical monitoring

Progress of treatment should be assessed by monitoring the following parameters
(1) Amylase—for the first 3-4 days
(2) Calcium—this correlates well with progress
(3) Methaemalbumin
(4) Hb. PCV WCC
(5) Indicators of coagulation disturbances (see Chapter 18).

Table 21.1 Summary of treatment of acute pancreatitis

I	Fluid and volume replacement
II	Naso gastric suction
III	Analgesia
IV	Correction of biochemical disturbances
	Calcium
	Magnesium
	Glucose
	Acidosis
V	Careful watch for serious complications
	Infection
	Coagulation disturbances
	Renal failure
	Respiratory insufficiency
VI	? Trasylol ? Glucagon ? Insulin/glucose infusion
VII	Peritoneal lavage

REFERENCES

Condon, J. R., Knight, M. and Day, J. L. (1973), Glucagon Therapy in acute pancreatitis. *Brit. J. Surg.*, **60**, 509.

Glucagon Therapy in acute pancreatitis (1973), Leader, *Brit. med. J.*, 4, 503.

Hallberg, D. and Theve, N. O. (1974), Observations during treatment of acute pancreatitis with insulin and glucose infusion. *Acta Chirugica. Scand.*, **140**, 138.

Hermon-Taylor, J. (1977), An aetiological and therapeutic review of acute pancreatitis. *Brit. J. Hosp. Med.*, **18**, 546.

Medical Research Council Multicentre trial of glucagon and aprotinin (1977), *Lancet*, ii, 632.

Murray, W. R. and Mackay, T. (1977), The amylase creatinine clearance ratio in acute pancreatitis. *Brit. J. Surg.*, **64**, 189.

Ranson, J. H., Turner, J. W. and Roses, D. F. (1974), Respiratory complications in acute pancreatitis. *Am. Surg.*, **179**, 557.

Rosato, E. F., Mullis, W. F. and Rosato, F. E. (1973), Peritoneal lavage therapy in haemorrhagic pancreatitis. *Surgery*, **74**, 106.

Trapnell, J. E., Rigby, C. C., Talbot, C. H. and Duncan, E. H. (1974), Trasylol in the treatment of acute pancreatitis. *Brit. J. Surg.*, **61**, 177.

TWENTY-TWO

Psychiatric problems of intensive care

Patients admitted to an intensive care unit are exposed to an environment that is strange, far from their concept of hospital, frightening and at times hostile. Furthermore, they will be ill and subjected to powerful therapy, often with distressing side-effects. Many will be unable to communicate, though fully conscious. Strange machines will emit monotonous noises and terrifying patterns will appear on oscilloscope screens. Under these circumstances, it is not surprising that specific alterations in behaviour have been described in intensive care units.

The staff of intensive care units are not immune from psychoreactive problems. Nurses working in such units are exposed constantly to the physical and emotional trauma of death and the severely ill patient.

The *Intensive Care Syndrome* was recognized in the early 1950's with the emergence of routine open-heart surgery and coronary care units. It is a product of two factors—Organic and Psychological. The presenting symptom can best be described as a confusional psychosis; the term delirium is usually held to refer to organically determined factors. The organic brain syndrome is by implication not only organic in origin, but essentially temporary. It is the fluctuating nature of the disturbance which differentiates the syndrome from other brain syndromes. It cannot be over-emphasized however that all relevant metabolic and respiratory causes must be excluded before the specific confusional psychosis of the intensive care environment is diagnosed.

MANIFESTATIONS OF CONFUSIONAL PSYCHOSIS

The basic disturbance is a reduction in the level of awareness and defects in orientation, comprehension and memory.

(1) Anxiety with hyperventilation, tachycardia and sweating.

(2) Confusion. This may be gross and obvious or much more subtle. Many patients will have only patchy defects in memory and orientation and will, to the superficial observer, appear normal. These patients will often claim to feel well but may quickly become agitated if pressed too hard. It should not be difficult to identify these patients by careful and tactful questioning.

(3) Lethargy. These patients frequently complain of feeling tired, are withdrawn and retarded. Questioning will reveal defects of memory and orientation.

(4) Sensory elaborations. Either visual or auditory illusions may be encountered. They characteristically fluctuate and are often related to noises from machines in the unit.

(5) Muttering incoherence.

These clinical pictures may be casually related to the underlying disease, and any pre-existing syndrome of cerebral insufficiency that may have been marked before the onset of an acute metabolic insult will be aggravated in the presence of severe systemic illness.

It is evident that disturbed states of this nature can, of themselves, be extremely hazardous to the patient and interfere with his treatment. It is therefore essential that early recognition of confusional states is an important aspect of medical and nursing responsibility.

Organic factors

These are related to the underlying disease and will often be self-evident. They are potentially reversible. The importance of hypoxia in this respect must be emphasized, especially in elderly patients and in patients who are receiving sedative drugs. Thus, blood gas estimations become an important part of the investigation of the confused patient. It is always unwise to assume that an elderly patient who becomes confused is suffering from cerebro-vascular insufficiency, unless such complications as gram-negative septicaemia or electrolyte disturbances have been excluded.

REACTIONS SPECIFIC TO THE ENVIRONMENT

Exhaustion

Deprivation of sleep and sensory deprivation are known to cause psychotic complications. This characteristically appears after a 'Lucid interval' of 4–5 days. Often it will improve within 48 h of transfer to a normal hospital environment. It is usually manifested as acute delirium at night and paranoid delusions by day. Many patients have written accounts of their stay in the intensive care unit, and described day merging imperceptibly into night with no way of knowing the passage of time, prolonged periods without sleep because of pain, regular therapeutic manoeuvres such as intragastric feeding, tracheal toilet, physiotherapy, blood pressure recordings, constant light, and the noise of not only the staff and other patients, but also the incessant mechanical noise of ventilators and cardiac monitors, on which they know their life depends.

It is essential that measures are taken to prevent sensory and sleep deprivation.

(1) Sleep pattern should be maintained in the normal night–day ratio. Clinical observations and therapeutic manoeuvres should be kept to a minimum in the night, unless absolutely necessary. Remote telemetry of vital functions should be employed wherever possible.

(2) Wherever possible, patients should be nursed in individual rooms where the light can be dimmed at night.

(3) Orientation should be maintained by placing a large clock and calendar visible to each patient.

(4) A window with an outside view.

(5) Television, radio and newspapers should be available to each patient. (Contrary to the belief of the planners, all patients in an Intensive Care Unit are not unconscious or unable to move their limbs.)

(6) Even patients on ventilators can sit in a chair and take an interest in the outside world.

(7) Open visiting by close relatives.

With the use of such measures, it has been claimed that a significant reduction in the incidence of confusional psychosis can be achieved.

Communication

The problem of communication assumes special importance in the context of an intensive care unit, where many patients will be fully conscious and lucid, but unable to speak because of mechanical ventilation through a tracheostomy or tracheal tube. The situation is analogous to that of an aphasic patient following a cerebrovascular accident where there is a tendency, however unintentional, of regarding a patient who cannot answer questions or speak voluntarily as a simpleton or child, who is not deserving of intelligent conversation.

Many nurses rapidly become adept at lip reading. It cannot be over-emphasized how important it is to speak to patients on ventilators regularly and reassure them that their loss of vocalization is only temporary.

Some use may be made of magnetic letters, re-usable writing boards with chinagraph pencils, etc. Frequently, it will then be noted that the patient writes jargon, and this may, therefore, be the only way to appreciate that patients on ventilators are suffering from a confusional state.

The broader aspects of communication must be extended to include relatives, who, themselves, are often undergoing severe emotional stress. Indeed, it is considered that one of the most important aspects of intensive care work is to keep both the patients and relatives fully in the picture all the time. This should be done by the medical staff whenever possible.

Psychological factors

Patients in the alien and hostile environment of the intensive care unit are frightened. This may be environmental or inherent. It should not be forgotten that very large quantities of tranquillizing drugs are prescribed for anxiety states, and, inevitably, many patients in this category will find themselves in the intensive care environment for other reasons.

It is essential that full explanations of the functions of any machines in use are explained to the patient. Although, to the staff, these machines are benign parts of a mechanized environment, to the patient they are alarming and constantly remind him of the nature of his illness and his total dependence on others for survival.

The use of psychotropic drugs

The use of psychotropic drugs in the intensive care unit will frequently depend on the nature of the underlying illness. Many patients will be receiving several drugs simultaneously, and the problems of drug interactions and incompatibilities must always be considered.

(1) *Benzodiazepines.* These drugs, which can be given orally, intramuscularly, or intravenously, are relatively safe and free from serious side-effects. They are the treatment of choice for anxiety and sedation. They are not powerful hypnotics, but a larger dose given at night from a background of basal sedation will often help the patient to sleep.

Diazepam (Valium) 5–20 mg daily; 10 mg at night.

Chlodiazepoxide (Librium) 30–50 mg daily.

Diazepam can also be used by intramuscular or intravenous injection. The intramuscular route is particularly important when many patients are unable to take oral therapy. When used intravenously, respiratory depression and hypotension may occur.

Their use in the intensive care unit is essentially short term, but it must be pointed out that dependence can occur, and, after prolonged courses, withdrawal fits have been described.

Although generally free of serious side-effects, in common with all sedative drugs, care should be taken in patients with actual or potential respiratory difficulties, as even mild sedation may cause significant respiratory depression, and a patient with chronic obstructive airways disease pushed over the precipice of acute respiratory insufficiency.

(2) *Phenothiazines*—chlorpromazine (Largactil), promazine (Sparine). This group of drugs exhibit good sedative properties, but are liable to cause hypotension and tachycardia. Although used routinely and in high dosage by psychiatric units, their use in the intensive care unit is likely to prove unpopular with anaesthetists, and, in general, the benzodiazepines are more useful. Jaundice may be an early complication of chlorpromazine therapy, and this could further complicate an already confused situation in a seriously ill patient. However, they are valuable drugs, and, despite their disadvantages, may be used, in particular, for night sedation.

(3) *Night sedation.* It has already been emphasized that sleep deprivation is an important cause of the 'Intensive Care Syndrome'. Conflicting interests will often rule out powerful hypnotics in a patient who urgently requires sleep. The barbiturates are nearly always contra-indicated, and the drugs of choice are diazepam (Valium) 10–15 mg, chlordiazepoxide (Librium) 10–20 mg, or nitrazepam (Mogadon) 5–20 mg, or, if a phenothiazine is required, chlorpromazine 25–50 mg, or promazine 50–100 mg. A chloral preparation, e.g. Dichloralphenazone (Welldorm) 1250 mg is occasionally helpful, but the bitter

taste is not acceptable to many patients. This preparation cannot be used by intramuscular injection.

The benzodiazepines and phenothiazines can be given intramuscularly.

(4) *Barbiturates.* This group will depress respiration and increase confusion, especially in elderly patients. Some are cumulative, and excretion will be delayed in renal impairment or liver disease.

More satisfactory drugs are usually employed.

(5) *The tricyclic antidepressant drugs.* This group of drugs exert profound pharmacological effects, and their therapeutic effects are delayed for two or three weeks. They are particularly hazardous in patients with cardiovascular disease, and if pressor agents are likely to be used. They are unlikely to be of much use in the intensive care unit.

(6) *Paraldehyde* is an unpleasant drug, which is given by painful intramuscular injection. Although it is now customary to decry its use, there are occasions when it can be the only agent available to quieten a violently confused patient. The intramuscular dose is 10–20 ml by deep injection, and plastic syringes must not be used to administer it.

The effects of intensive care work on the staff

The medical and nursing staff cannot be excluded from a discussion on the psycho-reactive aspects of intensive care. It is essential that the nursing administrators are made aware of the special demands on the nursing staff. Work in a general ward is generally punctuated by periods of freedom from anxiety. The atmosphere of recovery from illness and repartee with recovering patients is largely absent. Exhaustion and confusion, therefore, will arise commonly. It is essential that adequate rest periods are allowed for. Night duty is a particularly stressful situation, when experienced medical supervision may be less readily available. Conflicts of loyalty may arise when the experienced nurse is confronted by an inexperienced medical officer.

The psychiatric patient in the intensive care unit

Patients with severe psychiatric disorders are no more immune to serious illness than the general population, and severe drug overdosage forms an important reason for admission, so such patients will inevitably be admitted to intensive care units.

Generally, the physicians and anaesthetist will be well advised to ask their psychiatric colleagues for advice on the management of severely disturbed patients. An intensive care unit is no place for noisy violent patients, whose behaviour may well have disastrous effects on other patients in the same unit.

The management of drug overdose is discussed in Chapter 16.

FURTHER READING

Hackett, T. P., Cassem, N. H. and Wishnie, H. (1968), The Coronary Care Unit. An appraisal of its psychologic hazards. *N. E. J. Med.*, **279**, 1365.

Kornfeld, D., Zimberg, S. and Malm, J. (1965), Psychiatric complications of open heart surgery. *N. E. J. Med.*, **273**, 287.

Kornfeld, D. (1969), Psychiatric view of the Intensive Therapy Unit. *Brit. med. J.*, **1**, 108.

Lazarus, H. and Hagens, J. (1968), Prevention of Psychosis following Open-Heart Surgery. *Am. J. Psychiatr.*, **124**, 1190.

Schroeder, H. (1969), Psycho-reactive problems of Intensive Therapy. *Anaesthesia*, **26**, 28.

Shovelton, D. S. (1979), Reflections on an intensive therapy unit. *Brit. med. J.*, **1**, 737.

Tomlin, P. (1977), Psychological problems in intensive care. *Brit. med. J.*, **2**, 441.

West, L., Janszen, H., Lester, B. and Cornelisoon, F. (1962), The Psychosis of sleep deprivation. *Ann. N. Y. Acad. Sci.*, **96**, 66.

TWENTY-THREE

Regional blocks

Patients admitted to an intensive care unit following trauma or surgical operation often require analgesia. In selected cases it may be appropriate to employ regional techniques which offer results superior to those obtained by administration of centrally acting drugs without the disadvantage of producing clouding of consciousness.

Regional blocks are, however, not without disadvantages:

(1) The pain may not be related to nerve pathways which can be blocked easily. The effects of trauma may be widespread so that the quality of pain relief obtained from a single nerve block is disappointing.

(2) The effect of local analgesic drugs is limited in duration so that injections may have to be repeated at frequent intervals. Sometimes this disadvantage can be overcome by the use of an indwelling catheter as in the extradural space.

(3) The very excellence of the quality of pain relief which can sometimes be obtained can make the patient intolerant and demanding when these techniques have to be discontinued.

(4) Presence of analgesia may mask important clinical symptoms and signs.

EXTRADURAL BLOCK

The extradural space lies outside the subarachnoid space in the vertebral canal. It is of narrow width, lying between the dura mater and periosteum lining the inside of the vertebral canal, being only a few millimetres thick, but it extends the whole length of the vertebral column from the foramen magnum to the sacro-coccygeal hiatus widening inferiorly to occupy the cavity of the sacrum. The segmental nerves all traverse this space and can be blocked by local analgesic solutions deposited within it. The space can be entered by a needle introduced between the vertebral spines, in the manner of a lumbar puncture, but stopping short before the dura is pierced. The operator can be trained to recognize the 'loss of resistance' which occurs as the needle point emerges from the ligamentum flavum. The space can also be entered in the thoracic region, but with a little more difficulty owing to the way the spines of the thoracic vertebrae overlap. It can also be entered by a needle which pierces the sacro-coccygeal membrane to enter the sacral canal. In each case, if a suitable needle is used, a catheter can be introduced and fixed in position to allow repeated injection of analgesic solutions. Details of the technical management of

354

extradural block can be found in other texts (Atkinson, 1976; Moir, 1976; Lee and Atkinson, 1978; Bromage, 1979).

Extradural block requires careful management and supervision. The strength of analgesic solution and the volume injected should be chosen with care.

Experience will indicate the number of segments which require to be blocked to produce the desired analgesia, but block of motor nerves is undesirable and this is best avoided by the use of dilute solutions.

Bupivacaine is the most popular local analgesic agent for pain relief other than during operative surgery because of its relatively long duration of action. It may be used in a concentration of 0.25 or 0.375% in an effort to avoid the motor block associated with more concentrated solutions. It is not necessary to add adrenaline. Autonomic fibres will also be blocked by the local analgesic drug and if this occurs over a wide region, arterial blood pressure may fall. It is therefore always necessary to monitor arterial pressure closely in the half hour following injection.

An extradural catheter inserted in the thoracic region has for some time been well recognized as a method of postoperative pain relief after upper abdominal surgery (Simpson *et al.*, 1961). A relatively small volume of local analgesic solution will afford good pain relief without causing a fall in arterial pressure (7-10 ml). A similar technique is now widely used for pain relief in obstetrics, though the catheter is then usually inserted in the lumbar region.

Extradural analgesia may be appropriate in the intensive care unit for the management of postoperative pain in the patient with poor respiratory reserve.

The excellent pain relief obtained allows physiotherapy and prevents sputum retention. There is evidence that it is much more valuable in this respect than opiates (Spence and Smith, 1971). Respiration has a more normal character than when pain is associated with spasm of abdominal and intercostal muscles and the fall in functional residual capacity which normally follows abdominal surgery can be reversed leading to improved oxygenation of the blood leaving the lungs. This is particularly important in the elderly when the closing volume may be increased so that ventilation-perfusion inequalities occur.

Extradural analgesia is also useful in the management of pain following traumatic injuries to the thoracic cage and thus preventing the ill effects on respiratory function which result from pain. Careful selection of cases is, however, required. Extradural analgesia should not be carried out in the shocked patient until blood volume has been restored or hypotension may result from autonomic blockade. The clinical situation should be reasonably stable so that the diagnosis of complications is unlikely to be masked.

Extradural analgesia is contraindicated in the presence of a bleeding diathesis or when anticoagulant therapy is employed because of the risk of extradural haematoma causing cord compression. It is also to be avoided in the presence of septicaemia as infection may become established in an extradural haematoma with abscess formation.

INTERCOSTAL BLOCK

The intercostal nerves can be blocked as they pass around the chest wall beneath the inferior border of the rib. A few ml of local analgesic solution produce effective results which may last for some hours if a long acting agent such as bupivacaine 0.25 or 0.5% is used. The block is not without danger, however, as it is possible to insert a needle too far between the ribs to produce a pneumothorax. Air enters the pleural cavity either through the lumen of the needle itself, but, more dangerously, by causing a tear of the pleura covering the lung itself. Bilateral pneumothorax is a real risk if bilateral intercostal blocks are carried out and the operator must take great care both during the procedure and in observing the patient afterwards.

Intercostal block can be carried out for the relief of postoperative pain following abdominal surgery and it may also afford analgesia after rib fracture.

Intercostal block has its best effect in the patient with diminished respiratory function and minimal trauma to the thoracic cage. It can give a period of respite to the patient whose sleep is interrupted by pain or who has difficulty in expectoration. It is often, however, disappointing, because the trauma is widespread and haematoma extends outside the region supplied by the intercostal nerves blocked.

OTHER REGIONAL BLOCKS

The indications for these are few in intensive care practice, but occasionally pain relief is of great benefit to the patient. Procedures such as sciatic nerve block are easier to carry out than is generally realized and afford relief to patients with painful leg conditions. The technique of Bryce-Smith is recommended as being simple and effective (Bryce-Smith, 1966). Block of the nerves supplying the hip joint have recently been recommended for painful conditions of that joint (James and Little, 1976), while femoral nerve block is useful in the patient with fractured femur (Berry, 1977).

Tracheal intubation

Passage of a tracheal tube in the conscious patient is often indicated. Topical analgesia aids insertion and toleration of the tube. It often suffices to spray the patients pharynx and larynx with 4% lignocaine, or 2 ml can be injected directly into the trachea below the cords, by piercing the cricothyroid ligament.

Lignocaine has, however, potential toxic effects. It should be remembered that it is rapidly absorbed from the respiratory tract and the dose used should not exceed 3 mg/kg with a maximum of 200 mg. The toxic effects as a result of overdose include cardiac depression and convulsions, either of which may be catastrophic in the patient who needs intensive care.

REFERENCES

Átkinson, R. S. (1976), in Practical Regional Analgesia. eds Lee J. A. and Bryce-Smith, R., *Excerpta Medica*, Amsterdam, Oxford, New York.

Berry, F. R. (1977), Analgesia in patients with fractured shaft of femur. *Anaesthesia*, **32**, 576.

Bromage, P. R. (1979), *Epidural Analgesia*, Saunders, Philadelphia.

Bryce-Smith, R. (1966), Local and regional analgesia. *Postgrad. med. J.*, **42**, 367.

Janes, C. D. T. and Little, T. F. (1976), Regional hip blockade. *Anaesthesia*, **31**, 1060.

Lee, J. A. and Atkinson, R. S. (1978), *Sir Robert Macintosh's Lumbar Puncture and Spinal Analgesia—Intradural and Extradural.* Churchill Livingstone, Edinburgh.

Moir, D. D. (1976), *Obstetric Anaesthesia and Analgesia.* Bailliere Tindall, London.

Simpson, B. R., Parkhouse, J., Marshall, R. and Lambrechts, W. (1961), Extradural analgesia and the prevention of postoperative respiratory complications. *Brit. J. Anaesth.*, **33**, 628.

Spence, A. A. and Smith, G. (1971), Postoperative analgesia and lung function: a comparison of morphine with extradural block. *Brit. J. Anaesth.*, **43**, 144.

TWENTY-FOUR

Intravenous techniques

PERIPHERAL INTRAVENOUS LINES

Patients in intensive care units have often been the subject of several intravenous infusions and suitable peripheral veins are not always easy to find. A few minutes spent in careful examination, in association with mechanical stimulation to promote venous dilatation when appropriate, are invaluable in these circumstances. The chosen vein should be in a suitable site for cannulation, fixation and patient comfort. A vein in the arm is preferred. Veins in the leg should be used only as a last resort due to the harmful results of immobilization with risk of thrombophlebitis and embolism. Occasionally a central vein is the only one available.

A quick, clean skin puncture through a weal of local analgesic solution is followed by advancement into the vein, using a no-touch technique apart from the hub of the cannula. The infusion line is connected and the whole securely fixed.

The characteristics of the ideal cannula have been investigated (Bell and Farman, 1972), but there is no single commercial type which excells and the choice is often a personal one, the paramount factor being the confidence of the operator in his ability to enter difficult veins.

Thrombophlebitis, as a complication of intravenous infusion, is low when the drip runs for 24 hours or less (Carter, 1951) and it may be advisable to change the set itself daily. It is less when larger veins are used. Injection of drugs increases the incidence (Briscoe and Taylor, 1974) while addition of small doses of hydrocortisone (Jones, 1967) or heparin (Alford et al., 1972) diminish it.

Fibrin deposits occur along the wall of any plastic catheter lying in a vein. Metal needles and cannulae are less prone to this development. Fibrin deposition usually begins at the site of entry to the vein and then spreads centrally (Indar, 1959; Hoshal and Hoskins, 1971).

CENTRAL VENOUS LINES

These are required either for monitoring of central venous pressure (see Chapter 10) or for intravenous nutrition (Chapter 15). Occasionally it is the only route for intravenous fluids and electrolytes, but there are grave complications which can occur and a central route should never be undertaken unless the advantages to be gained justify such a choice.

The tip of the catheter should lie in the superior vena cava and access can be obtained by threading a catheter from a number of veins. Whatever route is chosen full aseptic precautions are necessary and the operator should scrub up and wear gown, gloves and mask. A percutaneous method is usually used today.

Arm veins

The catheter can be introduced via the median cubital or basilic vein and threaded up. The cephalic vein is not recommended because it dips in front of the shoulder to join the axillary vein and the catheter is often held up at this point and cannot be advanced into the larger vein. A long catheter is needed (60-70 cm) and it is by no means certain that the tip will end up in the required position. Radiological studies (Langston, 1971; Malatinsky et al., 1976) suggest that as many as 40% are incorrectly located and catheters may pass into neck veins.

Jugular veins

The external jugular vein, though more accessible than the internal, is less favoured as it is difficult to advance a catheter through it into the large intra-thoracic veins. The *internal jugular vein* (English et al., 1969; Defalque, 1974) is preferred and the right vein is used more often than the left because it is in more direct line with the superior vena cava. The patient should be placed in Tren-delenburg position, 20-30° head-down tilt, so that the pressure in the vein is increased and the hazard of air embolism diminished. The head is turned to the opposite side and an effort made to palpate the vein as it lies slightly lateral to a line joining the medial edge of the clavicular head of the sternomastoid muscle to the mastoid process. This is easier when the patients muscles are relaxed as during general anaesthesia. The needle is inserted from above at an angle of 30 to 40° to the skin and advanced caudally and laterally to enter the vein.

Another method is to identify the triangular space between the sternal and clavicular heads of the sternomastoid muscle. The needle is inserted at the apex of this triangle and advanced caudally and laterally at an angle of 30 to 40° to the skin, towards the inner border of the anterior end of the first rib to enter the internal jugular vein. This technique is preferred in emergency situations such as cardiac arrest or severe shock, in infants and whenever it is required in the conscious patient.

The internal jugular vein is appropriate to many situations, but particularly to the postoperative patients as the line can be set up in the operating theatre while the patient is anaesthetized. It is not satisfactory for patients with a tracheostomy or who are likely to require one, because of the proximity of the potentially infected wound.

Subclavian vein

This site of entry has advantages in that the patient has the arms free and the neck is avoided. The patient should be placed in the head-down position to fill the vein and reduce the danger of air embolism. The arms are adducted and the head turned to the opposite side.

The *infraclavicular route* is most commonly used. The needle is inserted 10 mm below the mid-point of the clavicle and advanced beneath it towards the sternal notch to enter the vein as it crosses the first rib.

The *supraclavicular route* (Yoffa, 1965) is more accessible to the anaesthetist in the operating theatre but has few real advantages. The needle is inserted at the tip of the angle between the medial margin of the sternomastoid and the upper border of the clavicle and advanced at 45° to the horizontal and sagittal planes and 15° forward of the coronal plane to enter the vein at a depth of about 1 to 1.5 cm (Thornton and Levy, 1974).

The subclavian route carries the serious hazard of pneumothorax. Repeated or deep thrusts in search of the vein are to be avoided and failure on one side should not be followed by attempts on the other because of the danger of bilateral pneumothorax. The experienced operator will advance the cannula only when the patient is apnoeic. Chest X-ray should be undertaken whether or not a successful line is set up.

Central venous catheters

These may be manufactured using polyethylene or polypropylene, materials which favour fibrin deposition. Tetrafluoroethylene (Teflon TFE) and Teflon FEP, a copolymer of hexfluoropropylene and tetrafluoroethylene are better from this point of view and the latter is widely used in the construction of cannulae, but the material is rather stiff for use in long catheters as difficulties arise during advancement and there is a tendency to kink (Farman, 1978).

Catheters may be advanced through a cannula or over a needle. Those which are passed inside a needle are subject to the danger of shearing of the catheter. The majority of catheters now manufactured are now radio-opaque.

Fixation

Once in position the catheter must be securely fixed. This can be done most effectively by suture to the skin. Tunnelling under the skin has also been recommended to improve fixation and reduce infection risk (Powell-Tuck, 1978).

Nursing care

The percutaneous site should be dressed carefully and inspected daily. One per cent iodine ointment has been recommended to reduce the incidence of local infection (Csanky-Treels, 1978). Injection of drugs should not be made into a central line because of the danger of contamination when 3-way taps or injection ports are used. Another peripheral vein should be used. When central venous lines are removed the cannula should be inspected carefully and the tip sent for culture.

COMPLICATIONS

Complications of central venous cannulation can be life-threatening. The incidence can be reduced when the operator is experienced and due care taken.

(1) *Air embolism.* Air can gain entrance to the venous system during insertion and removal. For this reason the patient should be in head-down position to increase pressure in the veins. The hub should not be left open to atmosphere and the catheter should be connected to a prepared filled infusion set during advancement.

(2) *Catheter embolism* (Bennett, 1963). A catheter should never be withdrawn through a needle because of the danger of shearing off of the distal part, an occurrence which can have fatal consequences. The type of needle where this is possible should never be used by the tyro.

(3) *Pneumothorax.* Tension pneumothorax has been reported (Cook and Dueker, 1976).

(4) *Injury to intrathoracic structures* (Csanky-Treels, 1978). Perforation of a major vessel can lead to haematoma or haemothorax. Hydrothorax and pericardial effusion have been reported. Cardiac tamponade has proved fatal (Dane and King, 1975).

(5) *Incorrect positioning of catheter.* It is important to confirm the correct position of the catheter tip. If correctly placed, respiratory pressure oscillations will be transmitted to a central venous pressure monitor. X-ray of the chest should always be carried out to ascertain catheter position. The tip should lie about 2 cm below a line joining the lower surfaces of the medial ends of the clavicles on a posterioanterior chest X-ray (Csanky-Treels, 1978).

(6) *Infection.* This may arise by contamination from outside or by blood-borne infection. Scrupulous aseptic technique must be observed when the line is set up. A fibrin plug commonly forms on the tip of a central catheter. This is an ideal culture site for bacteria and may act as a source for dissemination of organisms as the plug fragments. Central lines should, therefore, be used only after careful consideration in patients with septicaemia. Infection can also be prevented by removing a central line as soon as its purpose is served. Although such lines have been kept in place successfully for long periods of time, consideration should be given to their removal after one week or whenever unexplained pyrexia develops.

REFERENCES

Alford, F. P., Baker, H. W. G., Culross, J. and Chamley, W. A. (1972), Simple continuous blood-sampling double-lumen catheter. *Lancet*, i, 20.

Bell, G. T. and Farman, J. V. (1972), Disposable venous cannulae. *Brit. J. Hosp. Med.*, Equipment Supplement, 8, 49.

Bennett, P. J. (1963), Use of intravenous plastic catheters. *Brit. med. J.*, 2, 1251.

Briscoe, C. E. and Taylor, R. A. (1974), Morbidity following intravenous injections. *Anaesthesia*, **29**, 290.

Carter, J. F. B. (1951), Reduction in thrombophlebitis by limiting duration of intravenous infusions. *Lancet*, **2**, 20.

Cook, T. L. and Dueker, C. W. (1976), Tension pneumothorax following internal jugular vein cannulation and general anaesthesia. *Anaesthesiology*, **45**, 554.

Csanky-Treels, J. C. (1978), Hazards of central venous pressure monitoring. *Anaesthesia*, **33**, 172.

Dane, T. E. B. and King, E. G. (1975), Fatal cardiac tamponade and other mechanical complications of central venous catheters. *Brit. J. Surg.*, **62**, 6.

Defalque, R. J. (1974), Percutaneous catheterisation of the internal jugular vein. *Anaesthesia and Analgesia, Current Researches*, **53**, 116.

English, I. C. W., Frew, R. M., Pigott, J. F. and Zaki, M. (1969), Percutaneous catheterisation of the internal jugular vein. *Anaesthesia*, **24**, 521.

Farman, J. V. (1978), Which central venous catheter? *Brit. J. clin. Equip.*, **3**, 210.

Hoshal, V. L., Ause, R. G. and Hoskins, P. A. (1971), Fibrin sleeve formation on indwelling central venous catheters. *Arch. Surg.*, **102**, 353.

Indar, R. (1959), The dangers of indwelling polythene cannulae in deep veins. *Lancet*, i, 284.

Jones, P. F. (1967), Intravenous infusion techniques. *Proc. Roy. Soc. Med.*, **60**, 72.

Langston, C. S. (1971), The aberrant central venous catheter and its complications. *Radiology*, **100**, 55.

Malatinsky, T. (1976), Misplacement and loop formation of central venous catheters. *Acta anaesth. scand.*, **20**, 237.

Powell-Tuck, J. (1978), Skin tunnel for central venous catheter: non-operative technique. *Brit. med. J.*, **1**, 625.

Thornton, J. A. and Levy, C. J. (1974), *Techniques of Anaesthesia*. Chapman and Hall, London.

Yoffa, D. (1965), Supraclavicular subclavian venepuncture and catheterisation. *Lancet*, ii, 614.

TWENTY-FIVE

The control and management of infection

Intensive care units have acquired a justified reputation for a high incidence of infection. It is no coincidence that the dramatic increase in septicaemia, often due to Gram-negative organisms, has coincided with the efforts of the pharmaceutical industry to produce more wide-spectrum antibiotic agents. Not only are patients in an ITU particularly vulnerable to infection because of the nature of serious underlying disease, but the wide-spread proliferation and abuse of antibiotics is exposing them to the risk of acquired infection with organisms that often show multiple resistance to antibiotic agents. No programme designed to eliminate infection in the ITU can be successful unless a rational antibiotic policy is in operation.

ORIGINS OF INFECTION

Organisms may be spread in three ways:
(1) Airborne dissemination.
(2) Personal contact—including autogenous infection.
(3) Environmental sources.

Airborne dissemination

The staphylococci are particularly incriminated in this mode of dispersal. The organism readily becomes airborne and disseminated in dust which lodges on bedding, etc. where infection occurs by direct contact. The staphylococci survive drying and may persist in dust on ledges, etc. for considerable periods of time. The origin of these organisms may be healthy carriers—up to 30% of people carry *Stapholococcus aureus* in their noses or perineal areas—and dispersal may follow bathing. As staphylococci cause one-third of wound infections ready dispersal can occur when dressings are changed. However, in practice, Gram-positive infection with organisms of the staphylococcal group, has been eclipsed in importance by the increase in Gram-negative infection which is unlikely to be spread by airborne dissemination.

Personal contact and autogenous infection

Both Gram-positive and Gram-negative organisms can be spread by personal contact—most often via the hands or uniforms of the nursing and medical staff. Generally, Gram-positive organisms survive drying well, but do not multiply in hospital environment. It should however be remembered that gram-negative organisms can also survive drying, though only in small numbers.

Autogenous infection is of great importance in consideration of infection in the ITU especially as the increase in serious gram-negative infection is largely due to faecal organisms. *Pseudomonas aeruginosa* is often incriminated as an example of an organism which infects the patient from his own gastro-intestinal tract, and there are several studies which show this; it should however also be noted that this organism can be spread by personal contact and by environmental sources (Shooter *et al.*, 1966; Shooter, 1971). Organisms of the *Klebsiella group* are a classic example of autogenous infection promoted by the indiscriminate use of broad-spectrum antibiotics (Price and Sleigh, 1970).

Environmental sources

The ITU, with its multitude of equipment, propensity for the insertion of tubes and catheters, often crowded situation with chronic staff shortages and population of severely ill patients, is the ideal situation for the spread of organisms from environmental sources.

Environmental sources of infection are numerous some of the most important ones are given in Table 25.1.

Table 25.1 Environmental sources of infection

Respiratory
  Ventilators
  Humidifiers
  Nebulisers
  Suction apparatus
  Tracheal catheters
  Air-conditioning units

Intravascular
  Intravenous catheters
  Infusion fluids

External
  'Antiseptic' solutions and lotions
  Local anaesthetic jelly
  Eye drops
  Thermometers
  Shaving brushes
  Taps, sinks, overflows
  Food, food mixers

Urinary tract
  Catheters
  Cystoscopes

It is evident from this list that almost any item of equipment, or any therapeutic or diagnostic procedure, may be incriminated as a potential source of infection. These factors have most often been associated with Gram-negative infection—

organisms of this group not only survive, but multiply in a damp environment. Some caution, however, should be exercised when assessing bacterial swabs from such items as sinks and overflows because there is some evidence to suggest that, for example, *Pseudomonas aeruginosa* may be found in these sites only *after* infection in the patient. Although there can be no argument as to the significance of infected infusion fluids and deep intravenous lines it would be unwise to attach too much importance to routine cultures of sinks and water-traps, as it may be that the organisms travel from the patient to the environment rather than in the opposite direction (Gaya, 1974).

THE PATIENTS AT RISK

It should be emphasized that the spectrum of infection seen in the ITU includes infection with organisms that are not generally pathogenic, and will also include infection with opportunistic organisms. The role of the abuse of antibiotics will be discussed below. The patients at high risk in the ITU are, in general, there with conditions listed in Table 25.2.

Table 25.2 Special risk patients–acquired infection

Treatment with steroids, cytotoxic drugs or immunosuppressive agents
Malignant disease
Infancy and old age
Severe debilitating disease; major surgery
Mechanical interference with respiratory tract, e.g.
  IPPV
  tracheostomy
  endotracheal intubation
Renal failure
Burns
Diabetes
Diseases associated with altered immunity
Surgery of the GU tract
Deep intravenous lines
Previous treatment with broad-spectrum antibiotics

When considering this group of patients we must consider the organisms which are likely to cause problems in the ITU. It is, as has been explained above, the Gram-negative organisms, notably *Pseudomonas aeruginosa* and *Klebsiella aerogenes* which are the cause of the dramatic increase in infection, especially septicaemia in recent years (Finland *et al.*, 1959; Editorial, *Brit. med. J.*, 1974). Other faecal organisms including *Eschericia coli* and *Proteus* species will often be cultured, especially where broad-spectrum antibiotics have been used. However when assessing reports of swab cultures, etc. it is important to recognize that culture of an organism from a bacterial specimen does not necessarily mean that significant infection is present. The organisms mentioned above have achieved such significant pathological importance in recent years because of the relative

resistance of Gram-negative organisms to antibiotics. Prescribing more antibiotics on the basis of bacteriological reports rather than clinical assessment of
the patient often compounds the error, which is the abuse of antibiotics, and
produces a risk of increasingly difficult and resistant infection in the future.
Relevant to this are increasingly frequent reports of clinical infections by
organisms of the Bacteroides group (Leigh, 1974).

Special mention must be made of a group of patients who have a special risk
of infection by organisms that are only rarely pathogens in man.

Opportunistic infections have been defined as: 'Infections developing as a
result of (a) the predisposing role of other diseases (particularly systemic disease
of the lympho-reticular system, leukaemias, chronic anaemias and metabolic
disorders); or (b) the use of therapeutic agents' (Wolstenholme and Porter, 1968).
Some of the agents that have caused infection in this group of patients who
include those treated with immunosuppressive or cytotoxic agents are listed in
Table 25.3.

*Table 25.3 Opportunistic infecting agents in susceptible
patients*

Viral infections	*Varicella*
	Herpes simplex
	Vaccinia (Smallpox vaccination)
	Measles
	Cytomegalic inclusion disease
Bacterial infections	*Listeria monocytogenes*
	Atypical mycobacteriae
Protozoa	*Toxoplasma gondii*
	Pneumocystis carinii
Fungus	*Nocardia asteroides*
	Aspergillosis
	Candidiasis
	Cryptococcosis
	Histoplasmosis
	Mucormycosis

Therefore when patients in this group of high-risk develop an infection no
reliance must be placed on routine bacteriology. It is essential that the bacteriologists are informed of the nature of the underlying disease, and the clinical
state so that a search can be made for unusual organisms. Infection in patients
with altered immunity, due either to disease or drug therapy, may be unusual,
therefore, in three ways (Gowing, 1970; Smith, 1973).

It would not be appropriate here to discuss in any depth the therapy of
these opportunistic infections. The drugs used are toxic and the reader is
referred to specialist literature as to their use. Table 25.4 gives an indication of
some of the drugs used under these circumstances.

Table 25.4   The therapy of 'opportunistic infections'

Nocardia asteroides	Sulphadiazine
Aspergillus neoformans	Amphotericin B
Cryptococcus neoformans	Amphotericin B
	5-fluoro-cytosine (Alcobon)
Mucormycosis	Amphotericin B
Candidiasis	5-fluoro-cytosine
Herpes	Cytosine arabinoside
Cytomegalovirus	Idoxuridine
Toxoplasma	Spiramycin
	Pyrimethamine
Pneumocystis carinii	Pentamidine isothianate
Listeria monocytogenes	Penicillin/erythromyicin
Atypical mycobacteriae	Depending on sensitivities to antituberculous drugs.

(1) There is an increased incidence of 'rare' infections
(2) Common infections may be unusually severe or widespread
(3) Certain infections may show a shift in age distribution, e.g. measles in adults.

CONTROL OF INFECTION

Cross-infection in the ITU

Cross-infection implies the transfer of an organism from one human source to another. We will also consider the control of infection from environmental factors.

General principles

It is evident that seriously ill patients in an ITU must be protected against exposure to organisms that might be carried in by casual visitors. In this respect it should be emphasised that medical staff are not immune to the carriage of pathogenic organisms on their persons or clothing. Nursing staff are generally well disciplined as to the risks of cross-infection, but other personnel such as ward-maids, cleaners, radiographers, physiotherapists and dietitians may not be aware of the rules of carrying infection from one patient to another. The risks of cross-infection are greatly increased if the unit is short of staff and nurses have to tend to several patients, often in quick succession; under these circumstances the routine rituals of hand-washing can easily be neglected. Likewise, overcrowding of the unit is potentially hazardous and the temptation to erect extra beds must be resisted.

Clothing. Visitors to the ward should all wear a gown, either cotton or plastic. Overshoes are unnecessary. Face masks are not needed unless the visitor has a respiratory tract infection (under these circumstances he should not be in the unit at all) or is known to be carrying pathogenic staphylococci in the nose.

Skin care. The hands must be washed before entry to the ward and between patients. Dispensers of antiseptic hand creams have frequently been indicted as the source of infections. The best method is washing of the hands with hexachlorophane 2% bar soap. If a serious problem of infection is present this can be supplemented by a rinse with 70% ethyl alcohol.

Medical or nursing staff known to be carrying staphylococci in their noses should be given neomycin/bacitracin ointment to the nose and encouraged to add 1 oz of 10% hexachlorophane liquid to their bathwater. However, routine bacteriological studies on staff is not necessary unless there is an epidemic of staphylococcal infection; or if staff are suffering from recurrent skin infections.

General disinfection. Where possible disposable items should be used and in the most hospitals dressings will be supplied in pre-packed sterilized packages. It must be recognized that no chemical method of sterilising objects is satisfactory, organisms can only be killed with certainty by heat or ionising radiation.

Hepatitis. The transmission of viral hepatitis is a particularly grave risk where haemodialysis is performed, and in units where liver disease is treated. If there is any suspicion of the presence of viral hepatitis the greatest caution must be used to prevent spillage of tissue fluids and accidental innoculation of medical or nursing staff. All pathological specimens should be taken into specially labelled containers and transported in sealed packets. Venepuncture, setting up of intravenous infusions and intramuscular injections demand caution both in the mechanics of the technique and in the disposal of needles etc. It should also be remembered that the virus can be transmitted by saliva.

ANTIBIOTIC POLICY

It is essential that the principles of the rational use of antibiotics are clearly understood and that an antibiotic policy is operational in the ITU. It is evident that septicaemia, especially with gram-negative organisms of faecal origin, is increasing (Editorial, *Brit. med. J.*, 1974) and that this increase is associated with the indiscriminate use of broad-spectrum antibiotics. An antibiotic policy must be based on the following principles:

(1) Antibiotics should be used for bacterial infection.

(2) The antibiotic used must be the appropriate agent for the pathogenic organism isolated, or *likely* to be isolated.

(3) The correct antibiotic must be given in adequate dosage.

Infection

Fever does not necessarily indicate infection. The tendency to treat febrile patients with antibiotics without any thought as to the cause of fever must be resisted. The decision to given an antibiotic must depend upon the probability of a bacterial infection. Acute viral illnesses are unlikely to cause the same problems in the ITU as occur in general practice. Fever is common after myocardial infarction, both immediately and 8–12 days later if the post infarction syndrome develops. The collagen diseases and malignant disease, especially the reticuloses and leukaemia are characterized by fever; in these patients the abuse of antibiotics, in the presence of a compromised immunological syndrome, may lead to an opportunistic infection with rare organisms.

The diagnosis of infection, however, may not be easy, and bacteriological reports may be misleading. The report of *E. coli* or pseudomonas in the sputum, for example, does not necessarily indicate that the patients fever is due to these organisms. Most often this type of organism in the sputum merely reflects the previous over-enthusiastic use of inappropriate antibiotics (Philp and Spencer, 1974). A positive bacteriological culture does not prove, always, that a given organism is the pathogen, nor does it even necessarily indicate that significant sepsis is present (Burns, 1973).

Bacteriological reports must be interpreted in conjunction with the clinical indication of sepsis. The decision as to the presence of significant sepsis is therefore initially clinical, and will be based on such considerations as fever and white cell count. In general, difficulty in the interpretation of bacteriological reports arises when Gram-negative organisms are isolated and it is under these circumstances that the further use of antibiotics is likely to compound the error and make the situation potentially more dangerous in terms of super-infection with opportunistic organisms. It is swabs from wounds or tracheostomies and sputum cultures that are liable to be particularly misleading.

The organism

The choice of the appropriate antibiotic will be straightforward if clinical infection is present and bacteriological results with organism sensitivities are available. However under many clinical situations no bacteriology is available, or time cannot be wasted waiting for results. This particularly applies to the problem of septicaemic shock (see Chapter 3). It is often possible to forecast the likely organism, or group of organisms, which will be the most frequent pathogens in different situations. Under these circumstances an appropriate antibiotic can be selected and any alteration made as soon as culture and sensitivity reports are available. If it is decided to prescribe a broad-spectrum combination of drugs, any inappropriate agent must be withdrawn when sensitivities are available. There is no virtue in prescribing a broad-spectrum antimicrobial agent when a more specific drug is available for the pathogenic organism.

Table 25.5 gives an indication of some associations between infecting organisms and clinical problems.

Routine bacteriological monitoring is generally a waste of time and money. Environmental sampling is of principal importance to the epidemiologist.

Table 25.5 Clinical associations with infective organisms

E. coli	Urinary tract surgery or instrumentation Bowel surgery Abdominal sepsis
Klebsiella/Enterobacter	Bowel surgery Abdominal surgery Previous treatment with broad-spectrum penicillin
Pseudomonas	Blood dyscrasias Steroid therapy
C. Welchii	Septic abortion Severe trauma
Staphylococcus *Streptococcus*	Skin sepsis Bone or soft tissue infection

However some routine monitoring is essential. In particular patients undergoing peritoneal dialysis should have the dialysate cultured daily; urine should be cultured twice weekly in all patients with an indwelling catheter; intravenous catheters, especially deep lines that have been *in situ* several days should be cultured on withdrawal; tracheal aspirates should be cultured routinely every third day for evidence of infection.

Chemoprophylaxis

In general, there are very few indications for the use of prophylactic antibiotics in the intensive therapy unit. As has been emphasized above the abuse of broad-spectrum antibiotics not only exposes the patient under treatment to the toxic side effects of the drug, but increases the risk of superinfection by organisms not normally pathogenic, and enhances the ever increasing risk of the development of resistance to antibiotics.

The principal indications for prophylactic antibiotics are:

(1) Prophylactic penicillin should be given to patients following amputation of a limb for peripheral vascular disease, where there is a serious risk of gas gangrene infection. This policy also applies to major trauma affecting the limbs, where damaged muscle is present and the original wound contaminated.

(2) Following open heart surgery, where a combination of antibiotics should be given to prevent endocarditis by the organisms usually responsible for this complication. The usual combination is penicillin, streptomycin and cloxacillin; this should be commenced at the time of surgery and continued for seven days.

Other situations where chemoprophylaxis is accepted are unlikely to occur in the ITU, but it should be remembered that the risk of bacterial endocarditis in a patient with valvular heart disease, who has been subjected to surgery, including dental work, can be obviated by the use of an appropriate antibiotic.

Penicillin will be effective where the organism is likely to be a streptococcus viridans, e.g. in dental surgery, but where surgery to the bowel or urinary tract is to be performed an antibiotic with a broader spectrum will be necessary, e.g. ampicillin or a cephalosporin.

There is no indication for the routine use of prophylactic antibiotics in unconscious patients. Such patients are susceptible to chest infections but antibiotics should be reserved until there is clinical or bacteriological evidence of infection, when the appropriate drug is prescribed *after* bacteriological reports, with sensitivities are available.

Choice of antibiotic

The choice of antibiotic will depend upon the clinical situation and bacteriological sensitivity reports, when available. The object of antibiotic therapy is to obtain effective concentration of the appropriate chemotherapeutic agent at the site of infection without causing toxicity and without exposing the patient to the risk of superinfection or developing resistance to antibiotics. The right antibiotic must therefore be administered by the right route at the correct dosage. There are no 'strong' antibiotics, only appropriate ones.

Combinations of antibiotics are not generally indicated in specific infections but occasionally may be necessary pending sensitivity reports where the infection dictates immediate therapy, and the nature of the organism or its sensitivities are unknown.

The penicillins

The penicillins, despite being in clinical use for 35 years, still remain an important antibiotic, and generally, are free of serious side effects. The development of synthetic penicillins in recent years has broadened their area of use and also exposed risks, especially in a hospital environment.

Benzyl penicillin (Penicillin G)

Indications. Benzyl penicillin is effective against a broad spectrum of Gram-positive organisms, notably streptococci, including the β-haemolytic streptococci, pneumococci and some strains of staph. aureus. It is also highly effective against meningococcii, *Treponema pallidum*, *Clostridium welchii* and *Anthrax*.

Administration and dosage. It is given either intramuscularly or intravenously, when it can be given by slow infusion. Of all the antibiotics it has the widest range of dosage, between 1–40 megaunits/24 h. The dose will depend upon the infection and often the bacteriologists will be able to help by assaying the MIC (mean inhibitory concentration) for the organism. Dosage can then be monitored by measuring serum levels. This is of particular importance in the treatment of endocarditis when high doses have to be given for prolonged periods.

It should be noted that the intrathecal dose of penicillin-G must never exceed 20 000 units.

Side effects. The most serious side effect of penicillin is hypersensitivity. This can produce immediate severe, life-threatening, anaphylactic shock, or a more subacute syndrome of fever, joint pain and skin rash. A history of penicillin sensitivity should always be enquired for before administration.

In high doses, especially in the presence of renal impairment, neurotoxic side effects (fits, myoclonus, coma) have been reported. Very rarely penicillin has caused acute renal toxicity.

Disadvantages. The principal disadvantage of benzyl penicillin is its inactivity against the many strains of *Staph. aureus* which produce penicillinase.

Penicillinase—stable penicillins (Methicillin, Cloxacillin, Flucloxacillin)

Indications. These antibiotics are indicated for use against penicillin resistant *Staph. aureus.*

Dosage and administration. See Table 25.6.

Table 25.6

Drug	Route	Dosage
Methicillin	i.m. : i.v.	1 g 6 hourly
Cloxacillin	oral i.m. i.v.	500 mg 6 hourly
(Orbenin)		8 g daily
Flucloxacillin	oral i.m. i.v.	250 mg 6 hourly
(Floxapen)		4 g daily

Side effects. Occasional skin rashes.

Disadvantages. These drugs must be used only for the treatment of severe clinical infection with penicillin-resistant staph. aureus. The principal disadvantage is the packaging of cloxacillin and flucloxacillin with ampicillin (Magnapen, Ampiclox), which often leads to the indiscriminate use of an important therapeutic agent in an inappropriate clinical situation.

Broad-spectrum penicillins (Ampicillin, Amoxycillin, Talampicillin)

Indications. The spectrum of this group of penicillins includes many gram-negative organisms including coliforms and *H. influenzae.* They are also effective against the Salmonellae.

Dosage and administration. Ampicillin can be given orally or by intravenous or intramuscular injection. The dosage range lies between 1–4 g daily (given 6 hourly). The newer drugs of this group (Amoxycillin, Talampicillin) are claimed to produce higher blood levels when given orally, and 8 hourly dosage is recommended.

Side effects. The principal side effect of ampicillin is skin rash which may be delayed.

Disadvantages. (1) Ampicillin is not effective against penicillinase-producing strains of *Staph. aureus.*
(2) It is not effective against *Klebsiella* and *Pseudomonas.*

Other penicillins

Carbenicillin (Pyopen)

This drug, which has to be given intravenously in dosage of 20–30 g daily, should be reserved for use against some strains of *Pseudomonas*, and ampicillin resistant *E. coli.* Resistance to *Ps. aeruginosa* may develop during treatment and it is generally recommended to use gentamicin with carbenicillin for severe pseudomonas infection. The drug is ineffective against *Klebsiella.*

Mecillinam (Selexid)

This synthetic penicillin derivative—an amidinopenicillin—is selectively active against a broad spectrum of gram-negative organisms. Its activity extends against *E. coli, Klebsiella* spp., *Salmonella* and *Shigella*, and also some strains of *Proteus*, particularly *Proteus mirabilis* and *P. vulgaris.*

The drug appears to have a synergistic activity with other antibiotics, notably ampicillin.

The dose is 200–400 mg 6–8 hourly by mouth. An intravenous preparation is also available—doses up to 3.6 g in 24 h have been used for severe gram-negative infections, often with ampicillin in anticipation of a synergistic effect.

Ticarcillin, Mezlocillin, Azlocillin, Broad spectrum semisynthetic penicillins

Antibiotics (given parenterally) important in the treatment in life threatening infection, having an enhanced spectrum of antibacterial activity, including some anaerobes (see page 35).

Tetracycline group

The many members of this group share similar properties, generally there is no advantage in any particular preparation.

Indications. Although they have a wide spectrum of activity, many resistant organisms have developed, probably due to indiscriminate use. Their action is bacteriostatic. They are inactive against pseudomonas and proteus. Particular indications for the use of tetracycline are

(1) *Mycoplasma* infection
(2) Rickettsiae infection
(3) *Bacteriodes* infection

Administration and dosage. Tetracyclines can be given orally or intramuscularly. Intravenous preparations are available but this route of administration may produce acute hepatic toxicity. However i.v. oxytetracycline has been used particularly in acute toxic dilatation of the colon in ulcerative colitis. The dosage of tetracycline is 250 mg 6 hourly by mouth; 100 mg 6 hourly i.m.

(Some proprietary preparations are designed for twice daily, or even once a day administration.)

Side effects. Gastro-intestinal upsets are common, occasionally severe when staphylococcal entero-colitis develops. An important danger is in patients with renal impairment, when it causes a rise in the blood urea. (Doxycycline, Vibramycin is claimed to be non-nephrotoxic.)

Cephalosporins

The main use is in patients with gram-positive infection who are hypersensitive to penicillins. They have a wide spectrum of activity but must be used with great caution in the presence of renal impairment.

Polymyxins

(1) Clindamycin and Lincomycin

Clindamycin (Dalacin C) is the orally effective modification of Lincomycin (Lincosin). Their use in severe septicaemic states is described in Chapter 3.

Indications. The spectrum of activity is narrow, against gram-positive organisms, *H. influenzae* and *Bacteroides*. Their use should be reserved for gram-positive infection; or, in combination with gentamicin, for broad antibiotic cover in septicaemic states of uncertain bacteriological aetiology, pending results of sensitivity tests from the laboratory. The drugs penetrate bone well and are excreted in bile and urine.

Dosage. Clindamycin—150–300 mg 6 hourly by mouth; Lincomycin—600 mg 12 hourly by intravenous infusion in 250 ml of 5% dextrose.

Side effects. A severe pseudomembranous colitis has been described as a complication of clindamycin therapy, it is less likely to occur with lincomycin. Less severe gastro-intestinal side-effects are quite common.*

(2) Fucidic acid (Fucidin)

Indications. Infection with *Staph. aureus*, particularly in bone infection. Resistance, however, is acquired quite rapidly.

---

* The severe colitis precipitated by clindamycin, lincomycin and occasionally other antibiotics is associated with *Clostridium difficile* infection, and this may be treated with vancomycin. The oral dose is 1–2 g daily in divided doses.

Administration and dosage. it is very active when given orally, but an intravenous preparation is available. It should *not* be given intramuscularly.
The oral dose is 500 mg 8 hourly.

(3) Naladixic acid (Negram)

Indications. This antibiotic is used only for urinary tract infection. It is active against coliforms, some strains of proteus and *Strep. faecalis*. Most strains of *Pseudomonas* are insensitive.

Administration and dosage. Oral use only 1 g 6 hourly.

Disadvantages. Acquired resistance develops rapidly. Severe, light sensitive, skin eruptions have been reported. Gastro-intestinal side effects are frequent.

(4) Nitrofurantoin (Furadantin)

Indications. Urinary tract infection with coliforms and *Strep. faecalis*, only. *Proteus* and *Pseudomonas* are insensitive.

Administration. Oral 100 mg 6 hourly.

Side effects. Gastro-intestinal upsets prevent many patients from tolerating this drug.
It must *never* be used in uraemia as not only is it ineffective, but a severe motor polyneuropathy may develop.

Erythromycin

Indications. The spectrum is similar to benzyl penicillin but includes many penicillin resistant strains of *Staph. aureus*. It is also effective against *H. influenzae*. It should be regarded as an useful agent for the treatment of Gram-positive infection in patients hypersensitive to penicillin. Resistance however develops rapidly.

Dosage. Intravenous or oral erythromycin—250 mg 6 hrly.

Side effects. The base substance, erythromycin, is without serious side effects other than the mild gastro-intestinal symptoms common to many antibiotics, but the ester, erythromycin estolate, causes hepatic damage and should not be used.

Chloramphenicol

Indications. The only indications for the use of this toxic drug are
(1) typhoid fever
(2) meningitis due to *Haemophilus influenza*.
It is, however, a useful local agent for eye infections. It has a broad spectrum

375

of activity against gram-positive and gram-negative organisms. However its
activity against gram-positive cocci is less than penicillin or tetracycline. The
drug is also effective against the Rickettsiae and agents of the psittacosis-
Lymphogranuloma venereum group.

Dosage. 250 mg 6 hrly oral or i.m.

Side effects. The principal danger of chloramphenicol, which has restricted its
use to the two indications above, is of marrow aplasia. If the drug is to be used
daily blood counts must be performed.

The amino-glycosides
Gentamicin
Kanamycin
Tobramycin
Amikacin
Colomycin
Streptomycin
The use of this important and very valuable group of antibiotics, which are given
systemically, is described in Chapter 3.

Indications. Serious infection, especially with gram-negative organisms. The
spectrum of activity varies slightly within this group. Gentamicin, tobramycin
and amikacin have the broadest spectrum, particularly in respect of *Pseudomonas
aeruginosa*. The range of activity of the amino-glycosides does not include
streptococci, clostridia or bacteroides.

Dosage. See Table 25.7.

Table 25.7 Dosage of amino-glycoside antibiotics

Gentamicin	80–120 mg 8 hourly	i.m. or i.v.
Kanamycin	250 mg 6 hourly	i.m. or i.v.
Tobramycin	2–6 mg/kg body wt/24 h	i.m. or i.v.
Colomycin	2 000 000 units 8 hourly	i.m. or i.v.
Amikacin	15 mg/kg/day in 2 doses	i.m. or i.v.

(1) These doses must be reduced in the presence of renal failure (see
Chapter 3.
(2) Dosage given for adults.

Side effects. This group of drugs (which also includes streptomycin) all are
potentially toxic to the VIII Cranial nerve. Particular caution should therefore

be used in elderly patients, and in patients with renal failure (see page 33 Table 2.8). The nephrotoxic effect if used in combination with cephaloridine or high dose frusemide should also be considered.

Sulphonamides

The sulphonamides are not widely used in hospital practice, except for the treatment of meningococcal meningitis (see Chapter 19).

Co-trimoxazole (Septrin, Bactrim)

This drug consists of 80 mg trimethoprim with 400 mg sulphamethoxazole.

Indications. Broad spectrum bacteriocidal antibiotic given orally. Ineffective against pseudomonas. Particularly useful in chest and urinary tract infections.

Dosage. 2 tablets, 2 or 3 times daily.

Side effects. Non-toxic, but occasional transient nausea, vomiting or bone marrow depression.

ANAEROBIC SEPSIS

The increase in anaerobic infection is probably more apparent than real, depending upon improved laboratory techniques, but is of increasing importance.

Patients at risk include those undergoing surgery to the genital and intestinal tracts. The possibility of anaerobic sepsis should always be considered if the seriously ill patient who has had major abdominal surgery.

The only available antibiotic effective selectively against anaerobic organisms is *metronidazole* (Flagyl). Lincomycin and clindamycin are effective against bacteroides, and their spectrum of activity extends into gram positive organisms (see above). Mezlocillin and ticarcillin are effective against some anaerobes.

Metronidazole can be given orally, rectally and by the intravenous route.

In the seriously ill case the i.v. route is preferable, the dose is 500 mg/100 ml infused over 20 min every 8 hours.

The oral dose is 400 mg 8 hrly. (These doses should be halved for children) (Eykyn and Phillips, 1976).

A suspicion of anaerobic sepsis should be alerted if putrid pus is identified (if pus is subjected to chromatography peaks of volatile fatty acids will be seen when anaerobes are present).

Metronidazole should also be considered as an addition to the antibiotic 'cocktail' administered in cases of bacteraemic shock pending the results of specific bacteriological tests.

CLINICAL USE OF ANTIBIOTICS

The treatment of specific infections are dealt with in the other chapters of this book. The important principles of the correct use of antibiotics must be re-emphasized:

(1) Antibiotics should be given for clinically significant infection by an organism for which there is an effective antibiotic.

(2) Only very rarely should antibiotics be used in the absence of bacteriological investigations.

(3) The right antibiotic should be given, alone, in the correct dosage.

(4) Combinations of antibiotics may be dangerous and are rarely justified for prolonged use in bacterial infection.

REFERENCES

Burns, M. W. (1973), Significance of Pseudomonas Aeruginosa in sputum. *Brit. med. J.*, 2, 382.

Editorial (1974), Septicaemia on the Increase. *Brit. med. J.*, 4, 615.

Eykyn, S. J. and Phillips, J. (1976), Metronidazole and anaerobic sepsis. *Brit. med. J.*, 2, 1418.

Finland, M., Jones, W. F. and Barnes, M. W. (1959), Occurrence of serious bacterial infections since introduction of antibacterial agents. *J. Am. med. Ass.*, 170, 2188.

Gaya, H. (1974), The bacteriology of Intensive Care. *Brit. J. Hosp. Med.*, 11, 853.

Gowing, N. F. (1970), The Complications of Immunosuppression—morbid anatomical and histological features of unusual infections. *Proc. Roy. Soc. Med.*, 63, 1070.

Leigh, D. A. (1974), Clinical importance of infections due to bacteriodes fragilis and role of antibiotic therapy. *Brit. med. J.*, 3, 225.

Philp, J. R. and Spencer, R. C. (1974), Secondary Respiratory Infection in Hospital Patients: effect of antimicrobial agents and Environment. *Brit. med. J.*, 2, 359.

Price, D. J. and Sleigh, J. D. (1970), Control of infection due to Klebsiella aerogenes in a neurosurgical unit by withdrawal of all antibiotics. *Lancet*, ii, 1213.

Shooter, R. A. (1971), Bowel colonisation by Pseudomonas aeruginosa and Eschericae Coli. *Proc. Roy. Soc. Med.*, 64, 989.

Shooter, R. A., Walker, K. A., Williams, V. R., Parker, M. T. S., E. A. and Bullimore, J. F. (1966), Faecal carriage of Pseudomonas aeruginosa in hospital patients. *Lancet*, ii, 131.

Smith, H. (1973), Opportunistic infection. *Brit. med. J.*, 2, 107.

Wolstenholme, G. E. and Porter, R. (eds) (1968), Systemic Mycoses. *Ciba Foundation Symposium*, London.

FURTHER READING

Garrod and O'Grady (1973), *Antibiotic & Chemotherapy.* 4th ed. E. & S. Livingstone, 1973.

Index

Abruptio placentae, 300
Acid-base balance, **6-10**
Acidaemia, 8, 9
Acidosis, 8, 9, 10
Aconite, poisoning by, 272
Adult respiratory distress syndrome, 96-7
Airway, preservation of, **52-64**, 249-50
  tracheal intubation, **53-7**
  tracheostomy, **56-62**
Alcohols, poisoning by, 262-3
Alkalaemia, 8
Alkalosis, 8, 9, 10
Amikacin, 376
Amino-glycosides, *see also* individual antibiotics, 32, 376-7
Amitryptaline, poisoning by, 259
Amoxycillin, *see* Penicillins
Amphetamine, poisoning by, 252
Amphotericin B, 193
Ampicillin, *see* Penicillins
Anaphylactic shock, 38
Angiography, in acute renal failure, 180
Antibiotics, use of, *see also* individual antibiotics, **31-7, 368-78**
Anticholinesterase drugs, overdosage of, 308
Antidepressant drugs, poisoning by, **259-60**
Arsenic, poisoning by, 268
Arterial pressure monitoring, 133
Aspirin, poisoning by, *see* Salicylate, poisoning by
Asthma, **97-102**
  in child, 338-40

treatment, 98-100
Ativan, *see* Lorazepam
Atrial flutter, 119
Atrial pressure, monitoring of, 133-5

Bactrim, *see* Co-trimoxazole
Barbiturates, poisoning by, **253-5**
Benzodiazepines, *see* individual drugs
Bicarbonate, in acid-base deficits, 8-10
Blood
  gas, estimation of, 50-1
  oxygen, carriage of, 80-1
  replacement, in haemorrhagic shock, 22
  volume, monitoring of, 137
Blood pressure
  central venous pressure, 39, **133-4**
  lines, 358-61
  in shock, 19, 39
  in ventilation, mechanical, 70-1
Blood transfusion
  autotransfusion, in intrapleural haemorrhage, 166
  complications, **42-4**, 278-9, 304
Bradycardia, 114-6
Brain death, 162-3
Brain injury, effects of, 156-63
Bronchus, ruptured, 165
Buffering systems of the body, 6-8
Burns, **170-2**

Carbenicillin, 373
Carbon monoxide, poisoning by, 269-70
Carbon tetrachloride, poisoning by, 269

Cardiac arrest, treatment of, *see also* Defibrillation technique, **108-10**
Cardiac dysrhythmias, *see* Dysrhythmias
Cardiac output, measurement of, 136
Cardiac patient
  aftercare, 139-40
  surgical risks, 140-1
Cardio-pulmonary resuscitation, **108-10**
Cardiogenic shock, **124-9**
Cardiovascular system, monitoring of, **132-44**
  in diagnosis, 138
  methods, investigatory, 141-2
Carbenicillin, 373
Central venous lines, 358-361
Cephalosporins, 191, 374
Cerebral malaria, **328-9**
Cerebral oedema, 157, **329-30**
Chest, injuries to, **163-8**
  blunt trauma, 164-5
  diaphragm, traumatic rupture of, 167
  flail chest, 166-7
  great vessels, injuries to, 168
  haemothorax, 165-6
  heart, wounds of, 167-8
  pneumothorax, 165
Chloramphenicol, 375-6
Chlorate, poisoning by, 269
Chlordiazepoxide, poisoning by, 261
Chlordiazepoxide/amitriptyline, poisoning by, 259
Chloride balance, 11-12, 16
Chlorpromazine, poisoning by, 261-2
Cholinergic crisis, 308
Christmas disease, 302
Chronic respiratory disease, 93-95
Cirrhosis, *see* Liver disease, chronic
Clindamycin, 374
Clotting of blood, pathology of, *see* Diffuse intravascular coagulation
Cloxacillin, *see* Penicillins
Colisitin, 191
Colomycin, 376
Coma, differential diagnosis of, 319-20, 321

Congenital abnormalities in neonate, care of, 335
  preservation of airway, 52
Consumption coagulopathy, *see* Diffuse intravascular coagulation
Coronary care, *see* Cardiac arrest, treatment of; Myocardial infarction, acute; Heart failure
Co-trimoxazole, 377
Cresol, poisoning by, 269
Cyanide, poisoning by, 265-6

DDT, poisoning by, 268
Deadly nightshade, poisoning by, 272
Deep vein thrombosis, 144, 152-4
Defibrillation technique, *see also* Cardiac arrest, treatment of, 121-2
Defibrination syndrome, *see* Diffuse intravascular coagulation
Dehydration, *see* Water balance
Dextropropoxyphene, poisoning by, **258**, 261
Diabetes
  coma, *see* Diabetic coma, hyperosmolar non-ketotic; Diabetic keto-acidosis; Lactic acidosis
  nutritional problems, 242
  surgery in diabetic patient, 216-7
Diabetic coma, hyperosmolar non-ketotic, **213-4**
Diabetic keto-acidosis, **204-13**
  complications, 212-3
  management, 208-12
Dialysis, peritoneal, **187-91**
Diaphragm, traumatic rupture of, 167
Diazepam, poisoning by, 261
Diffuse intravascular coagulation, **296-301**
  diabetic keto-acidosis, complication of, 213
  renal failure, acute, complication of, 194-6
Digoxin, poisoning by, 264
Dihydrocodeine, poisoning by, 260
Diphenoxylate, poisoning by, 261
Disseminated intravascular coagulopathy, *see* Diffuse intravascular coagulation

Distalgesic, poisoning by, 257, 258
Disulfoton, poisoning by, *see* Insecticides, poisoning by
Doriden, *see* Glutethamide
Drowning, **105-6**
Drug overdose, *see* Poisoning
Drugs, psychotropic, 351-2
Duodenal ulcer and gastro-intestinal bleeding, 286
Dysrhythmias
    in myocardial infarction, **114-22**, 123
    in poisoning, 250, 259, 261, 262

Echocardiography, 141
Eclampsia, intravascular coagulation in, 194, 195
Electrolyte balance, *see* Fluid and electrolyte balance
Empyema, 104
Encephalitis, **326-7**
Endocarditis, in renal disease, 176, 198-9
Endosulfan, poisoning by, *see* Insecticides, poisoning by
Enterobacterial infection, 31, 32, 35, 370
Epiglottitis, acute, 337-8
Equanil, *see* Meprobamate
Equipment in the ICU, 2-3
Erythromycin, 375
Ethanol, poisoning by, 215
Ethylene glycol, poisoning by, 263
Exanthemata, and acute interstitial nephritis, 197
Extradural block, 164, 354-5
Extradural haematoma, 157
Extrasystoles, *see* Ventricular extrasystoles

Fat embolism, 168-70
Femoral nerve block, 356
Fibrosis, retroperitoneal, 199-200
Fits, *see* Status epilepticus
Flagyl, *see* Metronidazole
Flail chest, 166-7
Flucloxacillin, *see* Penicillins
Fluid and electrolyte balance, **11-17**

Fortal, *see* Pentazocine
Fucidic acid, 374-5
Fucidin, *see* Fucidic acid
Fungi, poisoning by, 271-2
Furadantin, *see* Nitrofurantoin

Gastric lavage, in treatment of poisoning, 251, 256, 262, 263
Gastro-intestinal bleeding, *see also* Oesophageal varices, 286-90
Gentamycin, 376
Glomerular thrombosis in renal failure, 182
Glomerulonephritis, 198-9
Glutethamide, poisoning by, 249, 262
Goodpasture's syndrome, 180, 201
Great vessels, injuries to, 168
Guillain-Barré syndrome, 47, 310-11

Haematoma, extradural, 157
Haemodialysis, in treatment of barbiturate poisoning, 252, 254-5
Haemoglobin, oxygen dissociation curve for, 80-1
Haemophilia, **301-2**
Haemorrhage
    in fat embolism, 168
    fibrinolytic therapy, as contraindication of, 151-2
    from eosophageal varices, 288-90
    pulmonary, 298
    subarachnoid, 328
Haemorrhagic disorders, **301-3**
Haemorrhagic shock, 18-29 *passim*
Haemothorax, 165-6
Haloperidol, poisoning by, 262
Head, injury to, **156-63**
Heart block in myocardial infarction, 114-5
Heart failure, **122-9**
    diabetic keto-acidosis, as complication of, 213
    structural abnormalities in, 124
    in thyrotoxic crisis, 217
Heart, wounds of, 167-8
Henbane, poisoning by, 272
Hepatic disease, *see* Liver disease
Hepatic encephalopathy, 281, 288

Hepatitis
  blood transfusion, complication of, 279
  transmission, prevention of, 368
'Hepato-renal syndrome', 196
Heroin, poisoning by, 260
Herpes encephalitis, *see* Encephalitis
Hip, block of nerves of, 356
Humidification, 68-9
Hydrogen sulphide, poisoning by, 270
Hyperbilirubinaemia, *see* Jaundice
Hypercalcaemia, 200, 220-2
Hyperkalaemia, **16**
Hypernatremia, **15-16**
Hypoadrenalism, 224-6
Hypocalcaemia, 222-3
Hyponatremia, **12-15**
Hypothermia, 219-20, 250
Hypovolaemic shock, 18-29 *passim*

IPPV, *see* Ventilation, mechanical
Imipramine, poisoning by, 259
Infection, control and management of, **363-78**
  opportunistic infections, 365-7
  origins, 363-5
Insecticides, poisoning by, 267-8
Intercostal block, 356
Intrahepatic cholestasis, 278
Intravenous lines, 358-61
Iron preparations, poisoning by, 264

Jaundice, **274-80**
  blood transfusion, complication of, 278-9
  halothane anaesthesia, complications of, 278
  in liver failure, acute, 281, 282
  post-operative obstructive, 279, 291
  surgery, contra-indications to, 276, 279-80
Jugular vein, catheterisation of, 359

Kanamycin, 376

Laburnam, poisoning by, 272
Lactic acidosis (diabetic coma), **214-5**

Largactil, *see* Chlorpromazine
Laryngomalacia, 337
Laryngo-tracheobronchitis, 337
Lead, poisoning by, 265
'Legionnaires' disease', 105
Leukaemia, lactic acidosis, association with, 215
Librium, *see* Chlordiazepoxide
Limbritol, *see* Chloridazepoxide/amitriptyline
Lincomycin, 374
Lincosin, *see* Lincomycin
Lithium, poisoning by, 260
Liver
  function, biochemical tests of, 274-5
  radiology, 275-6
Liver disease, acute, *see also* Jaundice
  central nervous system, effects on, *see* Hepatic encephalopathy
  foetor hepaticus, 282
  haemorrhagic signs, 282, 283, 285
  metabolic changes, 282, 284-5
  nutritional problems, 242
  treatment, 283-6
  uraemia, acute, associated with, 196-7
Liver disease, chronic, (cirrhosis), 287, **290-3**
  renal complications, 197
Liver trauma, **293-4**
Lomotil, *see* Diphenoxylate
Lorazepam, poisoning by, 261
Lung
  abscess, 101-2
  function, tests of, 50
  infections, acute, in babies, 337-41
  respiratory failure, 48
  in shock, **40-2**
  ventilation, mechanical, complications in, 74
Lymphoma, association of lactic acidosis with, 215

Malathion, poisoning by, *see* Insecticides, poisoning by
Mandrax, *see* Methaqualone/diphenhydramine

Maprotiline-Ludiomil, poisoning by, 259
Maxolon, *see* Metoclopramide
Mecillinam, 373
Meningitis, **322-6**
Meningoencephalitis, *see* Encephalitis
Meprobamate, poisoning by, 261
Mercury, poisoning by, 265
Metabromate, poisoning by, 252
Metals, heavy, poisoning by, 265
Methaqualone/diphenhydramine, poisoning by, 249, 262
Methicillin, *see* Penicillins
Methyl alcohol, poisoning by, 263
Metoclopramide, poisoning by, 262
Metronidazole, 377
Miltown, *see* Meprobamate
Mogadon, *see* Nitrazepam
Mono-amine oxidase inhibitory drugs, poisoning by, 259
Morphine, poisoning by, 260
Myasthenia gravis, **307-10**
Myelomatosis, 199
Myocardial infarction, acute, **110-22**
dysrhythmias, 114-22
management, 112-3
shock, association with, 124, 125
Myotonia, respiratory failure in, 48
Myxoedemic coma, **218-20**

Nalidixic acid, 375
poisoning by, 249
Negram, *see* Nalidixic acid
Neonate, intensive care of, 333, **335-6**
nutritional therapy, 242
oxygen therapy, 90
physiology, 332, 334-5
Nephritis, acute interstitial, 197-9
Nitrofurantoin, 375
Nuclear methods of monitoring, 142
Nutritional therapy, **230-47**
calorific requirements, assessment of, 239-40
complications, prevention of, 241
enteral nutrition, 237, 242-4
intravenous preparations, 236, 238
oral preparations, 235, 237, 238

Oedema, cerebral, 157
Oesophageal varices, *see also* Gastrointestinal bleeding, 288-90
Oxazepam, poisoning by, 261
Oxygen
carriage in blood, 80-1
estimation of, 83-4
tension in tissues, 79-81
Oxygen therapy, **79-92**
administering equipment, 86-8
hyperbaric, 89
in asthma, 99
in cardiogenic shock, 126
in infant and child, 340-1
in myocardial infarction, 113
oxygen toxicity, 83
respiratory disease, chronic, dangers in, 95
systems in use, 84-6
by ventilation, mechanical, 88

Paediatric intensive care, **332-40**
Pancreatitis, acute, **343-7**
lactic acidosis, association with, 215
Papilloedema, 314, 321
Papilloma of larynx, 337
Paracetamol, poisoning by, **257-8**
Paraquat, poisoning by, 266-7
Parathion, poisoning by, *see* Insecticides, poisoning by
Penicillins, 371-3
Pentazocine, poisoning by, 260-1
Pericarditis, in renal disease, 176
Pethidine, poisoning by, 260
Phaeochromocytoma, 223-4
Phenergan, *see* Promethazine
Phenobarbitone, poisoning by, 251, 254
Phenol, poisoning by, 269
Phenothiazines, poisoning by, 261-2
Phlebothrombosis, 241
Physiotherapy
in respiratory disease, chronic, 95
in ventilation, mechanical, 73
Plasma and substitutes, replacement of in haemorrhagic shock, 22-4
Plasma exchange in immunological diseases, 304-5

Pneumothorax, **102–4**, 165
Poison information centres, 252
Poisoning
  self-poisoning, 248–52
  treatment, immediate, 249–52
Poisons, index to specific, 253
Poliomyelitis, **327–8**
Polyarteritis, 196
Polymixins, *see also* individual anti-
  biotics, 374–5
Polymyosotis, **310**
Polyneuritis, 47
Polyneuropathy, *see* Guillain-Barré
  syndrome; Porphyrias
Porphyrias, **226–8**
Potassium balance, 11
  depletion, 15–16
  excess, *see* Hyperkalaemia
Potassium clonazepate, poisoning by,
  261
Privet, poisoning by, 272
Prochlorperazine, poisoning by, 261–
  2
Promazine, poisoning by, 261–2
Promethazine, poisoning by, 261–2
Pseudomonas infections, 31, 32, 35,
  364, 365, 370
Psychiatric patient in the ICU, 352
Psychosis, confusional, **348–53**
Psychotropic drugs, 351–2
Pulmonary embolism, **144–55**
  deep vein thrombosis, 152–4
  embolectomy, 149
  investigation, 145–6, 148
  and myocardial infarction, differen-
    tial diagnosis of, 112
  treatment, 148–9
Pulmonary oedema, high altitude,
  106
Pulse rate, monitoring of, 39
Pupil, size of, in evaluation of CNS
  function, 159–60, 319
Pyelonephritis, 199
Pyopen, *see* Carbenicillin

Rabies, 318–9
Radial artery, cannulation of, 133
Regional blocks, **354–7**

Renal failure, acute, **175–203**
  diabetic keto-acidosis, as complica-
    tion of, 212
  dietary management, 184–6
  diuretics, 183–4
  drug nephrotoxicity, 191–4
  liver disease, association with, 285,
    291–3
  peritoneal dialysis, 187–91
  pre-renal and intrinsic renal failure,
    differentiation between, 177–9
  radiology, 179–80
  renal biopsy, 180–1
  special situations arising, 194–201
  therapy, 183
  uraemia, acute, 175–7
Respiratory disease, chronic, (obstructive airways disease), **93–5**
Respiratory distress syndrome
  adult, **96–7**
  newborn, 335–6
Respiratory failure, 47–51, 94, **95–6**
Resuscitation, 90
Ribs, fracture of, 164, 166–7

Salicylate, poisoning by, 215, 251,
  255–7
Sciatic nerve block, 356
Sedatives and hypnotics, poisoning by,
  261–3
Selexid, *see* Mecillinam
Sensorium, in shock, 19
Septicaemia
  jaundice, cause of, 280
  lactic acidosis, association with,
    215
  in renal disease, 176
Septrin, *see* Co-trimoxazole
Serenace, *see* Haloperidol
Serenid, *see* Oxazepam
Shock
  anaerobic sepsis, 35
  anaphylactic, 38
  bacteraemic, **29–37**
  cardiogenic, 37
  clinical features, **18–21**
  diagnosis, 29–30
  diffuse intravascular coagulation,

associated with, 194
haemodynamic, 18, 19
lung in, 40-2, 169
monitoring, 38-40
neurogenic, 37
oxygen therapy, 90
pathophysiological changes, 30-1
renal failure, cause of, 182
treatment, 22-9
treatment: use of antibiotics, 31-7
with burns, 170-1
Sickle cell disease, 303
Skeletal injuries, fat embolism in, 168
Skin, burns of, 170
Skull, fractures of, 157
Snake bite, poisoning by, 270-1
Sodium balance, 11
depletion, see Hyponatremia
excess, see Hypernatremia
Sodium hypochlorite, poisoning by, 269
Sparine, see Promazine
Staff,
medical, 4
nursing, 4
physiotherapy, 5
psychological effects, 352
technical, 5
Staphylococcal infections, 363, 370
Starvation, metabolic responses to, 232
Status asthmaticus, see Asthma
Status epilepticus, 311-14
respiratory failure, 49
Stelazine, see Trifluoperazine
Stemetil, see Prochlorperazine
Stokes-Adams attacks, see Heart block
in myocardial infarction
Streptococcal infections, 370
Streptomycin, 376
Stridor, in small babies, 337
Subclavian vein, cannulation of, 133-4, 360

Tachycardia, 116-22
atrial flutter, 119
cardiac asystole, 122
conduction defects, 120

fibrillation, ventricular, 120-2
sinus tachycardia, 116
supraventricular, 116-7
treatment, 117
ventricular extrasystoles, 117, 118-9
Talampacillin, see Penicillins
Temperature monitoring, 39, 135
Tensilon test, 308
Tetanus, 314-8
respiratory failure, 49
Tetrachlorethane, poisoning by, 269
Tetracycline antibiotics, 193, 373-4
Thoracotomy, 166-7
Thornapple, poisoning by, 272
Thrombocytopenia, 302
Thrombosis, see Deep vein thrombosis
Thyroid disease, 217-8
Tobramycin, 376
Toframil, see Imipramine
Tracheal intubation, 53-7
in children, 338-40
Tracheostomy, 56-62
Tranxene, see Potassium clonazepate
Trauma, see specific cases
Tricylcic antidepressant drugs, poisoning by, 259-60
Trifluoperazine. poisoning by, 261-2
Tryptizole, see Amitriptyline

Unit, intensive care, 1-5
Uraemia, acute, 175-7, 183
lactic acidosis, association with, 215
liver disease, associated with, 196-7
renal biopsy in, 180-1
Urine
outflow
continuous measurement, 135-6
in hypotension, 181-2
obstruction in renal failure, 199-201
in shock, monitoring of, 39
-plasma ratios, in diagnosis of renal failure, 177-8
Uticillin, see Carfecillin

Valium, see Daizepam
Ventilation, mechanical, 65-78
activation, types of, 65

Ventilation (*cont.*)
in cardio-pulmonary resuscitation, 109
complications, 74-6
cycling, 66-7
discontinuation, 74-5
failure, procedure in event of, 75-6
generators, types of, 65
in head injuries, 157, **161-2**
humidifiers, 73, 76
in infant and child, 340
initiation, 70-1
maintenance, 71
monitoring, 73-4
oxygen therapy, 88
physiotherapy, 73

respiration, spontaneous, depression of, 69-70
respiratory disease, chronic, 95
after respiratory injury, 172
sterilization, 68-9
in tetanus, 317
tracheal suction, 72-3
Ventricular extrasystoles, 118-9
Ventricular fibrillation, 120-1

Water balance, 11, 12, 13, 14
Weedkillers, poisoning by, 266-7
Weil's disease, renal failure associated with, 198
'Wet lung' syndrome, 164

Yew, poisoning by, 272